Clinical Nursing Practices

For Churchill Livingstone:

Senior Commissioning Editor: Jacqueline Curthoys
Project Development Manager: Mairi McCubbin
Project Manager: Andrea Hill
Designer: Judith Wright

Clinical Nursing Practices

Elizabeth M. Jamieson BSc(Hons) MSc RGN ONC RCT RNT
Senior Lecturer/Programme Organiser, Department of Nursing and Community Health,
Glasgow Caledonian University/Primary Health Care Trust, Forth Valley Health Board, Glasgow, UK

Janice M. McCall BA RGN RCNT
Formerly Lecturer, Department of Nursing and Community Health, Glasgow Caledonian University/
Primary Health Care Trust, Forth Valley Health Board, Glasgow, UK

Lesley A. Whyte BA MPhil RGN DN RNT
Lecturer/Practitioner – District Nursing, Department of Nursing and Community Health,
Glasgow Caledonian University/Primary Health Care Trust, Forth Valley Health Board, Glasgow, UK

FOURTH EDITION

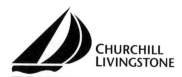
CHURCHILL
LIVINGSTONE

EDINBURGH LONDON NEW YORK PHILADELPHIA ST LOUIS SYDNEY TORONTO 2002

CHURCHILL LIVINGSTONE
An imprint of Elsevier Science Limited

First edition 1988
Second edition 1992
Third edition 1997
Fourth edition 2002

ISBN 0 443 07020 2

British Library Cataloguing in Publication Data
A catalogue record for this book is available from the British
Library

Library of Congress Cataloging in Publication Data
A catalog record for this book is available from the Library of
Congress

Note
Medical knowledge is constantly changing. As new information
becomes available, changes in treatment, procedures, equipment
and the use of drugs become necessary. The authors and the
publishers have taken care to ensure that the information given in
this text is accurate and up to date. However, readers are strongly
advised to confirm that the information, especially with regard to
drug usage, complies with the latest legislation and standards of
practice.

The
publisher's
policy is to use
**paper manufactured
from sustainable forests**

Printed in China by RDC Group Limited

Contents

Clinical advisors

Andrew Rideout BA(Hons) MPH DipN RGN RN(Child)
Public Health Practitioner, Annandale and Eskdale LHCC, Lochmaben, Dumfriesshire, UK

Sandra Stark BN MBA RGN
Head of Nursing and Quality, Ashbourne Limited, Glasgow, UK

Maggi Thomson BSc(Hons) RGN
Lecturer, Department of Nursing and Community Health, Glasgow Caledonian University, Glasgow, UK

Isabel Traynor BA(Hons) DipHEd&HP RGN FPC
Ward Sister, Gynaecology Department, Western Infirmary, Glasgow, UK

Preface to the fourth edition

The first edition of this book was published in 1988, subsequent editions having evolved in response to the many changes that have taken and are taking place in nurse education and practice. In response to favourable reviews, we have made only minor changes to the established format, which readers find easy to dip into and to apply to their particular patient and setting. We have tried to place an even greater emphasis on current evidence-based practice and to encourage our readers to reflect continually on their practice, to help to ensure the delivery of the highest-quality care to each individual patient.

Rona Blythe has retired and has not been involved in this edition, but we wish to acknowledge her contribution to the previous editions, much of which is still recognisable here. Rona has been a good friend and colleague, and we wish her many happy years of retirement.

For this edition we have benefited from the expertise of clinical advisors. These advisors, practitioners in a variety of settings, are interested in the profession of nursing and in trying to ensure that the highest possible standard of care is always delivered. In response to their suggestions, we have deleted some obsolete practices, expanded some existing ones and included new ones to reflect current practice. We are grateful to them for helping us to ensure that the information, artwork and research contained within this edition are relevant for today's practitioners in the wide variety of settings in which they may find themselves.

The authors are aware that, because of the evolving dynamic nature of health care in the 21st century, potential readers may be working outside, as well as within, the National Health Service, delivering care in private hospitals and clinics, residential homes, nursing homes and patients' own homes. We hope this book will be useful to all readers, whatever the setting.

Glasgow, 2002

Elizabeth M. Jamieson
Janice M. McCall
Lesley A. Whyte

Acknowledgements

The authors would like to thank Colette Dunn, Staff Nurse, ENT Department, Gartnavel General Hospital, Glasgow; Joyce MacLeod, formerly Moving and Handling Instructor, Greater Glasgow Health Board; and Emma Nelson, Staff Nurse, Glasgow Royal Infirmary, for their constructive comments.

Introduction

Worldwide, health-care systems are attempting to respond to the needs of their societies in the 21st century. In the UK, since Florence Nightingale and her peers set up training schools to educate nurses and improve the standard of care delivered, nursing has constantly evolved in response to the changes and demands of society. To respond effectively to these demands, nurses need to be well-educated practitioners aware of current research findings, able to assess situations, plan and deliver appropriate care and evaluate the results. A variety of models or frameworks has been developed over the years to enable nurses to do this.

This book does not relate to a particular model but should be broad enough in approach to enable it to be used within the context of many frameworks. There is, however, a section in the description of each practice that reinforces the need for each patient to be treated as a unique individual and emphasises some of the effects that the nursing practice may have on a patient's activities of living (ALs), as defined in the Roper et al (2000) framework. This framework has been deliberately chosen by the authors to help to reinforce in the reader's mind the relationship of each nursing practice to the individual patient and to the broader theoretical base of nursing. Activities of living are a concept familiar to a variety of disciplines within health care, for example occupational therapy, physiotherapy and social work, so this approach should remind readers that nurses are part of a team that, with good co-operation, communication and collaboration, should be capable of delivering optimum standards of care.

The nursing practices: the main headings

Knowing that this book would be 'dipped into' rather than read from cover to cover, we felt it important to present the information for each practice in a consistent format. The practices are set out in alphabetical order and are aimed at general clinical nurses rather than specialist practitioners; we are also aware that many practices that were traditionally carried out by nurses are now being delegated to health-care assistants and informal carers.

In each practice description, we have mentioned nurses' accountability for their practice in line with the UKCC's *Code of Professional Conduct* (1992) and *Guidelines for Professional Practice* (1996). The UKCC publishes and frequently updates specific guidelines for practice, for example, relating to medicines, records and record-keeping. These must be read in conjunction with local policies and protocols. It is hoped that this emphasis will also encourage health-care assistants and informal carers to consider their capability to carry out particular practices. There are an increasing number of nurse-initiated practices that have historically fallen within the medical profession's remit. Some practices within the book still acknowledge this and focus on the nurse's role in assisting in the practice. This is deliberate, as we recognise that many of our readers are students, and these nurse-initiated practices are carried out by qualified nurses. We again emphasise that each practice offers only guidelines and that readers must also refer to local policies and codes of practice.

Readers should be able to use the book easily and quickly once they have become familiar with the way in which the material is presented and, in particular, with what can be found under the main headings used for each practice. These are:

- Learning outcomes
- Background knowledge required
- Indications and rationale for ...
- Outline of the procedure
- Equipment
- Guidelines and rationale for this nursing practice
- Relevance to the activities of living
- Patient/carer education: key points
- References.

A brief summary is given below of the material covered under each of these headings.

Learning outcomes

The material under this heading indicates what nurses should know after reading and studying this practice, in combination with their existing personal knowledge and knowledge from other sources – the physical and social sciences, the humanities and the professional nursing literature.

It may of course be necessary for experienced nursing staff (both teaching and clinical) to demonstrate the manual aspects of the practice.

Background knowledge required

Included here are suggested areas of physiology and anatomy that should be reviewed to promote safe manual practice. A knowledge of physical aspects is emphasised because the practices described in the book are physical tasks and must be performed safely. (The relationship of psychosocial theory to the physical practice, and the importance of combining the two, are dealt with more fully under the subsequent heading 'Relevance to the activities of living'.)

In addition, cross-references to related nursing practices are given here, and the nurse's attention is also drawn to the need to consult health authority policy if it is likely to have a particular bearing on this practice in either a community or an institutional setting.

Indications and rationale for ...

Under this heading, a definition of the nursing practice is given where relevant, and common disease conditions, or other instances in which the practice might be undertaken, are mentioned. It was deliberately decided not to give a definition at the beginning of each practice but to place it instead in its context – that is, alongside examples of circumstances that might give rise to the practice. Definitions given in isolation may lead to the mistaken view that nursing practices are tasks with a beginning and an end rather than part of a nursing plan that requires thought and reflection. The rationale will be given where applicable in continuous text, but highlighted in *italics*.

Outline of the procedure

This heading appears for those few procedures normally performed by a medical practitioner, where the nurse is present to nurse the patient and/or assist the medical staff (a part of nursing that is 'doctor initiated'). The authors do acknowledge that some of these practices are now performed by qualified nurses who will have undertaken additional education and training in preparation for this extended role. A brief description of the sequence of events is given so that the reader can follow the steps intelligently; information on the position of the patient during the procedure is usually included, some of the commonly used tests are described, and the role of the nurse is emphasised. 'Outline of the procedure' may also appear if a particular theory needs to be highlighted.

Equipment

The material under this heading comprises a list of the equipment commonly used for the particular nursing practice. As far as possible, general terms such as 'local anaesthetic' or 'water-based lotion for cleansing the skin' are used, specific brand names being cited merely as an example. Where appropriate, some equipment is described: for example, the different types of catheter used in urinary catheterisation; the types of packaging used for intravenous infusions and how they are connected to the infusion system; and the various parts of the lumbar puncture needle.

In many instances, diagrams or drawings of actual pieces of equipment are provided to supplement the text.

Guidelines and rationale for this nursing practice

The general principles for the practice are outlined here and the rationale highlighted in *italics*. The following points should be noted.

- Early on in the guidelines, the nurse is alerted to 'observe the patient throughout the nursing practice'. Some suggested observations are given under the subsequent heading 'Relevance to the activities of living'.
- Later in the guidelines, the statement 'document the nursing practice appropriately, observe after-effects and report abnormal findings immediately'

appears. The meaning attached to these three phrases is discussed below:

— The wording '*document each nursing practice appropriately*' was chosen carefully; a discussion of methods of documentation would merit a separate book and has therefore not been attempted here. In each ward, clinic or community setting, a method of documentation will have been decided upon, ensuring that it meets with the requirements of UKCC record-keeping (UKCC 1998) and also local policy; indeed, in some authorities nursing data are recorded on computers.

— '*Observe the after-effects*' is really a follow-on from the earlier guideline 'observe the patient throughout the nursing practice'. It is part of the process of evaluating outcome – an integral phase of the process of nursing (individualising nursing). This is also a time to reflect on your own practice.

— '*Report abnormal findings immediately*' alerts the reader to the need not only to document the practice, but also to report abnormal findings immediately to the nurse in charge. Abnormal findings often require immediate action, for example altering the site of an intravenous infusion needle when there is evidence of fluid infiltrating the tissues around the site, discontinuing a drug because of the appearance of a rash, or investigating the cause of pain in the calf of the leg following surgery, where it can be indicative of deep venous thrombosis. As part of being able to 'do' the task, the reader needs to be aware of common complications to ensure competency according to the required UKCC competencies associated with nurse registration (NBS 2000).

▪ The last guideline for each practice is a reminder to readers of their accountability and legal responsibilities according to the UKCC's *Code of Professional Conduct* (1992), *Guidelines for Professional Practice* (1996) and *Guidelines for Records and Record Keeping* (1998). The authors have added this new guideline to each practice to help to emphasise the importance of these responsibilities for each practitioner.

Relevance to the activities of living

Observing is a crucial part of nursing, Florence Nightingale commenting on its importance in her famous publication *Notes on Nursing*. However, rather than providing a list of observations to be made before, during and after each nursing practice, the authors thought it would be much more helpful to present observations as and when they related – and only when they *directly* related – to the ALs suggested in Roper et al's (2000) model for nursing. The reference is usually to the patient's ALs, but when relevant, the nurse's responsibilities are also given by AL. Under 'Maintaining a safe environment', there is, for example, reference to nurses' responsibility to all patients, to themselves and to other members of staff in observing the general principles for preventing cross-infection.

Moreover, whereas under the second heading, 'Background knowledge required', material on the physical aspects of each practice is cited (because the content of the book is essentially concerned with observable physical procedures that must be carried out safely), this section *combines* physical science knowledge with the psychosocial and humanities knowledge that must be used before, during and after carrying out each nursing practice. It is this integrated thinking process that differentiates the performance of a routine physical task – even when performed dexterously – from a nursing practice. It demands assessment, planning and evaluation related to the specific practice within the context of the patient's total plan of care. Each nursing practice is an important part (but still only a part) of a total nursing plan.

Patient/carer education: key points

Health promotion and health education are key components in the development of a healthy community. With earlier discharge from hospital and increased care taking place in the community, the importance of educating patients and carers in relation to their own health and well-being cannot be overemphasised.

This section includes aspects of patient education that will help to give the patient or the carers increasing confidence in relation to particular nursing practices.

References

Listed here are books, articles and research reports relevant to each nursing practice that have been referenced in the text. Where possible, these have been selected from readily available material. This guided search and self-search is intended to encourage nurses to look at a variety of sources, to learn about research findings and to understand the reasons behind specific practices in the context of a total care plan. Research articles and reports are used whenever possible. Clinical reviews discussing research have also been useful references.

In conclusion, we hope that this introduction will provide a thought-provoking foundation for the nursing practices that follow. The practices are as succinct as possible for ease of reference, and we are confident that readers who assimilate the principles outlined in the introduction will be able to utilise the practices with individuality – while respecting the patient's special needs – and with the depth of thought that all nursing actions deserve and should indeed demand.

It is important to emphasise too that, apart from being needed to maintain a legal record, well-charted practices and observations are essential in developing nursing theory. In fact, Benner (1984) goes further and maintains that the practices and expertise of good nurse clinicians contain a wealth of untapped knowledge that will not expand unless nurses systematically record for themselves what they learn from their own practice experience.

References

Benner P 1984 From novice to expert: excellence and power in clinical nursing practice. Addison Wesley, Menlo Park, California

National Board for Nursing, Midwifery and Health Visiting for Scotland 2000 Partnerships in development and delivery. NBS, Edinburgh

Roper N, Logan W, Tierney A 2000 The Roper–Logan–Tierney model of nursing. Churchill Livingstone, Edinburgh

United Kingdom Central Council for Nursing, Midwifery and Health Visiting 1992 Code of professional conduct. UKCC, London

United Kingdom Central Council for Nursing, Midwifery and Health Visiting 1996 Guidelines for professional practice. UKCC, London

United Kingdom Central Council for Nursing, Midwifery and Health Visiting 1998 Guidelines for records and record keeping. UKCC, London

United Kingdom Central Council for Nursing, Midwifery and Health Visiting 2000 Guidelines for the administration of medicines. UKCC, London

1   Administration of Medicines

There are seven parts to this section:

1 Principles of medicine administration
2 Routes of medicine administration
3 Immunisation
4 Syringe driver pumps
5 Anaphylaxis
6 Patient-controlled analgesic devices
7 Patient compliance devices.

The concluding section, 'Relevance to the activities of living', refers to all practices.

Learning outcomes

By the end of this section, you should know how to:

- support and prepare the patient for this practice
- collect and prepare the equipment
- carry out the administration of medicines safely and accurately
- educate the patient on follow-up care.

Background knowledge required

A review of:

- the pharmacology of the medicine to be administered
- the metric system of volume and weight used in the dose calculation of a medication
- the Misuse of Drugs Act 1971 (HMSO, reprinted 1985), including all its amendments
- the contents of *The Scope of Professional Practice* (UKCC 1992a)
- the *Guidelines for the Administration of Medicines* (UKCC 2000)
- the Medicinal Products: Prescription by Nurses Act (HMSO 1992)
- the document *Immunisation Against Infectious Disease* (DoH 1996)
- health authority policy regarding the patient's medicine prescription and recording documents, the administration of drugs, the disposal of equipment and the management of anaphylactic shock.

Indications and rationale for the administration of medicines

A medication can be administered by a variety of routes and for many different reasons:

- *to prevent disease*
- *to cure disease*

- *to alleviate pain or other symptoms caused by disease, injury or surgery*
- *to alleviate a manifestation of disease.*

Outline of the procedure

The administration of medicine encompasses many different procedures depending on the needs of the patient. The UKCC (2000) lays great emphasis on issues of accountability for any nurse undertaking this practice. It is important that the following guidelines are used in conjunction with health authority policy as there may be policy or procedural differences (such as the grade and number of nurses required to undertake these practices) (Crown 1999).

Equipment

Means of identifying the patient
Patient's medicine prescription and recording documents
Trolley, tray or a suitable work surface for equipment
Medication to be administered
Equipment for use during medicine administration, e.g.:
— oral administration: medicine glass or spoon, glass of water
— injection: appropriately sized sterile needles and syringe, disposable gloves, alcohol-impregnated cleansing swab, cotton wool, adhesive plaster
Sharps box
Receptacle for soiled material
Equipment/medication for the treatment of anaphylactic shock (as per health authority policy).

1   Principles of medicine administration

Guidelines and rationale for this nursing practice

All forms of medicine administration

- discuss the procedure with the patient, asking whether he or she has any known allergy to this drug or other drugs or substances such as eggs, which are used as a carrier substance in some medications, and obtain consent (this may not always be possible, for example when the patient is unconscious) *to inform the patient about the procedure, discuss any concerns or queries, identify any known allergies and ensure that the patient is aware of his or her rights as a patient*
- wash the hands *to reduce the risk of cross-infection*
- select a suitable clean surface and lay out the equipment *to provide a suitable protected work surface*
- observe the patient throughout this procedure *to identify any potential reactions to the medicine*
- identify the medicine to be administered on the prescription document. The prescription should be complete and legible *to ensure that all details about the medicine can be clearly identified on the prescription documentation*
- check that the medicine has not already been administered *to ensure that only one dose of the medicine is given*

- select the appropriate medicine against the prescription documentation *to ensure that the correct medicine is administered*
- check the medicine's name, dosage, timing and expiry date. If the medication has been dispensed to a specific patient, check that his or her name is on the container *to ensure that all the relevant details are listed on the medicine container*
- remove the prescribed dosage from the container *to ensure that the correct amount of medicine is removed from the container*
- check the prescription and dosage against the medicine container *to ensure that the medicine details match*
- identify the patient to whom the medicine is to be administered. In an institution, this will normally be achieved by checking the details on the patient's identification bracelet. In a community setting, verbal verification should be obtained from either the patient or the carer *to ensure that the medicine is administered to the correct patient*
- administer the medicine by the route prescribed
- dispose of contaminated equipment according to health authority policy *to prevent the transmission of infection or the poisoning of other persons*
- ensure that the patient is comfortable following the administration of the medicine *to identify any reaction to the medication or to the chosen route of delivery*
- follow local policy regarding the time that a nurse must remain with a patient following the administration of certain medicines. This is particularly relevant when the medicine is being administered in the patient's own home or in a treatment room *to ensure prompt recognition and treatment of any reaction to the drug* (*see* 'Anaphylaxis', p. 13)
- record the medication details on the patient documentation, monitor any after-effects and report abnormal findings immediately *to ensure that there is a permanent record of the medicine administration and that any side-effects are reported to medical staff*
- in undertaking this practice, nurses are accountable for their actions, the quality of care delivered and record-keeping according to the *Code of Professional Conduct* (UKCC 1992b), *Guidelines for Professional Practice* (UKCC 1996) and *Guidelines for Records and Record Keeping* (UKCC 1998).

Controlled medicines

Institutional setting   The administration of a controlled medicine within an institutional setting must involve two nurses, or a nurse and another approved professional such as a medical practitioner or operating department practitioner. One nurse must be a registered nurse practitioner and may, according to local policy, need to be employed within that health-care setting. A controlled drug register is kept on each ward or department, giving details of the stock and administration of controlled drugs.

- as for 'All forms of medicine administration' up to the guideline 'check that the medicine has not already been administered'
- remove the appropriate medicine from the controlled drug store, check the stock number with the number detailed in the register, along with the other

nurse, *to ensure that the number of drugs in the container matches the number recorded in the register*
- check the date of the prescription *to ensure that the medicine is administered on the correct date*
- check the time of administration *to ensure that the medicine is given at the correct time*
- check the method of administration *to ensure the correct route of administration*
- remove the appropriate dose from the stock of controlled medicine, checking the name and dosage with the second nurse. Check and record the stock number of the remaining controlled medicine *to ensure that the correct dose is withdrawn from the container and the remaining balance recorded*
- enter into the controlled medicine record sheet the appropriate details *to ensure a permanent record of the administration details (date, time, patient's name, drug dosage and initials of staff)*
- continue as for 'All forms of medicine administration'.

Community setting   The administration of a controlled medicine within the patient's own home may be carried out by the patient or carer (this being the normal practice for medicines in tablet or liquid form). When medicines are given by injection, as a suppository or via a syringe driver, this is normally carried out by the community nurse(s). The number and grade of staff depend on health authority policy.

Controlled medicines belong to the patient and remain within his or her home. Advice should be given to the patient/carer on the safe storage of these medicines. A controlled medicine record sheet giving details of any medicine administered by the nurse and a balance of stock should be placed in the patient's house, along with a special prescription sheet for controlled medicines (completed and signed by the general practitioner or hospital consultant in charge of the patient's care).

- as for 'All forms of medicine administration' up to the guideline 'check that the medicine has not already been administered'
- check the stock number of medicines against the number detailed in the controlled drug record sheet *to ensure the number of medicines in the container matches the number recorded in the drug record*
- check the date of the prescription *to ensure that the medicine is administered on the correct date*
- check the time of administration *to ensure that the drug is given at the correct time*
- check the method of administration *to ensure the correct route of administration*
- remove the appropriate dose from the stock of controlled medicines, checking the name and dosage. Check and record the stock number of the remaining controlled medicines *to ensure that the correct dose is withdrawn from the container and the remaining balance recorded*
- enter into the controlled drug record sheet the appropriate details *to ensure a permanent record of the administration details (date, time, medicine dosage and signature of staff)*
- continue as for 'All forms of medicine administration'.

2 Routes of medicine administration

Oral preparation

- as for 'All forms of medicine administration' up to the guideline that begins 'remove the prescribed dosage ... .'
- remove the required number of tablets, pills or cachets from the medicine container without contaminating the preparation. Place into the medicine glass or medicine spoon *to ensure that the correct drug dosage is dispensed.*

or

- shake the liquid medicine preparation well. Pour into the appropriate container at eye level and on a solid flat surface, or draw up into a syringe *to ensure accurate drug dose measurement*
- check the medicine prescription and dosage against the container *to ensure that the correct medicine and dosage has been dispensed*
- identify the patient *to ensure that the medicine is administered to the correct person*
- administer the medicine and offer the patient water (if allowed) *to aid the swallowing of an oral preparation.* If the medicine is a powder that needs to be mixed with water, the instructions on the container should be followed *to ensure that the medicine moves efficiently down the oesophagus into the stomach*
- continue as for 'All forms of medicine administration'.

Injection preparations – intramuscular and subcutaneous routes

Equipment

Appropriately sized needles (21G, 23G and 25G) and syringes
Alcohol-impregnated swab
Drug ampoule or vial
Diluent if required
File
Disposable gloves
Gauze swab
Sterile adhesive plaster.

Guidelines and rationale for injections

- as for 'All forms of medicine administration', follow the guideline that begins 'check the medicine's name, dosage, timing and expiry date'
- put on gloves *to prevent contamination by the medicine and to protect against blood-borne infection.*

Ampoule

- snap the neck of the ampoule using a gauze swab *to protect the nurse from laceration by glass splinters should the medication be stored in a glass ampoule*
- if any glass enters the ampoule, discard the ampoule and start the process with a new one *as glass particles may have contaminated the medicine*
- if the solution is already present in the ampoule, draw up the required amount of medicine into the syringe
- if the medicine is in powder form, draw up the required amount of diluent and inject it slowly into the powder within the ampoule *to enable the medicine to be dissolved in diluent*
- gently rotate the ampoule and inspect it for any visible particles of undissolved powder *to ensure that the powder is fully dissolved*
- withdraw the required amount of drug solution into the syringe *to ensure that the correct amount of medicine is dispensed*
- gently tap the side of the barrel with the finger *to move any air bubbles to the neck of the syringe to enable them to be expelled prior to injecting the solution.*

Vial

- remove the protective cap and cleanse the rubber top with an alcohol-impregnated swab *to cleanse the entry point*
- insert the first needle, ensuring that the tip is above the fluid level *to release the vacuum within the vial*
- draw air into the syringe attached to the second needle to equal the amount of solution to be withdrawn from the vial *to enable the easier withdrawal of solution from the vial*
- insert the second needle attached to the syringe, and expel the air into the vial. Draw up the required amount of drug, expelling any air bubbles prior to removing the needle from the vial *to prevent spray of the drug solution into the atmosphere on withdrawal of the needle*
- if the medicine is in powder form, draw up the required amount of diluent and inject it slowly into the powder within the vial *to enable the medicine to be dissolved in diluent*
- gently rotate the ampoule and inspect for any visible particles of undissolved powder *to ensure that the powder is fully dissolved*
- change the needle to the required size for the route of administration; *if an intramuscular injection is to be given, a clean needle prevents irritation of the subcutaneous tissue as the needle is being inserted into the muscle* (Soanes 2000)
- place the prepared syringe and the empty ampoule or vial on a foil tray *to retain the original drug container so that a final check can be made prior to administering the medicine*
- identify the patient to whom the medicine is to be administered and recheck the prescription details with the medicine, container and dosage drawn up in the syringe *to ensure that the correct medicine is administered to the correct patient*

- ensure the patient's privacy
- cleanse the skin surface (if required); the policy on skin cleansing prior to injection varies according to the health authority concerned (Lawrence et al 1994). Patients receiving insulin injections should not have the area cleansed with an alcohol-impregnated swab as this will toughen the skin over time
- expose the chosen site and inject the drug.

Intramuscular injection

Sites for intramuscular injection are shown in Figure 1.1. Rodger & King (2000) suggest five injection sites, but this is as yet not common practice.

Using the non-dominant hand, stretch the skin over the site; with the dominant hand, insert the needle two-thirds in, at an angle of 90°, *to ensure that the needle is inserted into the muscle.*

Subcutaneous injection

Sites for subcutaneous injection are shown in Figure 1.2.

Using the non-dominant hand, gently grip the skin over the site. With the dominant hand, introduce two-thirds of the needle at a 45° angle. Release the skin once the needle is in position *to ensure that the drug is delivered into the subcutaneous tissue.*

For more information on insulin therapy, *see* 'Administration of insulin', p. 9.

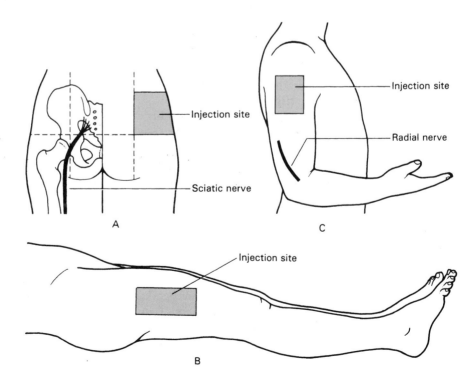

Figure 1.1
Administration of medicines: sites used for intramuscular injection
A Upper outer quadrant of the buttock
B Anterior lateral aspect of the thigh
C Deltoid region of the arm

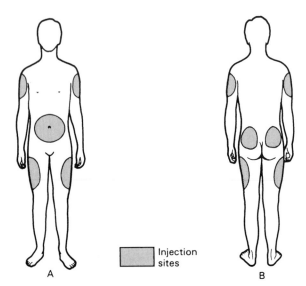

Figure 1.2
Administration of medicines: sites used for subcutaneous injection
A *Anterior aspect*
B *Posterior aspect*

All injections

- withdraw the piston of the syringe. If blood is drawn up into the syringe, withdraw the needle and syringe from the patient's tissue. Replace the needle, and start the procedure again *to prevent the drug being injected into a blood vessel*
- if no blood is withdrawn into the syringe, inject the solution slowly at a rate of 1 ml per 10 seconds (Soanes 2000) *to reduce patient discomfort and/or tissue damage*
- hold the needle in situ for 10 seconds *to allow the diffusion of the drug into the tissues*
- withdraw the needle smoothly and quickly. *To prevent the occurrence of a needle-stick injury,* do not resheath the needle
- apply pressure to the site of the injection using a cotton wool ball or swab. If bleeding occurs, apply a small adhesive plaster *to prevent blood leakage*
- continue as for 'All forms of medicine administration'.

Some medicines require a specialised technique, for example the subcutaneous injection of a goserelin implant. Specialised administration instructions provided by the manufacturer should always be followed.

A Z-track intramuscular injection technique may be required with certain medications that can stain the skin or are particularly irritant (Workman 1999):

- using the non-dominant hand, apply a shearing movement to the skin, causing the skin and subcutaneous tissue to slide over the underlying muscle. With the dominant hand, insert the needle two-thirds in, at an angle of 90°, *to ensure that the needle is inserted into the muscle*
- continue as for 'All injections' up to withdrawal of the needle

- withdraw the needle smoothly and quickly. Release the tension on the skin and subcutaneous tissue *to permit the tissues to return to their pre-injection position. This creates an internal seal over the muscle entry point preventing the leakage of the medication into the superficial tissues*
- withdraw the needle smoothly and quickly. *To prevent the occurrence of a needle-stick injury*, do not resheath the needle
- if bleeding occurs, apply a small adhesive plaster *to prevent blood leakage*
- continue as for 'All forms of medicine administration'.

The nurse should always be aware of the possibility of anaphylaxis following the administration of medicines. Health authority policy should be followed regarding the length of time for which the patient should be monitored following the administration of the medicine. This is particularly important for patients receiving medicines in the community. For further information, *see* 'Anaphylaxis', p. 13.

Administration of insulin

Insulin may be given via special insulin syringes or by an insulin pen device and is delivered subcutaneously. For patients who are self-administering insulin, the pen system is often more practical as the vial in the pen holds enough insulin for several doses. Some pen systems have a needle that is of a shorter length than the standard one used for subcutaneous injections. Various manufacturers advise that their pen be introduced at 90° angle, but there has been some debate over whether this technique causes insulin to be injected into the muscle rather than the subcutaneous tissue (in patients who have less than 10 mm of subcutaneous tissue), thus increasing the absorption rate (Engstrom 1994). Patients injecting insulin should be taught the technique advised by the diabetic specialist within the health authority.

A small American study has suggested that some diabetics find injecting insulin through one layer of clothing more convenient than the conventional technique requiring skin exposure (Brown 1998).

Intradermal route

This route is used only for selective vaccinations such as the BCG (Workman 1999), and the nurse must meet the criteria for immunisation prior to administering this or any other vaccine via this route. The injection of a medicine into the dermis is a skilled injection technique. The sites where the injections can be given may vary according to the type of vaccination being administered; local health authority policy should therefore be followed. More detailed information on this technique is provided by the Department of Health (1996).

Topical application

There is a growing trend for certain medicines to be administered via the transdermal route (Kelly 1994), usually in the form of a 'skin patch'.

Some drugs that can be given by this method include hormone replacement therapy and certain analgesics.

The patches should normally be applied to clean dry skin. The length of time they should be worn depends on the drug involved, so the manufacturer's instructions should be followed. The site of the patch should be rotated to reduce risk of a skin reaction, and care should be taken to ensure that only one patch is in place at a time, thus ensuring that the correct dose of medication is administered. Further information on drugs delivered via this route is available from individual manufacturers.

3   Immunisation

Nurses working in both community and institutional settings are increasingly undertaking immunisation. This may include child immunisation regimes, vaccinations for travel abroad, the administration of influenza vaccines and the giving of anti-tetanus or hepatitis B vaccinations within accident and emergency units or treatment rooms.

Jones (1994) examines some of the legal and professional aspects of immunisation by nursing staff and discusses the use of protocols for this practice. Nurses participating in any immunisation programme must meet the following criteria (DoH 1996). They must:

- undertake additional training on immunisation
- undertake training in the management of anaphylaxis
- be competent in the practice of immunisation and be able to recognise contraindications for vaccination
- be accountable for their practice.

4   Syringe driver pump

Indications and rationale for use of a syringe driver

A patient who requires a continuous dose of medicine may be given it via a syringe driver pump. A pump may be used:

- *when the patient is unable to tolerate oral medication* (for example, because of a pathological lesion, unresolved nausea or vomiting, or a reduced level of consciousness)
- *when adequate pain control cannot be achieved by oral medication*
- *when a medicine needs to be administered via the subcutaneous route over a period of time.*

Outline of the procedure

The syringe driver administers a continuous amount of a prescribed medicine via the subcutaneous route over a set period of time (for example, 24 hours). It may be used when a continuous infusion of a medicine is required, such as to manage postoperative pain or to control symptoms during the terminal stage of an illness. More than one medicine may be administered at a time via this route. It is of especial benefit for patients being nursed in the community as it enables a more accurate titration of drug doses and therefore more effective symptom control.

In many settings, this practice has to be undertaken by two people, although policy may vary in the community setting. Within an institutional setting, the medicine may already be made up in the syringe by the pharmacist or doctor. In a community setting, the medicine is likely to be made up by the district nurse in the patient's own home. Health authorities may have different policies, which should be followed (Quinn 2000).

Different models of syringe driver with differing operating instructions are available, so it is essential that any nurse working with them is fully familiar with the particular manufacturer's instructions (Smith 1997, Wilson 2000). It is therefore possible to provide here only general guidelines, which should be followed in conjunction with health authority policy and the manufacturer's instructions.

Equipment

Syringe driver and battery (if required)
Manufacturer's instructions for the syringe driver
Patient's medicine prescription and recording documents
Trolley, tray or suitable work surface for equipment
Medication to be administered (including diluent)
22 G butterfly cannula and giving set
Syringes (type and size as instructed by the manufacturer of the syringe driver)
Sterile needles
Disposable gloves
Cotton wool
Semi-permeable adhesive film dressing
Sharps box
Receptacle for soiled material
Adhesive label.

Guidelines and rationale for this practice

The following steps should be undertaken in conjunction with local policy and the instructions of the manufacturer of the syringe driver.

- as for 'All forms of medicine administration' (*see* p. 2), up to the guideline 'check that the medicine has not already been administered'. If a controlled drug is to be administered, the guidelines given under 'Controlled medicines' (*see* p. 3) should be followed
- ensure that the syringe driver is functioning by following the checking procedure advised by the manufacturer and health authority. This normally involves inserting the battery or attaching the pump to the mains supply and ensuring that the indicator light is lit. When applicable, a check on the inbuilt alarm system should also be carried out *to perform any recommended safety checks*

- in an institutional setting: collect the pre-prepared syringe containing the prescribed medicine and check the details on the syringe (patient's name and hospital number, date, medicine name(s) and diluent, dosage, total volume of fluid in the syringe, starting time of administration, expiry date). This information should be checked with the details given on the patient's prescription sheet *to ensure that the medicine details on the syringe match those on the prescription sheet*
- in a community setting: prepare the medicine for administration as per the patient's prescription sheet (although the medicine dosage will be the same irrespective of the pump, the amount of diluent may differ). A label should be attached to the barrel of the syringe giving information on the contents of the syringe (date, name and dosage of the medicine, volume of drug and diluent, starting time of administration, signature of nurse) *in order that the contents are clearly identified*
- attach the giving set to the syringe and prime the tubing *so that all air is expelled from the tubing*
- elicit the duration of administration *as this will affect the rate of administration*
- set the prescribed rate according to the manufacturer's instructions *to ensure the correct infusion rate*
- select the site for infusion (the same as for 'Subcutaneous injection', p. 7) and, using the same method as for giving a subcutaneous injection, insert the needle of the infusion set at a 45° angle
- secure the needle with the semi-permanent adhesive dressing *to prevent its becoming dislodged and to enable the entry site to be clearly visible*
- secure the syringe into the driver, ensuring that the plunger mechanism is correctly positioned and that any securing straps are in place to enable the administration of the medicine and *to ensure that the syringe does not become dislodged from the pump*
- start the syringe driver and observe it for the time specified by the health authority *to ensure that the driver is functioning*
- place the driver in a safe position (a carrying case is normally available for patients who are mobile) and ensure that it is kept away from water *to prevent the infusion set being dislodged from the syringe driver and to avoid damage to the machine*
- the syringe driver should be checked regularly and recordings such as fluid volume length (the length of fluid in the syringe barrel, measured normally in millimetres) documented (remembering that the checks to be carried out and their frequency may vary according to health authority policy) *to ensure that it is continuing to function correctly*
- check the infusion site regularly and report any signs of localised pain, inflammation or swelling; in the community, the patient or carer may be taught how to check the site. Any problems necessitate the resiting of the infusion set. Doyle & Benton (1994) advise that the site be changed routinely every 3–4 days *to identify and rectify at an early stage any localised skin reaction*
- observe the patient's symptoms *to monitor the effectiveness of the drug therapy*

- in undertaking this practice, nurses are accountable for their actions, the quality of care delivered and record-keeping according to the *Code of Professional Conduct* (UKCC 1992b), *Guidelines for Professional Practice* (UKCC 1996) and *Guidelines for Records and Record Keeping* (UKCC 1998).

The regular maintenance and calibration of the pump by the health authority or manufacturer is essential.

5   Anaphylaxis

Outline of the procedure

Anaphylaxis can result from an anaphylactic reaction (a reaction to a substance to which the body has previously been exposed and sensitised) or an anaphylactoid response (in which there has been no previous exposure). An anaphylactic reaction can lead to respiratory distress, shock, cardiac arrest or death and can occur at any time. It is essential that all nurses involved in the administration of medicines are familiar with the symptoms of an anaphylactic reaction. It is particularly important that nurses working in a community setting have the competence to both recognise and treat anaphylaxis (additional training being given to staff in order that they can undertake this procedure).

A reaction to a medicine may occur at any time following administration: it is not possible to give a time limit (DoH 1996). Ewan (1998) reports that a reaction frequently occurs within minutes of the patient receiving the injection (although it can also occur following the oral ingestion of medicines or certain foods, or through skin contact) but that it may also be delayed for up to several hours following administration.

The information provided in this section is based on the guidelines given by the Department of Health (1996) and the Resuscitation Council (Chamberlain 1999), but individual health authorities may provide additional guidance for staff.

Presenting characteristics

- airway obstruction presenting as wheezing from bronchospasm and laryngeal oedema, dyspnoea and stridor
- skin itching, flushing, urticaria and angio-oedema
- extreme anxiety and a feeling of 'impending doom'
- hypotension
- tachycardia followed by bradycardia (secondary to profound hypotension).

If untreated, the patient may eventually suffer respiratory and cardiac arrest.

Management of anaphylaxis

- if the patient still has an adequate cardiac output, place him or her in the recovery position and insert an artificial airway *to maintain an airway* if the gag reflex has been lost
- in an institutional setting: remain with the patient but get help urgently from other medical and nursing staff (in most units, it will be necessary to call the cardiac arrest team). When help arrives, inform the senior staff of the

Table 1.1   **Dosage of adrenaline (epinephrine) 1/1000 (1 mg/ml) in different age groups**

Age	Dose of adrenaline (ml)
0–1 year	0.05
1 year	0.1
2 years	0.2
3–4 years	0.3
5 years	0.4
6–10 years	0.5
Adults	0.5–1.0

From DoH (1996), with the permission of the Stationery Office.

medication that the patient received prior to collapse *to initiate treatment and sustain life*
- in a community setting: first summon help by dialling 999 and asking for an ambulance; then return to the patient and start treatment as soon as possible. When possible, send someone for medical help.

Administer adrenaline (epinephrine) 0.5 ml 1/1000 solution by deep intramuscular injection to all adult patients with shock or respiratory distress. This dose can be repeated after 5 minutes and given several times until the patient responds to treatment (*see* Fisher 1995, and Ewan 1998, for further information on the physiological changes associated with anaphylaxis). The suggested doses of adrenaline (epinephrine) for other age ranges are given in Table 1.1.

The Resuscitation Council (Chamberlain 1999) recommends giving intravenous antihistamine, and possibly hydrocortisone, intravenous fluids and salbutamol nebulisers.

- commence the resuscitation procedure if the patient has suffered a respiratory and/or cardiac arrest (*see* 'Cardiopulmonary resuscitation', p. 79) *to initiate treatment as quickly as possible and sustain the patient's life*
- any patient suffering an anaphylactic reaction should be admitted to hospital as soon as possible *in order that his or her condition may be monitored*. Fisher (1995) advises that a secondary reaction may occur up to 72 hours following the initial anaphylactic incident.

6   Patient-controlled analgesic devices

Devices that enable the patient to self-administer analgesia are becoming increasingly popular (Willis 1995). These work via a pump system that enables the patient to administer small doses of the prescribed analgesic, an inbuilt safety mechanism preventing overdosage of the drug. The main administration routes are intravenous, subcutaneous and epidural. The benefits of this system are that the patient is more empowered and less anxious about effective pain control

(McDonald 1994). The devices may be used by patients in both institutional and community settings (Roberts & Seaby 1995, Williams 1996).

Patient-controlled analgesia may be prescribed for patients:

- following surgical procedures such as hysterectomy and hip replacement. *It allows the patient to administer frequent small boluses of analgesia for pain relief without becoming oversedated. Good pain control enables the patient to mobilise earlier and enhances postoperative recovery*
- for pain relief as part of palliative care in terminal illness. This may be at home or in an institutional or hospice setting *and allows the patient to be alert and aware of the surroundings with adequate pain control* (Roberts & Seaby 1994).

Equipment

Venous or subcutaneous access

Specialised patient-controlled analgesia infusor (referring to the manufacturer's instructions)

The infusor consists of a reservoir balloon or a reservoir syringe that is prepared with the prescribed analgesic medication by the nursing staff. The fluid from the reservoir flows through a filter and a control nozzle on the demand button via its associated tubing (Fig. 1.3). Many devices are available, and the individual manufacturer's instructions must always be followed.

Patients administer their own dose of analgesia by pressing the demand button, which may take the form of a wrist button or a small hand-held demand set. When further analgesic is required, the demand button is again pressed, and a small amount of medication, usually 0.5–1 ml, is delivered. The equipment has an inbuilt safety mechanism that allows only a certain amount of fluid to be infused during 1 hour, so there is no possibility of a medication overdose. The strength of the individual bolus will be prescribed by the medical practitioner after assessing the patient's pain (Doverty 1994). The amount transfused each hour should be recorded, monitored and documented for evaluation of the patient's pain control.

7 Patient compliance devices

There are many types of device on the market to assist the patient to administer his or her medicines. These may comprise individual trays for each day of the week, each with different compartments for the different times of day when the patient must take the medication. The trays are usually filled (by the patient, carer or pharmacist) with all the patient's medicines up to 1 week in advance. If the nurse is required to fill these devices, the *Guidelines for the Administration of Medicines* (UKCC 2000) and *Administration of Medicines: Standards for the Use of Monitored Dosage Systems – Position Statement* (UKCC 1994, McGraw & Drennan 2001), as well as health authority policy, should be followed.

All patients should be fully assessed before a medicine device is given, and checks made that the medicines can be stored in it. Interactions between

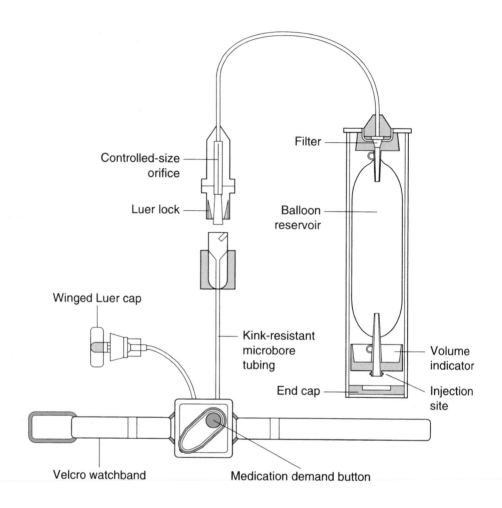

Figure 1.3
Patient-controlled analgesia infusor

Labels (clockwise):
- Controlled-size orifice
- Luer lock
- Winged Luer cap
- Filter
- Balloon reservoir
- Kink-resistant microbore tubing
- Volume indicator
- Injection site
- End cap
- Velcro watchband
- Medication demand button

medicines should also be checked, so it is essential that a pharmacist be involved at all stages. Packs prepared by the pharmacist that provide a 7 day supply of medicines in blister packaging are increasingly being used.

Relevance to the activities of living

Maintaining a safe environment

The nurse in charge of the ward, department, unit or treatment room at any time of the day or night is responsible for maintaining the safe and correct storage of all medicines, these storage requirements being enforced by law through the Misuse of Drugs Act 1971. Medicines kept in patients' own homes are their responsibility, but the community nurse has an important role in educating patients on all aspects of their regime. All protocols and records pertaining to medicine administration must be maintained, adhering to health authority legal requirements.

A learner nurse should be supervised by a qualified member of staff while administering medicines, and a nurse can administer a medicine only on the written instruction of a medical practitioner, dentist or a nurse prescriber. The formulary for nurse prescribing is at present limited, but the government intends to extend it following consultation with a number of health professionals. The use of evidence-based protocols may assist the nurse prescriber to keep within the allocated financial budget (Stilliard 2000). The UKCC *Guidelines for the Administration of Medicines* (UKCC 2000) and health authority policy should be followed with respect to this practice.

The medicine prescription should be written in indelible ink, giving the date, the patient's full name and age, the name (preferably generic title) of the medication, the dosage to be given and the time of administration, and the prescription then being signed by a medical practitioner, dentist or nurse prescriber. The whole prescription should be legible. Community nurses who have undertaken additional training may be able to prescribe items from a nurses' formulary.

The nurse is responsible for the correct administration and documentation of a prescribed medication. Recording the administration may be performed only once the nurse is satisfied that the patient has received the prescribed medication. Should any error occur during administration, this must be reported so that the appropriate action can be implemented (UKCC 2000).

The manufacturer's recommendations for the storage environment and expiry date should be adhered to or the composition of the medicine may be altered. Vaccines in particular require to be stored under very stringent conditions (recommendations being provided by both the manufacturer and the health authority).

The nurse should be familiar with the use, action, common side-effects and therapeutic dose of the medicine being administered. This will help in the education of patients and assists in identifying any adverse reaction that may develop.

The administration of oral medicine does not require an aseptic technique, but all equipment should be clean or disposable, and all precautions should be taken to prevent cross-infection. Nurses should wash their hands (and when indicated wear gloves) before commencing and after completing the administration of an oral medicine.

If the patient has difficulty swallowing an oral preparation, the nurse may request that the medicine be supplied in another form. The pharmacist should be consulted before any tablet is crushed or halved (as this may affect the composition or absorption of the medicine). Pills, capsules and cachets should be supplied in the dosage stated on the prescription sheet.

Liquids for oral administration should be shaken well to disperse the medicine thoroughly in the liquid base before pouring the prescribed amount. Spillage on the outside of the bottle should be wiped off to prevent disfiguration of the label.

An injection is an invasive procedure, so all principles of asepsis should be maintained. The equipment should be disposed of safely and immediately following the injection to reduce the potential hazards. To reduce the incidence of needle-stick injury and prevent the accidental introduction of a contaminated needle into the nurse, which may be a health hazard, needles should never be resheathed. Some clinical areas now purchase pre-assembled syringes and needles, which automatically retract the needle into the barrel of the syringe once the medication has been administered, thus preventing needle-stick injury. Certain medications (such as some used in the treatment of cancer) can be hazardous to staff during preparation and administration, so disposable gloves and/or other protection may be required.

An intramuscular injection should be administered only into the areas shown in Figure 1.1 above as this reduces the risk of damage to underlying tissue such as nerves and/or blood vessels.

If a patient is receiving subcutaneous injections over a period of time, the site of injection should be rotated to reduce subcutaneous tissue irritation and maintain the medicine's absorption rate.

Oral medications are dispensed in child-resistant containers unless a specific request has been made for a screw-top container. It is therefore necessary for the nurse to assess the patient's ability to remove medicines from the container (this being especially important for elderly or disabled people).

Communicating

The nurse should help to reinforce any information given to the patient by the medical practitioner and/or manufacturer about the prescribed medicine and its effect within the patient's body.

Information about any known allergy to medicine, food or topical application (such as adhesive tape) should be requested during the initial patient assessment.

It is important to observe the effectiveness of a medicine, for example following the administration of an anti-emetic or analgesic. Any sign of the development of a side-effect, of non-effectiveness or of dependence should be reported to the medical practitioner or prescriber.

Most medicines are known to have some side-effects, these varying from minor upsets to life-threatening events, so the nurse should have a knowledge of the side-effects of the medicine being administered. When an adverse effect is not life-threatening, it may be necessary for the patient to adjust to a change in his or her activity of living. The nurse therefore has a role as an educator and facilitator during the adjustment.

Eliminating

The patient should be told if the medicine is likely to discolour the urine. Some medicines, such as opiates, may cause constipation; education should therefore be given on diet, and a laxative can be prescribed if necessary.

Patient/carer education: key points

In partnership with the patient and/or carer, ensure that they are competent to carry out any required practices. Information should be given on an appropriate point of contact should any concerns arise.

Whatever the care setting, the nurse should use every opportunity to educate the patient on all aspects of the medication regime. A study carried out by Whyte (1994) found that a personal medication record card significantly increased the amount of information that elderly patients were able to recall about their medication regime. A more structured programme may involve a self-administration system implemented while the patient is still in institutional care (Fuller 1995).

Education is needed to ensure that medicines are kept safely within the patient's own home.

Patients and carers can be taught how to administer medicines such as insulin as well as to report any side-effects from medication. This is particularly important for those receiving chemotherapy, for whom a structured education programme relating to the therapy is essential.

References

Brown S 1998 Injecting insulin through clothing was safe and convenient. Evidence-based Nursing 1(1): 12

Chamberlain D 1999 Emergency medical treatment of anaphylactic reactions. Project Team of the Resuscitation Council (UK) Emergency Medical Journal 16: 243–247

Crown J 1999 Review of prescribing, supply and administration of medicines – final report. DoH, London

Department of Health 1996 Immunisation against infectious diseases. Stationery Office, London

Doverty N 1994 Making pain assessment your priority. Practitioner led management of pain in trauma injuries. Professional Nurse 9(4): 230–237

Doyle D, Benton TF 1994 Palliative medicine: pain and symptom control. St Columba's Hospice, Edinburgh

Engstrom L 1994 Technique of insulin injection: is it important? Practical Diabetes 11(1): 39

Ewan P 1998 ABC of allergies – anaphylaxis. British Medical Journal 316: 1442–1445

Fisher M 1995 Treatment of acute anaphylaxis. British Medical Journal 311(Sept 16): 731–733

Fuller D 1995 Simplifying the system. Professional Nurse 10(5): 315–317

Jones M 1994 Vaccination: the facts. Primary Health Care 4(1): 16–17

Kelly J 1994 Understanding transdermal medication. Professional Nurse 10(2): 121–125

Lawrence JC, Lilly HA, Kidson A 1994 The use of alcoholic wipes for disinfection of injection sites. Journal of Wound Care 3(1): 11–14

McDonald S 1994 Controlled environment. Nursing Times 90(47): 42–44

McGraw C, Drennan V 2001 Self administration of medicine and older people. Nursing Standard 15(18): 33–36

Quinn C 2000 Infusion devices: risks, function and management. Nursing Standard 14(26): 35–41

Roberts K, Seaby L 1995 Empowering patients. Journal of Community Nursing 9(6): 4–6

Rodger M, King L 2000 Drawing up and administering intramuscular injections: a review of the literature. Journal of Advanced Nursing 31(3): 574–582

Smith A 1997 The use of syringe drivers and Hickman lines in the community. British Journal of Community Health Nursing 2(6): 292–296

Soanes N 2000 Injection site safety. Nursing Standard 14(25): 55

Stilliard K 2000 Professional issues. Clinical and financial governance of nurse prescribing. Community Nurse 6(4): 63–64

United Kingdom Central Council for Nursing, Midwifery and Health Care 1992a The scope of professional practice. UKCC, London

United Kingdom Central Council for Nursing, Midwifery and Health Visiting 1992b Code of professional conduct. UKCC, London

United Kingdom Central Council for Nursing, Midwifery and Health Visiting 1994 Administration of medicines: standards of monitored dosage systems, position statement. UKCC, London

United Kingdom Central Council for Nursing, Midwifery and Health Visiting 1996 Guidelines for professional practice. UKCC, London

United Kingdom Central Council for Nursing, Midwifery and Health Visiting 1998 Guidelines for records and record keeping. UKCC, London

United Kingdom Central Council for Nursing, Midwifery and Health Visiting 2000 Guidelines for the administration of medicines. UKCC, London

Whyte LA 1994 Medication cards for elderly people: a study. Nursing Standard 8(48): 25–28

Williams C 1996 Patient-controlled analgesia: a review of the literature. Journal of Clinical Nursing 5(3): 139–147

Willis J 1995 Patient-controlled analgesia devices. Professional Nurse 10(9): 579–583

Wilson V 2000 Guidelines for use of the MS26 daily rate syringe driver in the community. British Journal of Community Health Nursing 5(4): 162–168

Workman B 1999 Safe injection techniques. Nursing Standard 13(39): 47–53

Web site: Online pain   http://www.pain.com/default.cfm

2 Apical–Radial Pulses

Learning outcomes	By the end of this section you should know how to: - prepare the patient for this nursing practice - locate, assess, measure and record the apical–radial pulses.
Background knowledge required	Revision of the anatomy, physiology and pathology of the cardiovascular system Competency in measuring and recording a peripheral pulse (*see* p. 297).
Indications and rationale for assessing the apical–radial pulses	The rate at the apex of the heart and a peripheral pulse rate, usually the radial pulse, are counted simultaneously and compared to ascertain whether there is a discrepancy in the rate. It may be assessed *to estimate the degree of dysfunction on admission and the effect of treatment on*: - patients who have cardiac impairment, for example frequent ventricular ectopic beats or atrial fibrillation - patients who are receiving medication to improve heart action - patients who have peripheral arterial disease. The assessment elicits a pulse–apex deficit and helps in decisions on the necessity for treatment (Alexander et al 2000).
Equipment 	Watch with a second hand Stethoscope.
Guidelines and rationale for this nursing practice 	- measurement is carried out by two nurses simultaneously over 1 minute *to allow accuracy in recording an irregular rate* - explain the nursing practice to the patient, including the reasons for the procedure and the manner in which it will be carried out *to gain consent and co-operation. Patients should be encouraged to be active informed partners in their care* - ensure the patient's privacy *to maintain dignity and a sense of self* - collect the equipment *for efficiency of practice and to reduce any unnecessary stress for the patient*

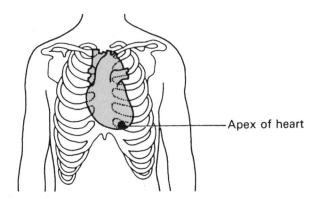

Apex of heart

Figure 2.1   *Position of the apex of the heart*

- assist the patient to a comfortable position, inclined slightly forward if possible *so that there is easy access to the chest wall and gravity will move the heart to the front of the thoracic cage. Patient comfort will also prevent an artificial elevation of the pulse rate*
- observe the patient throughout this activity *to detect any signs of discomfort*
- place the diaphragm of the stethoscope over the apex of the heart (nurse 1) (Fig. 2.1). This is usually located at the 5th intercostal space and 12 cm left of the midline
- locate the peripheral, usually radial, pulse (nurse 2)
- ensure that the watch is visible to both nurses, who begin counting the rates simultaneously for 1 minute
- at the end of 1 minute, the nurses compare results and document them appropriately, compare these with past recordings and report any abnormal findings immediately
- in undertaking this practice, nurses are accountable for their actions, the quality of care delivered and record-keeping according to the *Code of Professional Conduct* (UKCC 1992), *Guidelines for Professional Practice* (UKCC 1996) and *Guidelines for Records and Record Keeping* (UKCC 1998).

Relevance to the activities of living

Breathing

The patient who has a radial pulse deficit because of heart disease may also show an elevated respiratory rate because the inefficient action of the heart eventually leads to pulmonary oedema, which causes respiratory distress. The rate at the apex and at the radial artery should be compared. If there is a deficit in that of the radial pulse, it should be reported as it may indicate ongoing disease processes.

Eating and drinking

The patient with a recent onset of atrial fibrillation may need to be treated by cardioversion under sedation or general anaesthesia and fasting may be required until this procedure has been carried out. The increased autonomic nerve activity may cause dryness of the mouth, so frequent mouthwashes should be offered.

Controlling body temperature

An impaired blood supply to the limbs as a result of heart disease will probably result in complaints of cold hands and feet, and the wearing of gloves and socks should be encouraged. Because sensation is also impaired, caution should be exercised in the use of hot applications.

Mobilising

Mobilisation may be limited because of cardiac impairment and respiratory distress (Roper et al 2000). The medical practitioner may request that this practice is carried out with the patient in a standing position.

Working and playing

Patients with a radial pulse deficit may be unable to continue in their previous employment and hobbies.

Sleeping

The patient's normal sleeping pattern may be altered because of some of the physical features of cardiac impairment. Assisting the patient into a fairly upright position with plenty of pillows may help to relieve any discomfort.

Expressing sexuality

Recording the apical pulse may involve exposing the patient's chest, which for some patients, independent of gender, may be embarrassing.

Patient/carer education: key points

In partnership with the patient and carer, ensure that they are competent to carry out any practices required. Information should be given regarding an appropriate point of contact for any concerns that may arise.

Explanations given before, during and after the practice will help the patient to understand more about his or her health problems.

References

Alexander M, Fawcett J, Runciman P 2000 Nursing care – hospital and home: the adult. 2nd edn. Churchill Livingstone, Edinburgh

Roper N, Logan W, Tierney A 2000 The Roper–Logan–Tierney model of nursing. Churchill Livingstone, Edinburgh

United Kingdom Central Council for Nursing, Midwifery and Health Visiting 1992 Code of professional conduct. UKCC, London

United Kingdom Central Council for Nursing, Midwifery and Health Visiting 1996 Guidelines for professional practice. UKCC, London

United Kingdom Central Council for Nursing, Midwifery and Health Visiting 1998 Guidelines for records and record keeping. UKCC, London

3   Bathing and Showering

Learning outcomes

By the end of this section you should know how to:

- prepare the patient for this nursing practice
- collect and prepare the equipment
- help the patient with an immersion bath or shower, at home or in an institutional setting.

Background knowledge required

Revision of the anatomy and physiology of the skin, with special reference to its function as a barrier to infection

Review of health authority policy relating to moving and handling, in both an institutional and a community setting

Review of health authority policy relating to the use of aromatherapy

Review of local policy regarding preoperative skin preparation

Review of health authority policy regarding cleaning bathroom equipment and the control of infection.

Indications and rationale for immersion bath or shower

An immersion bath or shower enables the patient to have a total body wash and may be indicated:

- to maintain personal hygiene *and promote a feeling of well-being*
- to clean the skin prior to surgery *in order to help prevent infection in the wound area during the operation*
- to clean the skin following surgery *to prevent infection and promote healing.*

Equipment

Soap or emollient
Bath thermometer
Face cloth
Bath towel
Clean clothing
Chosen toiletries, e.g. deodorant, perfume, aftershave
Suitable bath or shower
Chair or shower stool
Disposable floor mat
Bathing/showering equipment aids as appropriate.

Guidelines and rationale for this nursing practice

Bathing

- discuss the arrangements for the bath with the patient *to gain consent and co-operation and encourage participation in care*. In the community, the patient should have a bathing assessment carried out; *this will assess the need for the use of equipment available from occupational therapy and whether help with bathing and showering should be given by the nursing or social services' staff* (as can be ascertained by referring to health board policy)
- help the patient to collect and prepare the equipment *so that everything is ready for use*
- help the patient to the bathroom; this may include the use of mechanical lifting aids or a wheelchair *if the patient has any difficulty with mobilising*
- ensure the patient's privacy as far as possible, *to respect individuality and maintain self-esteem*
- prepare the water in the bath, maintaining a safe temperature, and gain the patient's approval *as bathing is a very personal activity*
- help the patient to undress *if he or she needs help, giving encouragement for the patient to be as independent as possible*
- observe the patient throughout this activity *to observe any adverse effects*
- help the patient into the bath. For some patients, two nurses may be needed *to help the patient*; alternatively, mechanical aids may be used as appropriate according to the manufacturer's instructions (NBPA and RCN 1997)
- help the patient to wash himself or herself, commencing with the face and neck (*see* 'Bed bath', p. 32) *so that clean water is used first on these areas*
- help to wash the patient's hair *if required* (*see* 'Hair care', p. 169)
- help the patient out of the bath. The patient may sit on a chair that is protected with a towel *to prevent any unsteadiness and danger of falling*
- help the patient to dry *as required and encourage independence*
- help the patient to dress as required. *To promote patients' self-esteem and independence*, they should choose what they want to wear
- allow the patient time to clean his or her teeth or dentures at the basin, *to promote oral hygiene*, giving help as required
- help to brush or comb the patient's hair *to help self-esteem*
- help the patient to a chair or bed as is chosen, or as the condition allows, *for a period of rest after the exercise of bathing*
- ensure that the patient is left feeling as comfortable as possible *to promote relaxation*
- clean the bath *to promote a safe environment*
- dispose of equipment safely *to prevent any transmission of infection*
- document the nursing practice appropriately, monitor the after-effects and report abnormal findings immediately *to ensure safe practice and enable prompt appropriate medical or nursing intervention to be initiated*
- in undertaking this practice, nurses are accountable for their actions, the quality of care delivered and record-keeping according to the *Code of Professional Conduct* (UKCC 1992), *Guidelines for Professional Practice* (UKCC 1996) and *Guidelines for Records and Record Keeping* (UKCC 1998).

Showering

- discuss the arrangements for the shower with the patient *to gain consent and co-operation*
- help to collect and prepare the equipment *so that everything is ready for use*
- help the patient to the shower room. This may include the use of mechanical lifting aids or a wheelchair *if the patient has any difficulty with mobilising*
- help the patient to undress as required, *maintaining privacy to respect individuality*
- help the patient to sit on the shower chair or stool *so that there is no danger of falling*
- adjust the flow of water from the shower *to maintain a safe water temperature and gain the patient's approval*
- help the patient to wash while showering as required *so that he or she may have an enjoyable body wash*
- help the patient to wash his or her hair if required *to promote self-esteem*
- help the patient to dry
- proceed as in the guidelines for bathing, above.

Relevance to the activities of living

Observations and further rationale for this nursing practice will be included within each activity of living as appropriate.

Maintaining a safe environment

The nurse should ensure that patients have appropriate assistance to help them to bathe or shower safely. Self-care abilities may fluctuate, particularly in older people, and the nurse should constantly assess the situation and adapt the level of assistance to maintain maximum patient independence. A chair should be available so that patients can sit to dry or dress themselves without any danger of falling.

The water temperature should be checked to ensure that there is no danger of scalding; the maximum temperature should be 43°C. The ability to judge temperature may be impaired in elderly patients or those with diabetic neuropathy, so the water temperature should always be checked by a nurse or a responsible adult. The use of a bath thermometer will help with this.

The bath, shower area and bath hoist if used should be cleaned after each use. Bath hoists in particular may harbour harmful organisms (Boden 1999). If the nurse is not confident that this has been done, the bath should be cleaned before preparing it for the patient in order to prevent any cross-infection.

The patient's manual handling plan should be followed in order to prevent injury to the patient and the staff. For safety, it is advised that a frail, disabled or elderly person should always enter and leave a bath while sitting rather than by climbing over the side of the bath (NBPA and RCN 1997). Variable height or adjustable baths, for example, Parker baths, may be used.

To prevent the patient or staff slipping, the spillage of water onto the floor should be avoided; any spills that do occur should be dried immediately.

Communicating

The choice and timing of a bath or shower should as far as possible be arranged according to the patient's preference. The patient's condition and the ward or community situation may, however, affect this, and appropriate arrangements should be discussed with the patient to gain his or her co-operation. Cultural, ethnic and religious preferences should be observed (Roper et al 2000), as should the patient's preference for a male or female carer.

The development of a caring relationship between the nurse and the patient is often enhanced during the patient's bath or shower. The opportunity for communication is increased, so the nurse can encourage patients to talk about themselves, their family or their worries, providing information that may contribute to the nursing assessment. The time can also be used for patient education in personal hygiene, using good communication skills.

Eliminating

The patient should be given the opportunity to use the toilet or commode before bathing or showering.

Personal cleansing and dressing

While bathing the patient, the nurse should observe the condition of the skin for any abnormalities. Any redness, rashes, bruises, sores or lumps should be noted and reported (*see* 'Bed bath', p. 33). Soap and water may be harmful when used on fragile skin and may cause drying, eczema and dermatitis (Jeter & Lutz 1996). Alternatives such as emollients may be preferable to soothe and hydrate the skin (Courtnay 1998).

The skin should be dried carefully after bathing or showering, especially in the creases of the body such as under the breasts and in the groin. This helps to maintain the skin in a good condition to act as a barrier to infection. A light dusting with talcum powder may help to keep the skin dry, but too much may collect in the body creases and cause soreness.

Patients should wear their own clothes after a bath or shower to help to retain their individuality.

Controlling body temperature

The bath or shower room should be at a comfortable room temperature of 18–21°C. This will prevent the loss of body heat after a bath, when the patient may be exposed during drying and dressing.

Mobilising

Mechanical lifting aids should be used appropriately, according to the manufacturer's instructions, to help the patient in and out of the bath or shower (NBPA and RCN 1997). In the community, this will be in accordance with the individualised community bathing assessment.

Sleeping

A warm bath may relieve pain. In addition, the use of aromatherapy oils in the bath according to health authority policy may assist with relaxation, promote a feeling of well-being and encourage sleep (Buckle 1997, Price & Price 1996).

Expressing sexuality

If the patient is left alone to bathe or shower, it is often difficult to ensure the safety of the environment, so complete privacy cannot be assured; the patient will usually accept the nurse's presence if the safety implications are explained. The nurse's attitude and communication skills should help the acceptance of this invasion of privacy and prevent embarrassment. Apart from necessary attendant helpers, however, privacy should be ensured during this activity.

Male patients should be encouraged or helped to shave before or immediately after bathing or showering. They may like to apply some pleasant aftershave lotion to enhance their self-image. Women may be encouraged to apply make-up and perfume after bathing to help their individuality and self-esteem.

Patient/carer education: key points

In partnership with the patient and/or carer, ensure that they are competent to carry out any practices required. Information should be given regarding an appropriate point of contact for any concerns that arise.

The nurse should emphasise the role of personal hygiene in the prevention of infection. The importance of a safe water temperature for bathing and showering should be explained, and the height of the controls or taps may need to be adapted for safe use.

The use of aids, both simple and mechanical, should be explained to the patient. This helps to maintain a safe environment by preventing accidental falls and also ensures safe moving and handling techniques for nurses and carers. Advice and teaching on the availability of aids and the adaptation of the patient's home should be part of the responsibility of the community nursing team and the occupational therapist.

The patient should understand the importance of reporting any redness, swelling or breakdown of the skin to the nurse or medical practitioner so that any further deterioration in the condition of the skin can be prevented.

References

Boden M 1999 Contamination of moving and handling equipment. Professional Nurse 7: 484–487

Buckle J 1997 Clinical aromatherapy in nursing. Arnold, London

Courtnay M 1998 Preparations for skin conditions. Nursing Times 94(7): 54–55

Jeter FK, Lutz JB 1996 Skin care in the frail, elderly dependent, incontinent patient. Advances in Wound Care 9: 29–34

National Back Pain Association and Royal College of Nursing 1997 Washing and bathing. In NBPA and RCN Guide to the manual handling of patients, 4th edn. NBPA, Middlesex

Price S, Price L 1996 Aromatherapy for health professionals. Churchill Livingstone, Edinburgh

Roper N, Logan W, Tierney A 2000 The Roper–Logan–Tierney model of nursing. Churchill Livingstone, Edinburgh

United Kingdom Central Council for Nursing, Midwifery and Health Visiting 1992 Code of professional conduct. UKCC, London

United Kingdom Central Council for Nursing, Midwifery and Health Visiting 1996 Guidelines for professional practice. UKCC, London

United Kingdom Central Council for Nursing, Midwifery and Health Visiting 1998 Guidelines for records and record keeping. UKCC, London

4 Bed Bath

Learning outcomes

By the end of this section, you should know how to:

- prepare the patient for this nursing practice
- collect the equipment
- carry out a bed bath.

Background knowledge required

Revision of the anatomy and physiology of the skin tissue
Revision of 'Skin care' (*see* p. 309) and 'Mouth care' (*see* p. 225).

Indications and rationale for a bed bath

Bed-bathing assists a bed-fast patient *to maintain personal hygiene during a period of bed rest*. A patient may require a bed bath:

- postoperatively following major surgery when mobility is restricted
- following an acute illness, e.g. myocardial infarction
- while in an unconscious state
- following trauma, e.g. a patient in traction
- when extremely weak and debilitated as a result of the prolonged effects of a disease, trauma or a treatment being administered.

Equipment

Basin of hot water (35–40°C)
Lotion thermometer
Soap, preferably the patient's own
Patient's toiletries such as deodorant and talcum powder
Bath towels
Two face cloths/sponges or disposable wipes
Disposable paper towel or similar
Patient's brush and comb
Nail scissors and nail file if required
Clean nightdress or pyjamas
Clean bed linen
Trolley or adequate surface
Equipment for catheter care (*see* p. 102) if required
Equipment for skin care (*see* p. 309)
Equipment for mouth care (*see* p. 226)
Receptacle for the patient's soiled clothing
Receptacle for soiled bed linen
Receptacle for soiled disposable items.

Guidelines and rationale for this nursing practice

- explain the nursing practice to the patient *to gain consent and co-operation*
- collect and prepare the equipment *to ensure that all equipment is available and ready for use*
- ensure the patient's privacy *to reduce anxiety*
- observe the patient throughout this activity *to note any signs of distress*
- check that the bed brakes are in use *to prevent the patient or nurse sustaining an injury from a sudden uncontrolled movement of the bed*
- adjust the bed height *to ensure safe moving and handling practice* (NBPA and RCN 1997)
- help the patient into a comfortable position *permitting the nurse easy and comfortable access to the patient*
- arrange the furniture around the patient's bed space *to allow easy access to equipment on the trolley or surface*
- remove any excess bed linen and bed appliances if in use, *allowing easy access to the patient*, but leaving the patient covered with a bed sheet *to maintain modesty*
- help the patient to remove the pyjamas or gown in order *to reduce exertion as this can be a strenuous activity for a person who is in a weakened state*
- check the temperature of the basin of water using the lotion thermometer, and ask the patient to test the water temperature, *ensuring that the water is neither too hot nor too cold*
- check with the patient whether he or she uses soap on his face, *ensuring individualised care*
- wash, rinse and dry the patient's face, ears and neck; when possible, assist patients to do this for themselves *to encourage independence*
- if the face cloth is not going to be laundered after the procedure, the second face cloth should be used to wash the rest of the body *in order to reduce the risk of cross-infection*
- expose only the part of the patient's body being washed in order *to maintain the patient's modesty and self-esteem*
- change the water as it cools or becomes dirty, and immediately after washing the patient's pubic area, *preventing the cooling of the patient and reducing the risk of cross-infection respectively*
- wash, rinse and thoroughly dry the patient's body in an appropriate order, such as the upper limbs, chest and abdomen, back and lower limbs, *preventing excessive exertion on the part of the patient*
- change the water immediately after perineal hygiene or leave this action until last, *reducing the risk of cross-infection from the normal skin flora of the perineal region to the rest of the skin*
- when washing the patient's limbs, first wash the limb furthest away from you. *This will allow the assistant to dry that limb as the other limb is being washed, thus reducing the time during which the patient's body is exposed to the cooling effect of the environment.* When possible, assist the patient to immerse the feet and hands in the basin of water (Fig. 4.1)

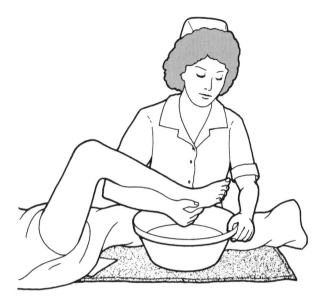

Figure 4.1 *Foot immersion: the patient's foot and leg should be supported. The upper limbs can be supported in a similar way*

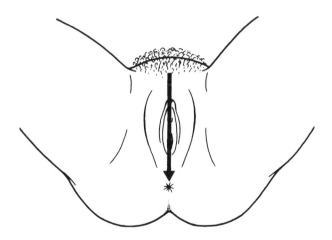

Figure 4.2 *Perineal hygiene: wash in one direction only, from the front to the back of the perineum*

- as each part of the patient's body is washed, observe the skin for any blemishes, redness or discoloration, ***which will alert the nurse to the potential problem of pressure sore development*** (*see* 'Skin care', p. 309)
- apply body deodorants and/or other toiletries as desired by the patient, ***ensuring individualised care***
- assist the patient to wash, rinse and dry the pubic area using the disposable wipes, washing from the front of the perineal area to the back ***to prevent cross-infection from the anal region*** (Fig. 4.2)
- carry out catheter care if required, ***which may prevent infection*** (*see* p. 102)
- help the patient to dress in clean pyjamas or gown ***to reduce exertion on the part of the patient***

- *to prevent injury, reduce the risk of cross-infection and promote self-esteem*, assist the patient to cut and clean the fingernails and toenails if required and unless otherwise instructed
- *to promote patient comfort*, remove any soiled or damp bed linen and remake the patient's bed
- assist the patient with mouth care (*see* p. 225) *to promote a positive body image*
- assist the patient to brush or comb the hair into its usual style, *promoting independence and self-esteem*
- ensure that the patient is left feeling as comfortable as possible while *maintaining the quality of this nursing practice*
- rearrange the furniture as wished by the patient *so that any articles needed are within easy reach and the patient is given control of the environment*
- dispose of the equipment safely *to reduce any health hazard*
- document the nursing practice appropriately, monitor any after-effects and report abnormal findings immediately, *providing a written record and assisting in the implementation of any action should an abnormality or adverse reaction to the practice be noted*
- in undertaking this practice, nurses are accountable for their actions, the quality of care delivered and record-keeping according to the *Code of Professional Conduct* (UKCC 1992), *Guidelines for Professional Practice* (UKCC 1996) and *Guidelines for Records and Record Keeping* (UKCC 1998).

Relevance to the activities of living	***Maintaining a safe environment***

It is necessary to wash at regular intervals to keep the natural flora of micro-organisms within manageable limits. When a patient is confined to bed, a bed bath is one of the nursing practices used to reduce the potential problem of cross-infection or self-infection during the period of vulnerability caused by illness (Roper et al 2000).

The nurse must check that the temperature of the water is at a safe level prior to starting the bed bath and must maintain this temperature throughout the bath to assist with patient comfort. The water should be changed as it becomes dirty or cooler, and immediately following perineal hygiene. When assisting the patient with perineal hygiene, wash from front to back to reduce the problem of cross-infection from the anal region.

All equipment used should be clean or disposable, and all precautions must be taken to prevent cross-infection. Nurses should wash their hands before commencing and on the completion of a bed bath. A disposable plastic apron should be used (Baker et al 1999a, b).

Both at home and in hospital, it is preferable that the patient has a personal washbasin during the period of confinement to bed. The nurse should wash the basin and trolley with a detergent and water solution, drying them thoroughly prior to and following a bed bath. The basin should be clean and dry when not in use, being stored inverted in an easily accessible area for the sole use of that patient. The use of abrasive materials to clean plastic wash bowls should be avoided as this roughens the surface, making it easy for micro-organisms to become trapped (Nicol et al 2000).

It is recommended that disposable flannels be used as fabric ones become colonised with micro-organisms when left damp (Baker et al 1999a, b). If the patient wishes to use a cloth flannel or a sponge, it should be rinsed in clean water and returned to the back of the patient's locker or to the bathroom, where it can be hung to dry. In this case, separate flannels should be used for the face and body, laundering taking place at a frequency agreed with the patient. Other toiletry items used and any soiled personal clothing that the relatives wish to take home for laundering during hospitalisation should be placed in the locker. Any appliances removed during the bed bath, such as a bed cage, bed table or cot side, should be returned to their previous position.

In some health authority areas, bathing at home is no longer the responsibility of the community health service but has become the task of social care workers. However, if the bed bath is part of an overall package of care, such as for a terminally ill patient, the community nurse will be involved in the management of the delivery of care.

Communicating

The nurse and patient should talk to each other during the bed bath, but this may have to be kept to a minimum when the patient is acutely ill. For acutely ill or unconscious patients, non-verbal cues can be used as a method of communication, and touch will become of increased importance.

The nurse should check that the patient who is suffering pain has had recent pain relief before starting a bed bath as the movement during bathing may exacerbate the pain.

Breathing

Patient movement during a bed bath should be kept to a minimum, especially when a patient suffers from dyspnoea; changing the bottom sheet should, for example, be planned to minimise movement and effort if the patient is acutely ill. When oxygen therapy is being administered, the mask or cannula can be removed for facial cleansing, hair care and mouth care at separate times during the bed bath.

Eliminating

The patient should be offered the facilities to empty his or her bladder prior to commencing a bed bath.

Personal cleansing and dressing

A patient who does not wash on a regular basis may require some assistance and education from the nurse on the benefit of this practice during his or her period of incapacity. Assisting a patient who has a pyrexia with personal hygiene can be comforting in terms of removing excess perspiration and providing clean, fresh clothing.

In hospital, it is usual to have disposable toiletries available in ward areas for patients who may have been admitted as an emergency, until their own personal equipment is brought from home. When possible, patients should be dressed in their own bed clothing for their comfort and to help maintain their individuality.

A patient who has the power, movement or sensation of a limb altered either temporarily or permanently, such as by the position of an intravenous infusion or following a cerebral vascular accident, will require some assistance and education on how to dress and undress during a bed bath. The weak or affected limb is undressed last and dressed first.

Soap should be used with caution as it has a drying effect on the skin (Mallett & Bailley 1997). A patient who has dry skin may have an emollient prescribed by a medical practitioner, this being added to the water for washing. The patient's skin must be rinsed well and thoroughly dried during the bed bath to reduce the potential problem of skin irritation. The nurse should carry out skin care (*see* p. 309) during a bed bath.

Patients should be assisted to keep their fingernails and toenails clean and manicured. A chiropody service may not be available for all patients but should be used when special care has to be taken of a patient's nails, for example with a diabetic patient or a patient suffering from peripheral vascular disease, to prevent injury to the nail or nailbed. The nurse may assist the patient to apply nail polish if desired.

When patients are confined to bed, the friction between their heads and the pillow can cause their hair to become tangled and matted. A patient's hair should therefore be brushed and combed into its usual style during a bed bath and at regular intervals throughout the day to prevent tangling and discomfort to the patient. The patient can have his or her hair washed while in bed (*see* p. 170) to maintain its cleanliness. Should a patient be confined to bed over a prolonged period, a hairdresser or barber may be required to cut and style the hair to improve morale.

Mouth care (*see* p. 225) may be required during a bed bath.

Controlling body temperature

Before starting the bed bath, the nurse should check that the environment around the patient's bed space is at a comfortable temperature and that no draughts are evident. During the bed bath, the nurse should ensure that the patient is kept warm as an excessive loss of body heat can lead to hypothermia. Pyrexial patients may be offered a cool-water bed bath to make them feel more comfortable, but there is no research demonstrating that applying cool water to the skin surface can alter a patient's physiological body temperature.

Expressing sexuality

In Western societies, feeling fresh and clean is known to create a positive body image and maintain self-esteem. A patient confined to bed will therefore not only feel more comfortable, but also benefit psychologically from a bed bath. The provision of privacy during this nursing practice is very important in the maintenance of the patient's self-esteem and individuality.

When possible, help patients to maintain their individuality and independence by allowing them to wash and dry any part of their body they wish, such as their face, hands and pubic area. As the patients have no choice of the method used for cleansing, instead allow them to make decisions in other areas, such as which clothing they wish to wear. The use of body deodorant, perfume and make-up is determined by personal preference, and the nurse should be guided by patients in their application.

Patient/carer education: key points

In partnership with the patient and/or carer, ensure that they are competent to carry out any practices required. Information should be given on an appropriate point of contact for any concerns that may arise.

The carer may be taught how to perform this nursing practice. Preventing infection because of the maintenance of skin hygiene by bed-bathing should be explained to the patient and carers. Advice on the direction of washing to reduce the risk of cross-infection from the anal region to the rest of the perineal area should be given to the patient and carers.

References

Baker F, Smith L, Stead L 1999a Giving a blanket bath. 1. Nursing Times 95(3, suppl): 1–2
Baker F, Smith L, Stead L 1999b Giving a blanket bath. 2. Nursing Times 95(4, suppl): 1–2
Mallett J, Bailley C (eds) 1997 Royal Marsden manual of clinical procedures. 4th edn. Blackwell Science, London
National Back Pain Association and Royal College of Nursing 1997 Guide to the handling of patients. 4th edn. NBPA, Middlesex
Nicol M, Bavin C, Bedford-Turner S, Cronin P, Rawlings-Anderson K 2000 Essential nursing skills. CV Mosby, London
Roper N, Logan W, Tierney A 2000 The Roper–Logan–Tierney model of nursing. Churchill Livingstone, Edinburgh
United Kingdom Central Council for Nursing, Midwifery and Health Visiting 1992 Code of professional conduct. UKCC, London
United Kingdom Central Council for Nursing, Midwifery and Health Visiting 1996 Guidelines for professional practice. UKCC, London
United Kingdom Central Council for Nursing, Midwifery and Health Visiting 1998 Guidelines for records and record keeping. UKCC, London

5   Blood Glucose Monitoring

Learning outcomes

By the end of this section, you should know how to:

- collect and prepare the equipment
- prepare the patient for this nursing practice
- carry out blood glucose measurement.

Background knowledge required

Anatomy and physiology of the endocrine system, with special reference to the regulation of blood glucose

Clinical knowledge of insulin-dependent and non-insulin-dependent diabetes

Target range of individual patient blood glucose level

Knowledge of the normal range of blood glucose concentration

Manufacturer's information on the selected reagent strip

Knowledge of different devices used to obtain the blood sample and to measure blood glucose level

Health authority policy or protocol for this practice

Principles of infection control with respect to blood-borne infection.

Indications and rationale for blood glucose estimation

Blood glucose estimation is the measurement of the level of blood glucose using a chemical reagent strip. This investigation may be carried out to:

- assist in the preliminary diagnosis of diabetes mellitus caused by pancreatic disease or other hormonal disorders *through the measurement of the level of glucose in the blood*
- monitor the blood glucose level in patients with established diabetes *in order to facilitate an acceptable blood glucose level*
- monitor patients receiving parenteral nutrition (*see* p. 263) *to ensure that the blood glucose level is kept within an acceptable range.*

Equipment

Sterile lancet or pricking device
Cotton wool balls
Blood-testing strip
Disposable gloves
Tray for equipment
Sharps box
Receptacle for soiled material
Patient documentation and personal diabetic diary (if appropriate)
Glucose meter device.

Guidelines and rationale for this nursing practice

There are several different blood glucose devices available in the UK, so the manufacturer's instructions for use must always be followed (Fig. 5.1).

- familiarise yourself with the instructions for the device you are using *to ensure a correct safe practice*
- check the expiry date of the reagent strip *to ensure that the strips are within the 'use by' date*
- confirm that the device is calibrated to the reagent strip *to reduce the risk of an error with the result*
- discuss the practice with the patient *to inform the patient about the practice and to discuss any concerns or queries*
- obtain consent from the patient to undertake the practice *to ensure that the patient is aware of his or her rights as a patient*
- select a suitable clean surface and lay out the equipment. If undertaking the practice in the patient's own home, protect the surface with a waterproof cover *to provide a suitable protected work surface and ensure that the equipment is ready for patient use*
- cleanse the hands using a bactericidal solution *to reduce the risk of cross-infection* (Gould 1995)
- ask or assist the patient to wash his or her hands with soap and warm water, ensuring that all traces of soap have been rinsed off and that the hands are dried thoroughly *to ensure that the skin surface is clean and that there is no residual soap, which may affect the accuracy of the reading* (Siegal 1993). *Heat will also help to dilate the small blood vessels in the fingertips*
- help the patient into a comfortable position (either sitting or lying supine) *to ensure patient comfort and prevent injury if the patient feels faint during the practice*
- select an appropriate puncture site (normally the soft flesh at the top of the fingers). If blood glucose monitoring is a regular practice, the site should be rotated *to avoid overuse of any one site and thus reduce discomfort for the patient*
- put on gloves *to protect the patient and nurse from potential blood-borne infection*

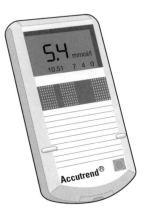

Figure 5.1   *Blood glucose monitoring device*

- using the lancet or pricking device (the latter now being the preferred option unless the patient objects to its use), prick the patient's finger *to pierce the skin with minimal discomfort*
- gently massage the finger to obtain an adequate drop of blood. *Obtain a suitable amount of blood to cover the reagent strip*
- allow the drop of blood to come into contact with the reagent strip without smearing and spreading the blood, *to ensure even coverage of the strip*
- continue as per the manufacturer's instructions for the specific device in use
- apply a clean cotton wool ball with firm pressure to the skin site for approximately 30–60 seconds or until bleeding has stopped (the patient may be able to undertake this activity) *to prevent any further bleeding after the sample has been obtained and prevent haematoma formation*
- read the result on the glucose meter device *to obtain the blood glucose level*
- note and document the results in both the nursing/medical notes and the patient's personal diabetic diary (where applicable). Informing the patient of the result should be carried out only in consultation with the medical practitioner who authorised the investigation. Opportunity should be given for the patient and/or carer to discuss anxieties or issues concerning any newly diagnosed disease *to ensure that the results are communicated to other health-care professionals and the patient. It may not be appropriate for the nurse to give the result to the patient at this point if further investigations are required before an accurate diagnosis can be made*
- report any abnormal results to a medical practitioner as soon as possible. If the practice is being carried out in the patient's own home, the nurse may be required to remain with the patient until the glucose level has stabilised *to ensure that prompt and appropriate treatment can be initiated. Some health authorities have a medically agreed treatment protocol to be followed when abnormal glucose readings are detected by nursing staff*
- dispose of any contaminated equipment according to health authority policy *to prevent the transmission of infection*
- remove the gloves and dispose of as above. Wash the hands or cleanse with bactericidal solution *to prevent cross-infection*
- ensure that patient is not feeling unwell after the practice (especially if the practice has been carried out in the patient's own home), *to ensure that the patient does not feel unwell as a result of the practice*
- discuss the points raised under 'Patient/carer education: key points', below. If the patient is unable to participate in follow-up self-care, this should be undertaken by the nurse or an appropriate adult carer *to ensure that the patient, carer and/or nurse are aware of, and understand, follow-up self-care*
- in undertaking this practice, nurses are accountable for their actions, the quality of care delivered and record-keeping according to the *Code of Professional Conduct* (UKCC 1992), *Guidelines for Professional Practice* (UKCC 1996) and *Guidelines for Records and Record Keeping* (UKCC 1998).

The frequency of blood glucose monitoring will be advised by the medical practitioner.

Relevance to the activities of living

Maintaining a safe environment

All reagent strip containers should be stored in a locked cupboard or drawer when not in use, in order to comply with health and safety at work regulations. The nurse in the community should encourage patients to keep all equipment in a safe place away from children. The manufacturer's recommendations for the conditions of storage and blood glucose monitoring technique must be observed; otherwise, inaccurate results may be obtained from the reagent strips. It is advisable to record the date when the strips have been opened as they may need to be used within a certain time. Regular checking of the glucose meter device with the control solution provided by the manufacturer is recommended (Hall 1999).

The nurse should assess the blood glucose level at the specific time requested by the medical practitioner.

Contamination of the reagent pad or the patient's blood could lead to inaccurate results. The patient's finger should not be cleansed with an alcohol-saturated wipe as the alcohol acts as a contaminant and causes the skin to harden with constant use. Any reagent strip accidentally contaminated by the nurse or patient must be discarded.

The nurse must be aware of the theory underpinning glucose monitoring practice and have a knowledge of the normal range of blood glucose level in order that any abnormal readings may be immediately recognised and treatment initiated according to health authority policy. The blood glucose levels are measured in mmol/l, the range of blood glucose in a healthy individual being between 4 mmol/l and 7 mmol/l (Cowan 1997). The acceptable range for each individual patient (particularly with long-standing diabetes) may vary slightly but should be identified by the medical practitioner and recorded in all patient documentation.

'Hypoglycaemia' is the term used to describe an abnormally low blood glucose. 'Hyperglycaemia' describes an excessively high blood glucose. Both require urgent treatment.

Communicating

The experienced nurse should be able to detect potential problems in a patient with a fluctuating blood glucose level and communicate that information to other colleagues involved in the patient's care.

The nurse should be aware of what information the patient needs on the practice of blood glucose estimation. Nurses should encourage patients to discuss their understanding of why blood glucose estimation is being carried out and be responsive to patients' needs for information on the reasons for blood glucose estimation. (This should be carried out in consultation with the medical practitioner who authorised the investigation.)

The nurse should initiate a patient education programme at a time that best suits the needs of the patient and his or her ability to learn. Patient education may need to continue on transfer from hospital, good communication being essential for its continuity.

Health promotion may be carried out in relation to an underlying disease, for example in a diabetic patient attending for blood glucose monitoring.

Breathing

The development of tachycardia or palpitation in the patient can be suggestive of impending hypoglycaemic coma.

Eating and drinking

The most common reason for estimating the blood glucose is in the management of diabetes mellitus. Patients will usually be given advice on a diet to suit their needs, and they will require ongoing support and education to help them to cope with any changes in eating pattern.

Eliminating

Blood glucose estimation provides a more accurate assessment of blood glucose level than does assessing the level of glucose in the urine. Each patient's renal threshold (the level at which the blood glucose spills over into the urine) varies, so measuring the glucose in the urine can be an inaccurate guide to the effectiveness of the hormonal control of glucose level in the body.

Patient/carer education: key points

In partnership with the patient and/or carer, ensure that they are competent to carry out any practices required. Information should be given on an appropriate point of contact for any concerns that may arise.

- blood sample results: if the results are not given immediately after undertaking the practice, the patient should be informed of when they will be available and of the process for obtaining them
- for newly diagnosed diabetic patients, the teaching of blood glucose estimation should be part of an individual education package on disease and symptom management. Teaching the patient about blood glucose estimation should incorporate the following main stages:
  — education on the practice (including the rationale and the treatment of any abnormal readings) using verbal and written information
  — demonstration of the blood glucose monitoring technique
  — supervision of the patient carrying out blood glucose estimation
  — regular monitoring of the technique as part of the ongoing management programme of care for the patient with diabetes
- patient education is likely to be shared between institutional and community staff
- patient education material is available from many of the manufacturers who produce reagent strips and devices (Strachan 2000)
- glucose meters can be purchased from the community pharmacist

- hospitalised insulin-dependent diabetics who are self-caring in this practice should be encouraged to continue with their monitoring as this provides an opportunity to assess their technique and reinforce good practice.

References

Cowan T 1997 Blood glucose monitoring devices. Professional Nurse 12(8): 593–597

Gould D 1995 Now please wash your hands. Practice Nurse 10(3): 188–190

Hall G 1999 Blood glucose monitoring. Practice Nurse 18(7): 469–471

Siegal J 1993 Teaching infection control in blood glucose monitoring. Diabetes Education 19(6): 489–492, 495

Strachan K 2000 Diabetes mellitus. In: Alexander MF, Fawcett JN, Runciman PJ (eds) Nursing practice – hospital and home: the adult. 2nd edn. Churchill Livingstone, Edinburgh

United Kingdom Central Council for Nursing, Midwifery and Health Visiting 1992 Code of professional conduct. UKCC, London

United Kingdom Central Council for Nursing, Midwifery and Health Visiting 1996 Guidelines for professional practice. UKCC, London

United Kingdom Central Council for Nursing, Midwifery and Health Visiting 1998 Guidelines for records and record keeping. UKCC, London

6 Blood Pressure

Learning outcomes

By the end of this section, you should know how to:

- prepare the patient for this nursing practice
- collect and prepare the equipment
- assess, measure, and record blood pressure.

Background knowledge required

Revision of the anatomy and physiology of the cardiovascular system.

Indications and rationale for recording blood pressure

Blood pressure is the force exerted by the blood as it flows through the blood vessels. It is the arterial blood pressure that is normally recorded, and this may be indicated:

- *to aid the diagnosis of disease*
- *to aid in the assessment of the cardiovascular system during and after disease*
- *to assess the efficacy of antihypertensive medication*
- *preoperatively to assess the patient's usual range of blood pressure*
- *to aid in the assessment of the cardiovascular system following surgery or trauma.*

Equipment

Sphygmomanometer: aneroid (Fig. 6.1A), electronic (Fig. 6.1B) or mercury (Fig. 6.1C)
Stethoscope (for use with only an aneroid or mercury sphygmomanometer)
Swabs to clean stethoscope ear pieces.

Sphygmomanometers

Because of the health and environmental hazards associated with the use of mercury, mercury sphygmomanometers are increasingly being phased out and replaced with aneroid or electronic sphygmomanometers to monitor patients' blood pressure. Should nurses encounter any sphygmomanometers that they have not previously used, competency in the use of the equipment must be assured before assessing any patient's blood pressure.

Guidelines and rationale for this nursing practice

- explain the nursing practice to the patient *to gain consent and co-operation*
- wash the hands *to reduce the risk of cross-infection*
- ensure the patient's privacy *to reduce anxiety and/or embarrassment*
- collect the equipment *to assist in the planning and implementation of the practice*
- observe the patient throughout this activity *to note any signs of distress*

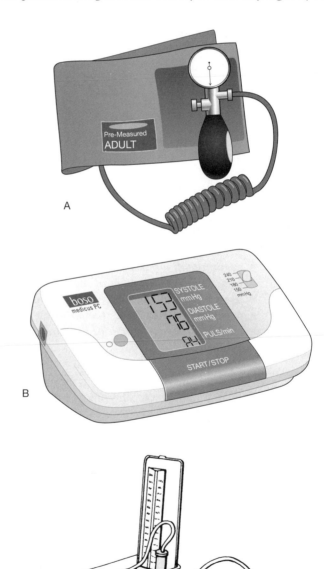

Figure 6.1
Sphygmomanometers used for blood pressure measurement
A Aneroid
B Electronic
C Mercury

- help the patient into a suitable position, either sitting or lying, and remove any restrictive clothing from the arm. Avoid tightly rolled-up sleeves *as these prevent constriction of the vessels of the limb immediately before the practice and may lead to an inaccurate recording.*

Electronic sphygmomanometer

- follow the manufacturer's instructions to achieving a recording, *thus ensuring an accurate measurement*
- continue as for 'All sphygmomanometers', below.

Aneroid sphygmomanometer

- apply the cuff 3–5 cm above the point at which the brachial artery can be palpated. The cuff should be applied smoothly and firmly, covering 80% of the arm circumference (Croft & Cruickshank 1990), the middle of the rubber bladder lying directly over the brachial artery *to permit access to the brachial artery by the stethoscope and even pressure around the circumference of the limb. A bladder that is too large or too small will result in a respective under- or overestimation of the blood pressure* (O'Brien 1995)
- ask the patient to rest the arm on a suitable firm surface *to ensure patient comfort and prevent movement of the limb, which may lead to inaccurate results*
- palpate the radial pulse and inflate the cuff until the pulse has been obliterated. Inflate for a further 20 mmHg. Release the valve slowly, taking note of the reading on the dial when the radial pulse returns. Allow all the air to escape from the cuff. *This will provide an initial assessment of the systolic pressure*
- palpate the brachial pulse, place the stethoscope over the site, and inflate the cuff to 20 mmHg above the previous reading. Release the valve of the inflation ball at a rate of 2–3 mmHg per second. When the first pulse is heard, the reading on the dial should be noted – this is the systolic pressure (Petrie et al 1990a). *This provides an accurate assessment of the systolic pressure without excessive discomfort to the patient*
- continue to deflate the cuff, the pulse sounds changing to muffled sounds until it finally disappears. The mercury level should be noted – this is the diastolic pressure (Petrie et al 1990a). *This provides an accurate assessment of the diastolic pressure*
- continue controlled deflation until a value 20 mmHg below the diastolic pressure has been reached *as this will eradicate the chance of a 'silent interval' leading to a false recording.*

Mercury sphygmomanometer

- position the sphygmomanometer at approximately heart height, ensuring that the mercury level is at zero and that the mercury column can be easily read. *This will reduce the incidence of over- or underestimation of the blood pressure* (Petrie et al 1990b)
- apply the cuff 3–5 cm above the point at which the brachial artery can be palpated. The cuff should be applied smoothly and firmly, covering 80% of

the arm circumference (Croft & Cruickshank 1990), the middle of the rubber bladder being placed directly over the brachial artery *to permit access to the brachial artery by the stethoscope and even pressure around the circumference of the limb. A bladder that is too large or too small will result in under- and overestimation of the blood pressure respectively* (O'Brien 1995)

- ask the patient to rest the arm on a suitable firm surface *to ensure patient comfort and prevent movement of the limb, which may lead to inaccurate results*
- connect the cuff tubing to the manometer tubing and close the valve of the inflation ball, *creating a sealed unit within the equipment*
- palpate the radial pulse and inflate the cuff until the pulse is obliterated. Inflate for a further 20 mmHg. Release the valve slowly, taking note of the reading on the mercury column when the radial pulse returns; the mercury level is read at the top of the meniscus. Allow all the air to escape from the cuff. *This will provide an initial assessment of the systolic pressure*
- palpate the brachial pulse, place the stethoscope over the site, and inflate the cuff to 20 mmHg above the previous reading. Release the valve of the inflation ball at a rate of 2–3 mmHg per second. When the first pulse is heard, the mercury level should be noted – this is the systolic pressure (Petrie et al 1990a). *This provides an accurate assessment of the systolic pressure without excessive discomfort to the patient*
- continue to deflate the cuff; the pulse sounds will become muffled until they finally disappear. The mercury level should now be noted – this is the diastolic pressure (Petrie et al 1990a). *This provides an accurate assessment of the diastolic pressure*
- continue controlled deflation until a value 20 mmHg below the diastolic pressure has been reached *as this will eradicate the chance of a 'silent interval' leading to a false recording.*

All sphygmomanometers

- completely deflate the cuff, disconnect the tubing and remove the cuff from the patient's arm *to prevent further compression of the limb*
- ensure that the patient is left feeling as comfortable as possible *to ensure the quality of this nursing practice*
- if a communal stethoscope has been used, clean the ear pieces with an alcohol-saturated swab *to reduce cross-infection between staff*
- dispose of the equipment safely *to comply with health and safety criteria and prolong the use of the equipment*
- document the nursing practice appropriately, comparing with past recordings: note any differences, detect trends, monitor the after-effects and report abnormal findings immediately. *This provides a written record and assists in the implementation of any action should an abnormality or adverse reaction to the practice be noted*
- in undertaking this practice, nurses are accountable for their actions, the quality of care delivered and record-keeping according to the *Code of Professional Conduct* (UKCC 1992), *Guidelines for Professional Practice* (UKCC 1996) and *Guidelines for Records and Record Keeping* (UKCC 1998).

Relevance to the activities of living

Maintaining a safe environment

It is recommended that any sphygmomanometer be calibrated at regular intervals by trained personnel to maintain the accuracy of the equipment.

The size of the cuff is important in achieving accurate recordings (Croft & Cruickshank 1990). Different cuffs are available for use on a baby, a child or an obese person, or for taking recordings using the patient's thigh.

By listening 20 mmHg above and below the points of appearance and disappearance of sounds, the possibility of a 'silent interval' falsifying the reading is overcome.

Repeated measurements, i.e. more than twice in 5 minutes, should be avoided as venous congestion can cause a rise in pressure.

All equipment should be clean, and all precautions should be taken to prevent cross-infection. Nurses should wash their hands before commencing and on completion of the nursing practice. When a communal ward stethoscope has been used, the ear pieces should be cleaned with an alcohol-saturated swab before and after blood pressure assessment. A nurse may wish to purchase his or her own stethoscope to prevent any ear cross-infection.

Recent research has demonstrated that manual mercury sphygmomanometers are poorly maintained in hospitals (Carney et al 1999, Markandu et al 2000), which may be part of the reason for the change to automated measurement. Other research has, however, shown that the accuracy of automated instruments is poor (Carney et al 1999, Natarjan et al 1999). The measurement of blood pressure is clearly in a period of change, and the nurse must have an understanding of all three methods.

Communicating

Blood pressure measurements can be recorded on a graded chart or abbreviated by placing the systolic pressure reading over the diastolic:

130/80 mmHg

'Hypertension' is the term used when the systolic or diastolic blood pressure is elevated above the normal range. 'Hypotension' is said to occur when the blood pressure lies below the normal range.

Stressful situations such as admission to hospital or a visit to a health-care professional are known to have an effect on a person's blood pressure, so the nurse should allow the patient to relax before taking the recording.

Patient/carer education: key points

In partnership with the patient and/or carer, ensure that they are competent to carry out any practices required. Information should be given on an appropriate point of contact for any concerns that may arise.

Inform the patient of the results and any action required should an abnormality be detected.

Information regarding the common lifestyle factors that are known to affect blood pressure should be discussed with the patient. This may allow the patient to make an informed choice about whether or not to continue such practices.

References

Carney S, Gillies A, Green S, Paterson O, Taylor M, Smith A 1999 Hospital blood pressure measurement: staff and device assessment. Journal of Quality in Clinical Practice 19(2): 95–98

Croft P, Cruickshank J 1990 Blood pressure measurement in adults: large cuffs for all? Journal of Epidemiology and Community Health 44: 170–173

Markandu N, Whitcher F, Arnold A, Carney C 2000 The mercury sphygmomanometer should be abandoned before it is proscribed. Journal of Human Hypertension 14(1): 31–36

Natarjan P, Shennan A, Penny J, Halligan A, De Sweit M, Anthony J 1999 Comparison of auscultatory and oscillometric automated blood pressure monitors in the settings of pre-eclampsia. American Journal of Obstetrics and Gynecology 181(5/1): 1203–1210

O'Brien E 1995 Blood pressure measurement. In: O'Brien ET, Beevers DG, Marshall HJ (eds). ABC of hypertension. 3rd edn. BMJ Publishing Group, London

Petrie J, Jamieson M, O'Brien E, Littler W, Padfield P, de Swiet M for the Working Party on Blood Pressure Measurement 1990a Blood pressure measurement [videotape]. BMJ Publishing Group, London

Petrie JC, O'Brien ET, Littler WA, de Swiet M, Dillon MJ, Padfield PL 1990b Recommendations on blood pressure measurement. 2nd edn. BMJ Publishing Group, London

United Kingdom Central Council for Nursing, Midwifery and Health Visiting 1992 Code of professional conduct. UKCC, London

United Kingdom Central Council for Nursing, Midwifery and Health Visiting 1996 Guidelines for professional practice. UKCC, London

United Kingdom Central Council for Nursing, Midwifery and Health Visiting 1998 Guidelines for records and record keeping. UKCC, London

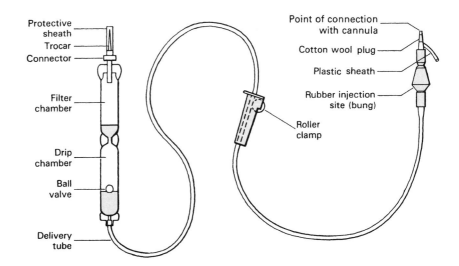

Figure 7.1

Administration set for blood transfusion. An extra filter may be introduced between the blood pack and the blood administration set

Labels on figure: Protective sheath; Trocar; Connector; Filter chamber; Drip chamber; Ball valve; Delivery tube; Point of connection with cannula; Cotton wool plug; Plastic sheath; Rubber injection site (bung); Roller clamp

- help the patient into a comfortable position following the commencement of the transfusion *to help the patient accept the transfusion for a period of time*
- regulate the input *to maintain the flow of blood at the prescribed rate*
- monitor the patient's temperature and pulse every 15 minutes for the first hour of the transfusion (Atterbury & Wilkinson 2000, Duke 2000). Thereafter, continue assessing the temperature, pulse, respiration and blood pressure hourly *to identify any change that might indicate the development of an adverse reaction*
- accurately record the volume of blood transfused. Note that the volume of 1 unit of whole blood is 500 ml and that of 1 unit of concentrated red cells 300 ml. *Any adverse effects may be related to the amount transfused*
- ensure that the patient is left feeling as comfortable as possible *to help to reduce anxiety*
- dispose of the equipment safely *to prevent the transmission of infection*
- document this nursing practice appropriately, monitor the after-effects, and report any abnormal findings immediately *to ensure safe practice and enable prompt appropriate medical and nursing intervention to be initiated as soon as possible*
- in undertaking this practice, nurses are accountable for their actions, the quality of care delivered and record-keeping according to the *Code of Professional Conduct* (UKCC 1992), *Guidelines for Professional Practice* (UKCC 1996) and *Guidelines for Records and Record Keeping* (UKCC 1998).

Guidelines and rationale for withdrawal of blood from the bank

- refer to health authority policies for access to the blood bank and local procedure *as there may be slight variations in documentation*
- withdraw blood from the blood bank 1 unit at a time immediately before transfusion into an individual patient *so that each unit of blood is stored at the correct temperature until just before use*

- check the information on the label of the blood container against the appropriate documentation for that particular patient *as incompatible blood causes adverse reactions*
- complete the documentation of withdrawal for the blood transfusion service and the patient's medical records, *ensuring accurate record-keeping*
- in undertaking this practice, nurses are accountable for their actions, the quality of care delivered and record-keeping according to the *Code of Professional Conduct* (UKCC 1992), *Guidelines for Professional Practice* (UKCC 1996) and *Guidelines for Records and Record Keeping* (UKCC 1998).

Guidelines and rationale for checking blood for transfusion

Blood for transfusion is normally checked by two people, one of whom must be a medical practitioner or a registered nurse. *This is safe professional practice for ensuring that the correct patient receives a compatible unit of blood.* This practice has, however, recently been questioned as it may lead to a diffusion of responsibility of the checking procedure, and recommendation has been made that it may be more appropriate for one registered nurse to perform the checking procedures at the patient's bedside (BCSH 1999).

- identify the prescription for blood transfusion and check the following information:
  - the date and time of commencement
  - the name of the patient
  - the unit or hospital number of the patient
  - the type of blood prescribed, e.g. whole blood or concentrated red cells
  - the number of units prescribed
  - the rate of transfusion ordered
  - the signature of the medical practitioner
- check the following information against the patient's own documentation and each labelled unit of blood:
  - the name of the patient
  - the unit or hospital number of the patient
  - the age and date of birth of the patient
  - the address of the patient
  - the blood group of the patient
  - the rhesus factor of the patient
  - the expiry date of the blood pack
  - the unit number of the blood pack
- establish the patient's identity by appropriate means, for example an identification bracelet, and if possible by verbal confirmation from the patient
- sign the label on the checked blood unit; this is normally done by the two people involved, *acknowledging professional responsibility*
- transfer the duplicate unit pack number to the patient's records according to health authority policy; *if adverse effects occur, the blood unit transfused can then be investigated to identify any problems* (Williamson et al 1999)

- in undertaking this practice, nurses are accountable for their actions, the quality of care delivered and record-keeping according to the *Code of Professional Conduct* (UKCC 1992), *Guidelines for Professional Practice* (UKCC 1996) and *Guidelines for Records and Record Keeping* (UKCC 1998).

Relevance to the activities of living	Observations on and further rationale for this nursing practice will be included within each activity of living as appropriate.

Maintaining a safe environment

Gloves should be worn at all times when handling blood products and associated equipment to prevent cross-infection from blood-borne viral infections such as hepatitis B or HIV/AIDS (Roberts 2000) and to protect staff from invasive contact (*see* 'Isolation nursing', p. 201).

All precautions for the prevention of infection and of air emboli should be maintained (*see* 'Intravenous infusion', p. 181).

The accurate checking of individual units of blood will help to ensure that only compatible blood is transfused. From April 2001, a worldwide bar coding system for each blood donation was adopted in the UK.

Despite careful cross-matching, some patients develop a transfusion reaction, but accurate observation will help to detect this as early as possible. All observations should be continued for at least 4 hours after the last unit of blood has been transfused, and thereafter as appropriate (Glover 1995).

If a transfusion reaction is suspected, the transfusion must be discontinued and the medical practitioner informed immediately. The haematologist should also be informed, and used blood containers returned to the blood transfusion laboratory for testing.

In some centres, the practice of transfusing a patient's own blood has been employed, usually when elective surgical procedures such as joint replacement are planned.

The intravenous access site and cannula should be monitored for signs of infection such as phlebitis, or for infiltration of the tissues by the transfusion fluid.

Communicating

Any complaint of pain, for example headache or loin pain, should be reported. These may indicate emboli caused by a transfusion reaction.

Breathing

Pulse, respiration rate and blood pressure should be monitored, normally hourly, during the transfusion. Respiratory function should not be affected unless a transfusion reaction occurs or the blood is transfused at a rate that causes fluid overload (*see* 'Intravenous infusion', p. 181).

Patients who have congestive cardiac failure should be transfused at an appropriately slower rate to prevent fluid overload with its associated pulmonary oedema and dyspnoea; diuretics are sometimes prescribed for the duration of the transfusion to prevent this complication. The use of concentrated red cells instead of whole blood can also help.

Eating and drinking

An accurate chart of fluid intake should be maintained. The patient may need help with placing and preparing food if one hand is immobilised (*see* 'Intravenous infusion', p. 181).

Personal cleansing and dressing

Skin colour should be noted and any abnormalities such as pallor, flushing or a rash reported as these may indicate a transfusion reaction.

The patient may need some help with personal cleansing and dressing if one arm is immobilised. The need for light clothing to allow access to the transfusion site should be explained.

Eliminating

Urinary output should be accurately measured to allow fluid balance to be maintained. Diuresis may occur if diuretic medication has been ordered; this should be explained to the patient.

If any incompatibility occurs, the kidneys may be the first organs to be affected because emboli form in the renal capillaries as a result of the clumping of incompatible blood. The patient may complain of back pain, and there may be frank haematuria, which should be reported immediately.

The patient may need help, when using a commode, to support the administration tubing while the transfusion is in progress.

Controlling body temperature

Body temperature should be monitored every 15 minutes for the first hour and then hourly (Duke 2000) as one of the early signs of an adverse reaction may be a sudden rise in body temperature. This is often associated with rigor, and either chilling or flushing is experienced by the patient.

Appropriate clothing and covering will help the patient to feel more comfortable. Donor blood remains stable only at 1–6°C and should not be warmed prior to transfusion. In emergencies, when a rapid transfusion is needed, special blood-warming equipment is used, as ordered by the medical practitioner. This is usually confined to transfusions occurring in accident and emergency units, operating theatres and intensive care areas.

In non-acute situations, transfusions are normally prescribed at a flow rate of 1 unit every 4 hours. This slower rate of transfusion allows the body to adjust to the initially low temperature of the donor blood. Maintaining an accurate flow rate will help the patient to control body temperature.

Mobilising

The degree of mobility may depend on other factors. It may initially be appropriate for the patient to rest comfortably; this allows more accurate recordings and observations to be maintained.

The patient may move around the bed, sit in a chair and use a commode with help, as the condition allows.

Sleeping

Any change in the patient's general state of consciousness, for example confusion, restlessness or disorientation, should be noted as it may indicate a transfusion reaction.

Patients may find it difficult to lie in their normal sleeping position because of the transfusion lines, and help may be needed in adjusting to a suitable and comfortable position.

Necessary observations may waken the patient. Continuous recording of body temperature with an electronic probe may be less disturbing than intermittent recording with a mercury thermometer. The blood pressure may be recorded less frequently during the sleeping period, as the patient's condition allows, if the less disturbing pulse recording is continued.

Patient/carer education: key points

In partnership with the patient and/or carer, ensure that they are competent to carry out any required practices. Information should be given on an appropriate point of contact for any concerns that may arise.

- explain the reason for the transfusion as part of the patient's treatment, and state the time expected for the completion of each unit. This makes it easier for the patient to tolerate the practice
- explain the importance of maintaining the cannula and lines safely in situ and the need to keep the cannulated limb as still as possible. The dangers of disconnection should be emphasised so that the lines and dressing are not dislodged
- the patient should understand the importance of immediately reporting any soreness or redness at the site of the transfusion, which may be a sign of local infection, even after completion of the transfusion
- the patient should understand the importance of reporting any headaches, sweating, dizziness or feeling of distress to the nursing staff who will be monitoring his or her progress, as this may indicate an adverse reaction to the blood being transfused
- patients who have had a blood transfusion will have had their blood group identified. They should be given information on this, preferably documented, for future reference.

References

Atterbury C, Wilkinson J 2000 Blood transfusion. Nursing Standard 14(34): 47–54

Bradbury M, Cruickshank JP 2000 Blood transfusion: crucial steps in maintaining safe practice. British Journal of Nursing 9(3): 134–138

British Committee for Standards in Haematology (BCSH) Blood Transfusion Task Force 1999 The administration of blood and blood components and the management of transfusion patients. Transfusion Medicine 9(3): 227–238

Dodworth H 1995 Making sense of ... blood and blood products. Nursing Times 91(1): 25–29

Duke F 2000 Blood disorders. In: Alexander M, Fawcett J, Runciman P (eds) Nursing practice – hospital and home: the adult. 2nd edn. Churchill Livingstone, Edinburgh

Glover G 1995 Blood transfusion. Nursing Standard 9(33): 31–35

Higgins C 1994 Blood transfusions: risks and benefits. British Journal of Nursing 3(19): 986–991

Higgins C 1995 Haematology blood testing for anaemia. British Journal of Nursing 4(5): 248–253

Roberts C 2000 Universal precautions: improving the knowledge of trained nurses. British Journal of Nursing 9(1): 43–47

United Kingdom Central Council for Nursing, Midwifery and Health Visiting 1992 Code of professional conduct. UKCC, London

United Kingdom Central Council for Nursing, Midwifery and Health Visiting 1996 Guidelines for professional practice. UKCC, London

United Kingdom Central Council for Nursing, Midwifery and Health Visiting 1998 Guidelines for records and record keeping. UKCC, London

Williamson L, Lowe S, Love E et al 1999 Serious hazards of transfusion (SHOT) initiative: analysis of the first two annual reports. British Medical Journal 319: 16–19

8   Body Temperature

Learning outcomes

By the end of this section, you should know how to:

- prepare the patient for this nursing practice
- collect and prepare the equipment
- measure and record the body temperature at the axilla, in the oral cavity, ear canal or in the rectum, in both a community and an institutional setting.

Background knowledge required

Revision of the anatomy and physiology of the skin in relation to the control of body temperature and the temperature-regulating centre, and of the related body mechanisms associated with heat production and heat loss.
Revision of the anatomy of the area where the temperature is to be measured.

Indications and rationale for recording body temperature

A temperature recording is a measurement of body temperature in degrees Celsius (°C) using a disposable thermometer, a calibrated electronic probe or a tympanic thermometer. The axilla, the oral cavity, the rectum or the ear canal may be the site chosen for recording. For each patient, the preferred site should be used consistently so that any change in temperature can be accurately monitored.

The normal range of body temperature is 36–37.5°C, but this may vary, by as much as 0.6°C, according to the site used for measurement. The core temperature can be more than 0.4°C higher than the oral temperature and more than 0.2°C lower than the rectal temperature. The upper and lower limits of survival are not precisely known but are thought to be a body temperature of 44°C and 27°C respectively (Fig. 8.1).

The recording of body temperature may be required:

- *to establish a baseline temperature*, for example when patients are admitted to the hospital or clinic
- *to monitor fluctuations in temperature*, as may occur during the postoperative period, *as temperature fluctuations can indicate developing infection or the presence of a deep venous thrombosis*
- *to monitor signs of incompatibility when patients are receiving a blood transfusion*
- *to monitor the temperature of patients being treated for an infection*
- *to monitor the temperature of patients recovering from hypothermia.*

The frequency of the recording will depend on the reason for monitoring the body temperature and on the patient's condition (Gould 1994).

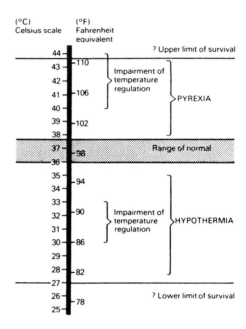

Figure 8.1 *Range of normal/abnormal (oral) body temperature. From Roper et al (1990), with permission*

Equipment

Tray

Appropriate thermometer, e.g.:

— disposable thermometer

— electronic thermometer plus probe and disposable cover

— tympanic thermometer and disposable cover

NB Clinical thermometers with mercury should not be used in health-care settings, thereby complying with health and safety guidelines to reduce the exposure to mercury

Alcohol-impregnated swabs

Watch with a second hand

Tissues

Receptacle for disposable items.

Disposable thermometers

A variety of disposable thermometers are available for purchase, two of the more common ones being the chemical dot thermometer and the liquid crystal heat-sensitive synthetic strip (Fig. 8.2). These are for single use only, and the manufacturer's instructions for use must be followed to ensure an accurate recording. These thermometers tend to be used in a community or domestic setting.

Electronic thermometers

These either have probes that will be protected by a disposable cover before being placed at the recording site or use a disposable probe.

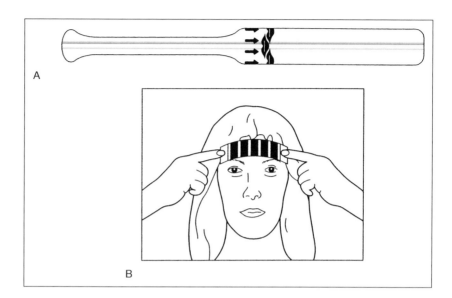

Figure 8.2
A *Disposable chemical dot thermometer*
B *Liquid crystal disposable thermometer*

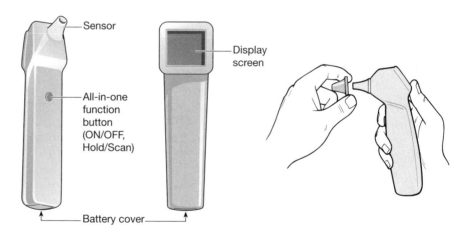

Figure 8.3   *A tympanic thermometer*

They are connected to equipment that gives an electronic readout of the temperature in 25–35 seconds. The mode of the recording equipment must be correctly selected depending on the site of measurement. The manufacturer's instructions must be followed carefully in order to obtain a valid recording.

Tympanic thermometers

Tympanic thermometers (Fig. 8.3) have a probe with a disposable cover that is inserted into the ear canal. They detect infrared energy that is emitted from the tympanic membrane and surrounding tissue, this then being displayed digitally as a temperature reading. The tympanic temperature correlates well with the core temperature, which is thought to be because the tympanic membrane shares its blood supply with the hypothalamus (Bezinger 1969).

The thermometer must be covered by a disposable cover in order to function, and the detection window must be kept clean in order to obtain an accurate result. False readings may arise from incorrect technique, a damaged lens or an inaccurate timing between measurements (Jevon & Jevon 2001).

Guidelines and rationale for this nursing practice

The manufacturer's guidelines must always be followed, so only general guidelines are given here for temperature recording as the principles can normally be adapted for any type of thermometer (Fulbrook 1993).

The patient should be assessed carefully to identify the most appropriate site for temperature measurement, which will ensure an accurate and safe result.

Axilla

- wash the hands *to prevent cross-infection* (Horton 1995)
- explain the nursing practice *to gain consent and co-operation, and encourage participation in care.* Ensure that the patient has not recently had a hot bath or been engaged in strenuous exercise *as these will cause a temporary rise in body temperature*
- ensure the patient's privacy *to respect individuality*
- help the patient into a comfortable position, either sitting or lying, with the back and shoulders well supported *so that the position can be maintained for a few minutes*
- help the patient to remove or adjust the clothing *to expose one axilla*
- observe the patient throughout this activity *to monitor any adverse effects*
- dry the skin of the axilla by wiping with a tissue: *a film of moisture between the skin and the thermometer probe can cause an inaccurate reading*
- place the probe of the thermometer in the axilla where the skin surfaces will surround it *to gain an accurate temperature reading*
- help the patient to hold the arm across the chest *to retain the thermometer in the correct position*
- leave the thermometer in position as per the manufacturer's instructions *to ensure an accurate technique*
- remain with the patient if required *to reassure the patient and ensure that the thermometer remains in the correct position*
- remove the thermometer *when the optimum time for accurate recording has been reached*
- read the temperature measured by the thermometer *for an accurate recording to be monitored and documented*
- ensure that the patient is left feeling as comfortable as possible *to reassure the patient and reduce anxiety*
- dispose of equipment safely *to prevent cross-infection*
- document the temperature reading in the patient's records, compare the reading with previous recordings, and report any abnormal findings immediately. *This will ensure safe practice and enable prompt, appropriate medical and nursing intervention to be initiated*

- in undertaking this practice, nurses are accountable for their actions, the quality of care delivered and record-keeping according to the *Code of Professional Conduct* (UKCC 1992), *Guidelines for Professional Practice* (UKCC 1996) and *Guidelines for Records and Record Keeping* (UKCC 1998).

Oral cavity

- wash the hands *to prevent cross-infection* (Horton 1995)
- explain the nursing practice *to gain consent and co-operation*. Ensure that the patient has not recently had a hot or cold drink, or a hot bath, or been engaged in strenuous exercise *as this may temporarily raise the body temperature*
- help the patient into a comfortable position *so that he or she will more readily tolerate the thermometer probe*
- prepare the thermometer as per the manufacturer's instructions
- apply a disposable sleeve if required *to prevent the transmission of infection*
- place the thermometer probe under the patient's tongue so that the probe lies adjacent to the frenulum at the junction of the floor of the mouth and the base of the tongue, on either the right or left side. *A maximum temperature recording will be obtained from one of these two 'heat pockets' in the mouth* (Fig. 8.4). This is also the position for disposable oral thermometers
- explain to the patient the importance of closing only the lips round the thermometer, and not biting it, *so that the oral temperature is maintained and not distorted by the inspiration of air through the mouth*
- leave the thermometer in position for the required time *for accurate recording to occur*
- remove the thermometer probe and proceed as for an axillary temperature recording.

Rectum

- wash hands and apply gloves *to prevent cross-infection* (Horton 1995)
- explain the nursing practice to the patient *to gain consent and co-operation*
- ensure the patient's privacy *to respect individuality and maintain self-esteem*
- help the patient into a comfortable position lying on his or her side with the knees bent *so that access is easier and the patient is least distressed*
- prepare the thermometer probe as per the manufacturer's instructions
- if suggested by the manufacturer, lubricate the end of the thermometer probe *to make insertion easier and prevent any damage to the mucosa*
- gently insert the thermometer probe into the patient's anus for 2–4 cm and hold it in position for the required time *for an accurate recording of the temperature to occur*
- remove the thermometer probe, dispose of the probe and soiled glove, and proceed as for an axillary temperature recording.

Ear canal – tympanic thermometer only

- wash the hands *to prevent cross-infection* (Horton 1995)
- explain the nursing practice *to gain consent and co-operation*. Ensure that the patient has not recently had a hot or cold drink, or a hot bath, or been

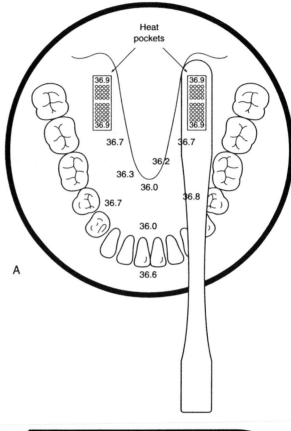

Figure 8.4   A *Heat pockets in the oral cavity* B *Recording area of a disposable thermometer*

engaged in strenuous exercise *as this may temporarily raise the body temperature*

- help the patient into a comfortable position *in order to gain safe access to the ear canal and so that the patient will tolerate the practice more readily*
- prepare the thermometer as per the manufacturer's instructions *to ensure an accurate measurement*
- apply a disposable sleeve *to prevent the transmission of infection and allow the device to function*
- switch the device on *to ensure that it is calibrated and ready to take an accurate measurement*

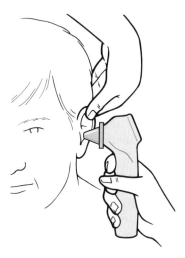

Figure 8.5 *Using a tympanic thermometer*

- stabilise the patient's head *to ensure the safe introduction of the thermometer probe*
- gently pull the ear lobe downwards and position the probe so that it occludes the canal; this will *straighten the ear canal and permit the probe a view of the tympanic membrane without interference from ambient air temperature* (Fig. 8.5)
- hold the thermometer steady and take the recording as per the manufacturer's instructions *for accurate recording to occur*
- remove the thermometer probe, dispose of the cover, and return equipment to its storage case *to prevent breakage and prolong usage*
- proceed as for an axillary temperature recording.

Relevance to the activities of living	Observations on and further rationale for this nursing practice will be included within each activity of living as appropriate.

Maintaining a safe environment

The mercury and glass thermometer may still be found in some settings, but its continued use should be questioned in light of the dangers associated with exposure to mercury and the common inaccurate use of these thermometers (Blumenthal 1992). O'Toole (1997) suggests that hospitals should make health-care environments mercury free.

Temperature recording is a non-invasive practice, but nurses should still wash their hands before and after the recording to prevent cross-infection. The equipment should be kept clean and stored as recommended by the manufacturer. The accuracy of temperature recording depends, however, not only on a fully functioning instrument, but also on the clinical skill of the nurse (Childs 2000).

Oral temperature recording should be used only for adult patients who are alert, well orientated and able to co-operate in carrying out the procedure.

The equipment of choice for all children is the tympanic thermometer. It is non-invasive and fast, which makes it well tolerated.

The probe of a rectal thermometer will normally be covered by a disposable cover or sleeve before lubrication and insertion. This not only prevents cross-infection, but also prevents damage to the surrounding mucosa.

In a general ward, fans should not be used to cool patients who have a pyrexia caused by infection as the increased movement of air may increase the risk of cross-infection in the area.

Communicating

The patient should not speak while the oral temperature is being recorded. Apart from the danger of damage to the thermometer probe, the passage of air through the mouth while talking affects the temperature reading, and this should be explained to the patient.

Eating and drinking

Patients with a raised body temperature are prescribed an increased fluid intake to compensate for the increased loss of fluid caused by perspiration. Fluid intake should be encouraged and accurately recorded, and fluid balance charts should be maintained for all patients with a pyrexia in order to monitor hydration.

Eliminating

Fluid output should be recorded and fluid balance charts accurately maintained for all patients with an abnormal body temperature.

Pyrexia may result in a decreased urinary output, the urine being concentrated and dark in colour. This may be a result of dehydration caused by an increased fluid loss resulting from perspiration.

Personal cleansing and dressing

Clothing may have to be adjusted for the recording of both the axillary and the rectal temperature. The nurse should gain the patient's help and co-operation during this nursing practice. The amount of clothing and bed covering may be adjusted depending on the patient's reaction to a change of body temperature. A patient with a pyrexia may feel very warm or very cold.

A bed bath should be given as frequently as required to ensure the patient's comfort as patients with a raised body temperature perspire profusely. Tepid sponging is not recommended as a method of lowering the patient's temperature as this will counteract the heat conservation mechanisms already in action (Bruce & Grove 1992).

Patients with a pyrexia may become dehydrated as a result of excess insensible fluid loss. Frequent mouth care should be given to maintain a healthy mucosa and to help to alleviate the 'dry mouth' effect associated with pyrexia.

Controlling body temperature

Any change in body temperature may indicate the patient's response to an adverse environment. Under normal conditions, the body's internal temperature remains remarkably constant at around 37°C, the range of normal in the adult being 36.0–37.5°C (*see* Fig. 8.1). Children have a correspondingly wider range of body temperature than adults because of their higher metabolic rate.

For a healthy person, the axillary temperature lies at the lower end of the normal range, the rectal temperature at the upper end and the oral temperature somewhere in between. For each patient, the site chosen for temperature recording should be used consistently in order to enable changes in body temperature to be accurately monitored.

Both core temperature and peripheral temperature may be recorded for seriously ill patients suffering from, for example, cardiogenic, bacteraemic or haemorrhagic shock. Under normal conditions, there should be no more than a 3°C difference between the core temperature and the peripheral temperature.

The **core temperature** should be recorded at a site where the reading will be as near as possible to the temperature of the blood. An electronic probe may be inserted into the rectum or the oesophagus and attached to an electronic monitor to give a continuous core temperature reading.

The **peripheral temperature** may be recorded by a small, flat probe taped or clipped to the patient's big toe to give a continuous readout of the peripheral temperature on the electronic monitor.

'Pyrexia' is the name given to a rise in body temperature above 37.5°C; this should be reported. 'Hyperpyrexia' refers to a body temperature of above 40°C. A body temperature of over 41°C or prolonged hyperpyrexia may damage brain cell function and result in associated fits or rigors. Hyperpyrexia should therefore be treated as an emergency and reported immediately.

'Hypothermia' is the term given to a fall in body temperature to below 35°C. Warming a patient suffering from hypothermia should be carried out gradually (a rise of 0.5°C per hour being suggested) under medical guidance. Any sudden heating of the periphery of the body can divert the blood from the vital centres and cause further shock.

Expressing sexuality

The recording of a rectal temperature can be an uncomfortable and undignified procedure, and the reason for this choice of site should be explained to the patient. A nurse who has good communication skills can help to maintain the patient's dignity.

Sleeping

When an electronic thermometer is in situ, there is no need to disturb a patient who is sleeping. When other types of thermometer are used, clinical judgement is needed to decide whether or not to wake a patient, especially during the night, in order to record the temperature.

Patient/carer education: key points

In partnership with the patient and/or carer, ensure that they are competent to carry out any required practices. Information should be given on an appropriate point of contact for any concerns that may arise:

- explain the importance of monitoring the body temperature for evaluating the progress and treatment of the patient's condition
- the patient should understand the importance of the thermometer remaining in position for the correct period of time
- explain the importance of reporting headaches, excess sweating, shivering or general feelings of distress, which may indicate a change in body temperature
- patients with pyrexia should understand the importance of drinking an adequate amount of fluid in order to prevent dehydration
- elderly patients should be given advice on how to prevent heat loss at home and told of the dangers of hypothermia. This should be reinforced with written advice and specific information about the resources available, and should involve family and carers as applicable.

References

Bezinger T 1969 Clinical temperature: a new physiological basis. Journal of the American Medical Association 209: 1200–1206

Blumenthal I 1992 Should we ban mercury thermometers? Discussion paper. Journal of the Royal Society of Medicine 85: 553–555

Bruce J, Grove S 1992 Fever: pathology and treatment. Critical Care Nurse 12(1): 40–49

Childs C 2000 Temperature control. In: Alexander M, Fawcett J, Runciman P (eds) Nursing practice – hospital and home: the adult. 2nd edn. Churchill Livingstone, Edinburgh

Connell F 1997 The causes and treatment of fever: a literature review. Nursing Standard 12(11): 40–43

Fulbrook P 1993 Core temperature measurement: a comparison of rectal, axillary and pulmonary artery blood temperature. Intensive and Critical Care Nursing 9(4): 275–286

Gould D 1994 Controlling patients' body temperature. Nursing Standard 8(35): 29–31

Horton R 1995 Handwashing: the fundamental infection control principle. British Journal of Nursing 4(16): 926–933

Jevon P, Jevon M 2001 Using a tympanic thermometer. Nursing Times 97(9): 43–44

O'Toole S 1997 Alternatives to mercury thermometers. Professional Nurse 12(11): 783–786

Rogers M 1992 A viable alternative to the glass/mercury thermometer. Paediatric Nursing 4(9): 8–11

Roper N, Logan W, Tierney A 1990 The elements of nursing. 3rd edn. Churchill Livingstone, Edinburgh

Sidebottom J 1992 When it is hot enough to kill (hyperthermia, heat related illness). Registered Nurse 55(8): 48–57

United Kingdom Central Council for Nursing, Midwifery and Health Visiting 1992 Code of professional conduct. UKCC, London

United Kingdom Central Council for Nursing, Midwifery and Health Visiting 1996 Guidelines for professional practice. UKCC, London

United Kingdom Central Council for Nursing, Midwifery and Health Visiting 1998 Guidelines for records and record keeping. UKCC, London

9   Bone Marrow Aspiration

Learning outcomes	By the end of this section, you should know how to:
	▪ prepare the patient for this procedure
	▪ collect and prepare the equipment
	▪ assist the medical practitioner during bone marrow aspiration.

Background knowledge required	Revision of the anatomy and physiology of the blood, with special reference to the source and development of the red blood corpuscles
	Revision of 'Wound care' technique (*see* p. 405).

Indications and rationale for bone marrow aspiration	Bone marrow aspiration is the aspiration of a specimen of red bone marrow:
	▪ *to aid the diagnosis of some anaemias, leukaemias and lymphomas*
	▪ *to aid an assessment of the effect of treatment during the course of a disease.*

Outline of the procedure	This procedure is carried out by a medical practitioner using an aseptic technique. The patient may have some form of sedation prescribed prior to the procedure. After handwashing, the medical practitioner administers the local anaesthetic into the chosen site and then prepares his or her hands for the application of the sterile gloves. The patient's skin is cleansed using the antiseptic, a small stab incision may be made, and the marrow needle is inserted into the red bone marrow cavity.
	The needle is specially designed and fitted with an adjustable protective guard to control its level of penetration (Fig. 9.1), thus preventing injury to the underlying vital organs. The stilette of the needle is removed and the syringe attached to the hub of the marrow needle. Following the aspiration of a specimen of red bone marrow, the syringe is disconnected, the stilette replaced and the needle withdrawn.
	The microscope slides are prepared by the medical practitioner or a haematology technician if present. As the microscope slides are prepared, pressure should be applied to the puncture site until bleeding ceases.
	The puncture site should be covered with a sterile adhesive dressing.
	The position of the patient during the procedure is dependent on the site chosen for aspiration of the red marrow. The main sites are:
	▪ **the sternum:** the patient lies supine with one pillow under the head. Care is required to prevent cardiac tamponade

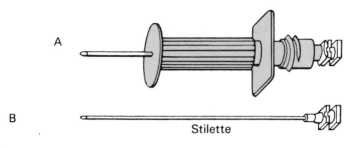

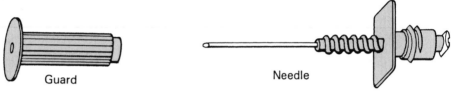

Figure 9.1 *Bone marrow aspiration needle (disposable) showing the adjustable guard*
A Complete needle
B Needle taken apart

- **the iliac crest**: this can be an anterior or a posterior approach from either side (Duke 2000). If the anterior approach is used, the patient can lie prone or on the side. When the posterior approach is used, the patient must lie on his or her side. The iliac crest has the advantage that there are no vital organs near the puncture site.

Equipment

Sterile gloves
Sterile dressings pack
Alcohol-based antiseptic for cleansing the skin
Local anaesthetic and equipment for its administration
Sterile disposable scalpel or similar equipment
Sterile marrow aspiration needles
Sterile 20 ml syringe for aspiration of the marrow
Plastic spray dressing
Sterile adhesive dressing
Disposable plastic aprons
Trolley for equipment
Receptacle for soiled disposable items
Microscope slides, appropriately labelled, coverslips and slide fixative if the haematology technician service is not available. Sterile specimen containers appropriately labelled with a completed laboratory form and plastic specimen bag for transportation.

Guidelines and rationale for this nursing practice

- help the medical practitioner to explain the procedure to the patient *to gain consent and co-operation*
- wash the hands *to reduce the risk of cross-infection* (Horton 1995)
- give the patient sedation if prescribed *to assist in the reduction of anxiety*
- prepare the equipment and trolley as required *to ensure that all the equipment is available and ready for use*
- ensure the patient's privacy *to assist in the reduction of anxiety*

- help the patient into the correct position depending on the chosen site *as this will permit easy access to the site and promote a positive outcome for the procedure*
- observe the patient throughout this activity *to note any signs of distress*
- assist the medical practitioner as necessary during the procedure *to ensure a safe and competent completion of the procedure*
- remain with the patient and help to maintain his or her position as required during the procedure, *giving physical and psychological support during what is an unusual experience*
- ensure that the patient is left feeling as comfortable as possible, *maintaining the quality of this nursing practice*
- dispose of the equipment safely *to reduce any health hazard*
- dispatch the labelled specimens to the laboratory immediately with the completed laboratory forms *to allow the microscopic examination of fresh body cells*
- document the nursing practice appropriately, monitor the after-effects, and report any abnormal findings immediately. *This provides a written record and assists in the implementation of any action should an abnormality or adverse reaction to the practice be noted*
- in undertaking this practice, nurses are accountable for their actions, the quality of care delivered and record-keeping according to the *Code of Professional Conduct* (UKCC 1992), *Guidelines for Professional Practice* (UKCC 1996) and *Guidelines for Records and Record Keeping* (UKCC 1998).

Relevance to the activities of living

Maintaining a safe environment

As this is an invasive procedure, all precautions and observations to prevent infection should be maintained by the medical practitioner and the nurse. The adhesive dressing can be removed 2–3 days after the procedure unless a complication has arisen.

For safe transportation of the specimen collected, see p. 317.

If the patient received sedation prior to the procedure, the effects of this should have worn off before he or she is allowed to mobilise. The patient may choose to attend as an outpatient, day patient or inpatient for this procedure if the daily lifestyle is not significantly affected by the undiagnosed condition (Duke 2000).

A bone marrow aspiration is contraindicated in a patient who is unable to co-operate or in whom there is a coagulation defect such as an extended blood clotting time as serious complications may occur (Mallett & Dougherty 2000).

Communicating

It is important that an easily understood explanation is given to the patient before the procedure. This is provided primarily by the medical practitioner, but the nurse may be required to repeat the explanation. If the sternal site is used, the thought of a needle being introduced into one's chest can be extremely alarming; if the patient is very anxious, the doctor may prescribe light sedation prior to the procedure.

The patient should be told to expect a momentary sharp pain during the procedure as a result of the suction created as the syringe piston is withdrawn (Long et al 1995).

The patient may require mild analgesia once the effect of the local anaesthetic has worn off.

Breathing

The patient's blood pressure, pulse and respiration rate should be taken prior to and following a bone marrow aspiration. The puncture site should be observed for continued bleeding or haematoma formation as some patients may have a bleeding disorder.

Any sudden change in the patient's general condition, especially in breathing if the sternal site is used, should be reported as this may signify injury to the underlying vital organs (Duke 2000). A cardiac tamponade can develop when bleeding from a ruptured blood vessel in the myocardium causes pressure on the pericardial sac (Mallett & Dougherty 2000). Pericardial bleeding can occur when the aspiration needle has passed through the sternum; the use of a needle guard can reduce this complication.

Mobilising

Patients should be allowed to rest quietly for approximately an hour following the practice, thereafter resuming their previous level of mobilisation. If sedation has been given prior to the practice, allow the effects to wear off before the patient is mobilised.

Patient/carer education: key points

In partnership with the patient and/or carer, ensure that they are competent to carry out any practices required. Information should be given on an appropriate point of contact for any concerns that may arise.

The medical practitioner and the nurse should provide information on the necessity for this procedure. The patient and relatives will need time to ask questions and discuss any aspect of the planned procedure that concerns them.

Before the procedure, the nurse should provide information on and the rationale behind the position the patient needs to adopt during and following the aspiration, as well as on the aftercare that will be delivered.

Should the patient be going to be discharged after the procedure, information should be provided on the care of the puncture site, what level of discomfort may be experienced, whom to contact should any adverse reaction occur, when the results will be available and the date and time of the next outpatient appointment (Duke 2000).

References

Duke F 2000 Blood disorders. In: Alexander M, Fawcett J, Runciman P (eds) Nursing practice – hospital and home: the adult. 2nd edn. Churchill Livingstone, Edinburgh

Horton R 1995 Handwashing: the fundamental infection control principle. British Journal of Nursing 4(16): 926–933

Long B, Phipps W, Cassmeyer V (eds) 1995 Adult nursing: a nursing process approach. Mosby-Times Mirror International, London

Mallett J, Dougherty L 2000 The Royal Marsden Hospital manual of clinical nursing procedures. 5th edn. Blackwell Science, Oxford

United Kingdom Central Council for Nursing, Midwifery and Health Visiting 1992 Code of professional conduct. UKCC, London

United Kingdom Central Council for Nursing, Midwifery and Health Visiting 1996 Guidelines for professional practice. UKCC, London

United Kingdom Central Council for Nursing, Midwifery and Health Visiting 1998 Guidelines for records and record keeping. UKCC, London

10 Bowel Washout/Colonic Irrigation

Learning outcomes

By the end of this section, you should know how to:
- prepare the patient for this nursing practice
- collect and prepare the equipment
- carry out a bowel washout/colonic irrigation.

Background knowledge required

Anatomy and physiology of the lower alimentary tract
Solutions that may be safely used for bowel washout/colonic irrigation.

Indications and rationale for a bowel washout/colonic irrigation

A bowel washout is the introduction of fluid through a tube into the rectum and the siphoning off of the contents to help to empty the rectum and sigmoid colon. It is used rarely and then only when patients cannot tolerate the oral preparation that is normally used to prepare the bowel for:
- *special radiological examinations*
- *sigmoidoscopy*
- *surgery on the rectum or descending colon*
- *urinary diversion surgery* (Selfe 2000).

It is also used in severe cases of constipation caused by reduced or absent peristalsis, such as with irritable bowel syndrome or certain neurological conditions. It helps *to relieve constipation and prevent the development of bowel obstruction*. In the latter, colonic irrigation is the method of washout. It is also used in some health spas and clinics as a method to detoxify the body.

Equipment

Trolley or tray
Protective covering for the bed and floor
Disposable gloves and apron
Large reusable irrigation bag (2 L capacity) attached to long tubing
Barium enema catheter
Lubricant: KY jelly
Solution as ordered – usually plain water, sodium chloride 0.9% at room
   temperature or the oral preparation used prior to surgery, e.g. Clean Prep
   (up to 8 L)

Medical wipes/tissues
Receptacle for soiled disposable items
Bedpan or commode.

Guidelines and rationale for this nursing practice

- explain the nursing practice to the patient *to gain consent and co-operation*
- wash the hands *to reduce cross-infection* (Horton 1995)
- collect and prepare the equipment *for efficiency of practice*
- if necessary, assist the medical staff to sedate the patient and then monitor the patient appropriately throughout the practice. The patient may be given regular intravenous doses of midazolam
- assist the patient into the left lateral position in bed, with the buttocks exposed, *but ensure that the patient is adequately covered*
- place the protective covering on the bed under the patient's buttocks
- put on the disposable gloves
- join the long tubing to the barium enema catheter
- prime the tubing with the irrigation fluid to expel air from the system *as this can cause discomfort to the patient*
- lubricate the barium enema catheter and gently insert it into the rectum for 10–12 cm in an upward and backward direction following the line of the rectum. When it is in place, gently inflate the retaining balloon
- allow about 1.5 L of fluid to run in over about 10 minutes. Then close the clamp to encourage the fluid to travel gently into the sigmoid colon. It may be helpful to tilt the foot of the bed up at this stage
- ask the patient to retain the fluid for as long as possible (usually around 15–30 minutes) to allow the softening and loosening of the faecal material
- after this time, lower the irrigation bag to below the level of the bed, loosen the clamp, and allow the tubing to drain until all the irrigation fluid has returned
- observe the character of the return flow
- empty and refill the bag after each irrigation and repeat until the return flow runs clear. This may take 4–6 hours and use up to 8 L of irrigation fluid
- gently deflate the retention balloon, withdraw the catheter, and offer the patient a commode or the facilities of an ensuite toilet, the choice depending on the patient's condition and whether or not he or she has received sedation. There may still be some leakage of fluid from the anal sphincter at this time
- assist the patient to wash and dry the perineal area carefully as faecal matter may cause skin breakdown
- allow the patient to recover from sedation if this has been administered, and monitor the vital signs and level of consciousness until these have returned to the values seen before the procedure
- ensure that the patient is left feeling as comfortable as possible. A protective pad may be placed under the patient if he or she is worried about any leakage
- dispose of the equipment safely *for the protection of others*
- document this nursing practice, monitor the after-effects and report any abnormal findings immediately *to provide a written record and assist in the implementation of any action should an abnormality or adverse reaction to the practice be noted*

- in undertaking this practice, nurses are accountable for their actions, the quality of care delivered and record-keeping according to the *Code of Professional Conduct* (UKCC 1992), *Guidelines for Professional Practice* (UKCC 1996) and *Guidelines for Records and Record Keeping* (UKCC 1998).

Relevance to the activities of living

Maintaining a safe environment

Although this practice does not require an aseptic technique, all the equipment involved should be clean or disposable. Nurses should wash their hands before commencing and on completion of the practice. Gloves and an apron should be worn for protection.

This nursing practice is contraindicated when the patient is known to have any disease or previous surgery on the anus, rectum and/or bowel (Mallett & Dougherty 2000) as these conditions may predispose to friable rectal mucosa, which could be easily damaged as a result of the mechanical effects of this practice.

This procedure is carried out by qualified nurses who have had appropriate education and training to carry out the practice safely.

Communicating

A careful explanation of the necessity for this nursing practice should be given to the patient to help to reduce embarrassment.

Eating and drinking

This procedure is often carried out prior to surgery on the bowel. After the procedure, the patient may be limited to fluids or a low-residue diet.

Eliminating

Ensure that the patient can get to a bedpan, commode or toilet after this nursing practice.

Mobilising

The effectiveness of the washout may be increased if the patient can move around in bed to distribute the solution.

Expressing sexuality

This is a very embarrassing practice for the patient, so an adequate explanation should be given and as much privacy as possible provided (Roper et al 2000). The procedure should ideally be carried out in a treatment room away from other patients and near a toilet.

Patient/carer education: key points

In partnership with the patient and/or carer, ensure that they are competent to carry out any practices required. Information should be given on an appropriate point of contact for any concerns that may arise.

A clear explanation of the necessity for this practice must be given to the patient.

The patient should be warned to expect some leakage of fluid after the procedure and should be given a supply of some type of protection.

References

Horton R 1995 Handwashing: the fundamental infection control principle. British Journal of Nursing 4(16): 926–933

Mallett J, Dougherty L 2000 The Royal Marsden Hospital manual of clinical procedures. 5th edn. Blackwell Science, Oxford

Roper N, Logan W, Tierney A 2000 The Roper–Logan–Tierney model of nursing. Churchill Livingstone, Edinburgh

Selfe L 2000 The urinary system. In: Alexander M, Fawcett J, Runciman P (eds) Nursing practice – hospital and home: the adult. 2nd edn. Churchill Livingstone, Edinburgh

United Kingdom Central Council for Nursing, Midwifery and Health Visiting 1992 Code of professional conduct. UKCC, London

United Kingdom Central Council for Nursing, Midwifery and Health Visiting 1996 Guidelines for professional practice. UKCC, London

United Kingdom Central Council for Nursing, Midwifery and Health Visiting 1998 Guidelines for records and record keeping. UKCC, London

11 Cardiopulmonary Resuscitation

Learning outcomes

By the end of this section, you should know how to:

- diagnose cardiac arrest quickly
- call the emergency team promptly
- initiate resuscitation effectively
- locate the necessary equipment.

Background knowledge required

Revision of the anatomy and physiology of the cardiovascular and respiratory systems

Review of the health authority and trust policy pertaining to the procedure of cardiopulmonary resuscitation.

Indications and rationale for cardiopulmonary resuscitation

Cardiopulmonary resuscitation is a dramatic, emergency exercise *to restore effective circulation and ventilation following cardiac arrest*. Of the three levels of skill detailed under the activity of living of communicating (*see* p. 83), the second is the level of knowledge expected of all nurses, although many will be able to carry out all the procedures involved in advanced life support (the third level).

Cardiac arrest is the abrupt cessation of cardiac function; it may be induced by any of the following:

- respiratory failure or asphyxia as the cardiovascular and respiratory systems are interdependent
- cardiac arrhythmias caused by cardiac disease, electrolyte imbalance or hypothermia
- surgery
- mechanical problems with the circulatory system, such as result from an embolus or cardiac tamponade
- accidents such as drowning or electrocution.

The diagnosis of cardiac arrest is confirmed by:

- a sudden loss of consciousness
- the absence of respiration
- the absence of signs of circulation (including the carotid pulse and perfused skin).

Immediate cardiopulmonary resuscitation consists of three procedures. The mnemonic 'ABC' acts as an aide-memoire:

A – Airway: providing and maintaining a clear airway
B – Breathing: supplying oxygen to the blood by means of expired air respiration or artificial ventilation
C – Circulation: forcing the blood into the coronary and cerebral circulation by means of external chest compression.

Equipment

Suction equipment
Airway adjuncts such as an oropharyngeal (Guedel) airway, nasopharyngeal airway or laryngeal mask airway
Disposable face mask, e.g. Laderal pocket mask (for community use)
Ambubag and face mask or similar equipment, with oxygen supply
Defibrillator
Equipment for intubation (including endotracheal tubes, laryngoscope, bougie and connectors)
Emergency cardiac medications and equipment for intravenous access (*see* 'Intravenous therapy', p. 181)
Receptacle for soiled disposable items.

Guidelines and rationale for this nursing practice

- once cardiac arrest has been diagnosed, note the time. *A knowledge of the time elapsed is very important as the brain cells will begin to die from a lack of oxygen within 3 minutes*
- in hospital, order someone to alert the cardiac arrest team and bring the relevant emergency equipment; in the community, order someone to contact the emergency services *to make best use of the elapsing time and gain support from skilled personnel*
- place the patient in a supine position on a firm surface *to permit easy access to the patient's airway and chest*
- in an institutional setting, remove the bed head from the patient's bed *to further enhance access to the airway.*

Support for breathing and circulation must be carried out simultaneously to be effective.

A – Airway

- use suction if it is available to clear the airway or clean the mouth of debris *to remove any obstruction.* Dentures should remain in situ if they are well fitting *as this creates a good seal during assisted ventilation*
- tilt the head backwards and pull the mandible upwards *to open the airway.* Maintain this position (Fig. 11.1). If an injury to the cervical spine is suspected, open the airway using the jaw thrust technique *as this will reduce any movement of the cervical spine*
- insert an airway if available *to maintain the airway in an open position by preventing the tongue falling back into the oropharynx* (Baskett 1993).

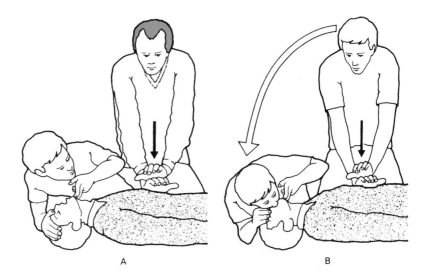

Figure 11.1
*Cardiopulmonary
resuscitation*
A *Two resuscitators*
B *One resuscitator*

B – Breathing

- two slow ventilations at 2–4 seconds per breath should be administered using mouth-to-mouth respiration or a disposable face mask *to provide supportive breathing* (Resuscitation Council UK 2000)
- note the rising of the chest wall *to confirm ventilation*
- ventilate at a rate of at least 12 per minute *as this imitates the physiological rate of an average breathing pattern* (Baskett 1993).

C – Circulation

- place the heel of one hand over the lower half of the sternum, two finger breadths from the xiphoid process, and place the other hand on top of it. While keeping the arms straight and the elbows locked, depress the sternum 4–5 cm towards the spine (*see* Fig. 11.1 above). *This compresses the heart between the spinal column and the posterior surface of the sternum, increasing the interthoracic pressure and creating a circulation*
- repeat this movement at a rate of 100 depressions per minute *as this sets up an adequate circulation to maintain perfusion of the essential body organs*
- continue chest compression and artificial ventilation at the rate of 15 chest compressions to 2 lung inflations (Resuscitation Council UK 2000). *These rates will provide a very modest level of oxygenation of the brain tissue* (Baskett 1993)
- check for the return of the pulse and breathing if the patient shows signs of breathing or respiratory effort, which may occur if a cardiac arrest has been caused by choking, drowning, drug overdose or trauma, *as these basic life support measures only **maintain** life*. Otherwise continue without checking until help arrives.

With the arrival of skilled personnel, the role of the nurses may alter. Breathing support is usually then provided by a medical practitioner (anaesthetist) or, in the community, by a paramedic, but external chest compression is not always taken over. Staff may continue:

- in a cardiac arrest caused by a primary cardiac event, defibrillation is normally the only way of restoring normal cardiac function by stopping a susceptible cardiac arrhythmia such as ventricular fibrillation or tachycardia. The defibrillator transmits an electric current through the patient's chest wall. All personnel must stand clear of the bed while the patient is being defibrillated as they will otherwise act as an 'earth' for the electric current, endangering the lives of those present and negating the technique's usefulness (Thompson & Hopkins 1987)
- assist a skilled practitioner or paramedic with the passage of an endotracheal tube *through which ventilation is continued*
- assist a skilled practitioner or paramedic with the commencement of an intravenous infusion *to provide a route for the administration of emergency medications and the taking of blood samples in order to detect any abnormality in blood chemistry*
- assist if required with the application of limb or chest electrodes *to provide a continuous monitoring of cardiac function*
- draw up emergency cardiac medications as needed. A brief record of all medications administered should be kept, *permitting written prescriptions to be made at a later time*
- ensure that the patient is left feeling as comfortable as possible following successful resuscitation, *maintaining the quality of this nursing practice*
- in the community, ensure the safe transportation of the patient to hospital, *maintaining the quality of this nursing practice*
- dispose of equipment safely *to reduce any health hazard*
- document the nursing practice appropriately, monitor the after-effects and report any abnormal findings immediately, *providing a written record of the practice, which should accompany the patient*
- in undertaking this practice, nurses are accountable for their actions, the quality of care delivered and record-keeping according to the *Code of Professional Conduct* (UKCC 1992), *Guidelines for Professional Practice* (UKCC 1996) and *Guidelines for Records and Record Keeping* (UKCC 1998).

Relevance to the activities of living	***Maintaining a safe environment*** Many nurses may face the ethical dilemma of the 'do not resuscitate' (DNR) order (BMA and RCN 1993). The decision not to resuscitate a patient is crucial to providing good-quality care as the experience of resuscitation is not pleasant for the patient, the family or the health-care professionals involved (Mason 1997). A transparent decision-making process involving all concerned must be used, and this process must be documented in the medical and nursing notes (Mallett & Dougherty 2000).

The tissue most sensitive to the lack of blood and oxygen is that of the brain; if an adequate cerebral circulation is not restored within 3 minutes, irreversible brain damage will occur. Nurses, when commencing work in a new ward or patient area, should quickly familiarise themselves with the position of the equipment used in that area during cardiopulmonary resuscitation.

Following cardiopulmonary resuscitation procedures, and at regular intervals, for example weekly, the equipment should be checked to ensure that it is in working condition and that stocks have been replenished.

In the community, the nurse should carry a disposable face mask for emergency use. In the UK, the emergency services provided by ambulance and paramedical personnel commonly deal initially with cardiac arrest situations outside health-care institutions. Once a patient has been stabilised, he or she will then be transported to an acute hospital environment.

The Resuscitation Council UK (2000) has published recommended protocols for advanced life support that have been adopted by staff in the UK health-care setting (Fig. 11.2).

Communicating

It is now accepted that three levels of skill in cardiopulmonary resuscitation should be taught (Chamberlain 1989). The first is 'basic life support', which the population as a whole should learn. No equipment is necessary as the victim's airway is maintained, and breathing and circulation supported, by simple skills that can be easily taught.

The second level is 'basic life support with adjuncts', which all nurses should learn. The basic principles of life support are utilised, with the additional use of an airway, Ambubag and mask. Nursing personnel working in high-dependency units frequently assume an extended nursing role by receiving further education and practice in the use of a defibrillator (Last et al 1992).

The third level is 'advanced life support', which all cardiopulmonary resuscitation teams should be competent to deliver. This involves the implementation of internationally recognised recommendations for treatment regimes following a cardiac arrest (Resuscitation Council UK 2000).

Other patients or bystanders witnessing any part of cardiopulmonary resuscitation will be alarmed and distressed. During the procedure, nurses who are not involved can give comfort and reassurance to these patients or bystanders and, wherever possible, continue with their normal work pattern. In some areas, such as the accident and emergency department, the patient's relatives are invited to be present during resuscitation attempts and will require an explanation of each activity and support through this experience (Resuscitation Council UK 2000).

Following this emergency, the patient's next of kin should be contacted and informed.

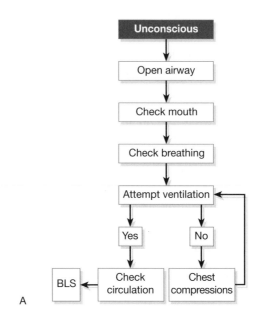

Unconscious

↓

Open airway

↓

Check mouth

↓

Check breathing

↓

Attempt ventilation

Yes   No

Check circulation   Chest compressions

BLS

A

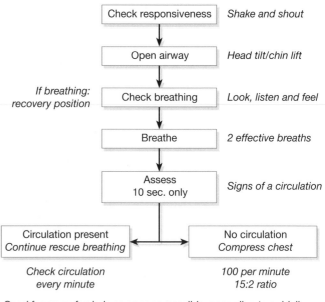

| Check responsiveness | Shake and shout |

Open airway — Head tilt/chin lift

If breathing: recovery position — Check breathing — Look, listen and feel

Breathe — 2 effective breaths

Assess 10 sec. only — Signs of a circulation

Circulation present *Continue rescue breathing*   No circulation *Compress chest*

Check circulation every minute   *100 per minute 15:2 ratio*

B   *Send for, or go for, help as soon as possible, according to guidelines*

Figure 11.2 *Revised advanced resuscitation protocols. From Resuscitation Council (2000), with permission*
A *Management of choking in adults*
B *Adult basic life support*

When resuscitative measures are successful, the patient will require a brief, easily understood explanation of what has happened and the reasons for using the equipment involved.

Following such a dramatic emergency procedure, junior nursing staff may be distressed and can be helped by supportive colleagues.

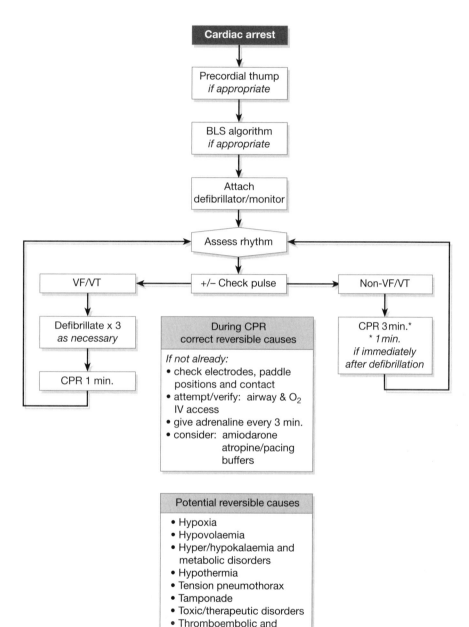

```
                        ┌─────────────────┐
                        │  Cardiac arrest │
                        └─────────────────┘
                                 │
                                 ▼
                        ┌─────────────────┐
                        │ Precordial thump│
                        │  if appropriate │
                        └─────────────────┘
                                 │
                                 ▼
                        ┌─────────────────┐
                        │  BLS algorithm  │
                        │  if appropriate │
                        └─────────────────┘
                                 │
                                 ▼
                        ┌─────────────────┐
                        │      Attach     │
                        │defibrillator/monitor│
                        └─────────────────┘
                                 │
                                 ▼
                        ⬡  Assess rhythm  ⬡
```

Cardiac arrest

Precordial thump *if appropriate*

BLS algorithm *if appropriate*

Attach defibrillator/monitor

Assess rhythm

VF/VT	+/− Check pulse	Non-VF/VT

Defibrillate x 3 *as necessary*

CPR 1 min.

CPR 3 min.*
* 1 min.
if immediately after defibrillation

During CPR correct reversible causes

If not already:
- check electrodes, paddle positions and contact
- attempt/verify: airway & O_2 IV access
- give adrenaline every 3 min.
- consider: amiodarone
    atropine/pacing
    buffers

Potential reversible causes

- Hypoxia
- Hypovolaemia
- Hyper/hypokalaemia and metabolic disorders
- Hypothermia
- Tension pneumothorax
- Tamponade
- Toxic/therapeutic disorders
- Thromboembolic and mechanical obstruction

Figure 11.2 (continued)
C *Advanced life support*
BLS, basic life support;
VF, ventricular fibrillation;
VT, ventricular
tachycardia; CPR,
cardiopulmonary
resuscitation;
IV, intravenous   C

Resuscitation is essentially a practical skill that requires regular practice to maintain the skill level (Ferguson 1990).

Nurses have a responsibility to ensure that they maintain their level of skill in resuscitative practices; this will involve regular practice at simulation sessions (Wynne 1990).

Breathing

A fractured rib may result from external chest compression. If the patient experiences pain on inspiration following external cardiac massage, this should be reported immediately.

When resuscitation is unsuccessful, the relatives may be approached regarding the possibility of organ donation. Nurses need to have a knowledge of the various physiological, psychological, social, cultural and spiritual aspects surrounding organ donation to give them greater confidence when faced with this issue (Orzel 2000).

Eating and drinking

During cardiac arrest and resuscitation procedures, a patient may vomit and create problems of maintaining a clear airway. When appropriate, sheets and clothing should be changed as soon as possible for the patient's comfort and dignity.

Eliminating

There may be incontinence of urine or faeces immediately following a cardiac arrest, which adds to the patient's distress, so sheets and clothing should be changed as soon as possible for the patient's comfort and dignity.

Personal cleansing and dressing

As cardiopulmonary resuscitation is an emergency procedure, during which immediate exposure of the patient's chest and limbs is required, some damage to the patient's clothing may occur, and this should be explained to the patient at a later time.

Immediately after successful resuscitation, the patient will require nursing intervention related to this activity of living to ensure that he or she is as comfortable as possible.

Sleeping

After being resuscitated and regaining consciousness, the patient may have difficulty in resuming his or her normal sleep pattern because of the fear of suffering a further cardiac arrest, and the nurse should take appropriate measures to help to induce sleep.

Dying

As a cardiac arrest is an emergency and may not be reversible, the patient's next of kin may suddenly have to be told of their relative's death and will display any of the many grief reactions; the nurse's empathy and support are then required.

Patient/carer education: key points

In partnership with the patient and/or carer, ensure that they are competent to carry out any practices required. Information should be given on an appropriate point of contact for any concerns that may arise.

Following a successful resuscitation, the patient and relatives must be given information about the event and be permitted to discuss their feelings and anxieties about the emergency. Other patients within the clinical area will also require to be given an explanation of the events to assist in relieving some of their own anxieties.

As suggested by the Resuscitation Council UK (2000), the nurse has a role in encouraging and teaching the general population to develop skills in basic life support.

References

Baskett P 1993 Resuscitation handbook. 2nd edn. Wolfe, London
British Medical Association and Royal College of Nursing 1993 Cardiopulmonary resuscitation: a statement from the RCN and BMA. Issues in Nursing and Health No. 20. BMA/RCN, London
Chamberlain D 1989 Advanced life support. British Medical Journal 299(6696): 446–448
European Resuscitation Council 1998 ERC guidelines. Resuscitation Council, London
Ferguson A 1990 Cardiopulmonary resuscitation – a teaching guide. Nurse Education Today 10: 50–53
Last T, Self N, Kassab J, Rajan A 1992 Extended role of the nurse in ICU. British Journal of Nursing 1(13): 672–675
Mallett J, Dougherty L 2000 The Royal Marsden Hospital manual of clinical nursing procedures. 5th edn. Blackwell Science, Oxford
Mason S 1997 The ethical dilemma of the do not resuscitate order. British Journal of Nursing 6(11): 646–649
Orzel M 2000 The patient who experiences trauma. In: Alexander M, Fawcett J, Runciman P (eds) Nursing practice – hospital and home: the adult. 2nd edn. Churchill Livingstone, Edinburgh
Resuscitation Council UK 2000 Advanced life support course provider manual. 4th edn. Resuscitation Council UK, London
Thompson D, Hopkins S 1987 Making sense of defibrillation. Nursing Times 83(49): 54–55
United Kingdom Central Council for Nursing, Midwifery and Health Visiting 1992 Code of professional conduct. UKCC, London
United Kingdom Central Council for Nursing, Midwifery and Health Visiting 1996 Guidelines for professional practice. UKCC, London
United Kingdom Central Council for Nursing, Midwifery and Health Visiting 1998 Guidelines for records and record keeping. UKCC, London
Wynne G 1990 Training and retention of skills. In: Evans T (ed.) ABC of resuscitation. 2nd edn. British Medical Journal, London
Web site: Resuscitation Council UK   http://www.resus.org.uk

12   Care of the Deceased Person

Learning outcomes	By the end of this section, you should know how to: ▪ care for a deceased person.
Background knowledge required	Review of the health authority policy pertaining to the care of a deceased person Review of the religious and spiritual rites of care of a deceased person Revision of 'Bed bath' (*see* p. 31) and 'Mouth care' (*see* p. 225).
Indications and rationale for care of a deceased person	Before transfer to the mortuary or undertaker's premises, a deceased patient requires care that may be delivered by a professional carer, an undertaker or the appropriate person identified by the spiritual beliefs of the deceased. This care may also be referred to as the 'Last Offices'.
Equipment 	Disposable gloves Equipment as for 'Bed bath' (*see* p. 31) Equipment as for 'Mouth care' (*see* p. 225) Incontinence pad or disposable napkin Dressing pack Waterproof dressing for open wounds if necessary Hypoallergenic tape Shroud Disposable bowl Two patient identification bands ⎫ appropriately completed with the Patient identification cards and/or ⎬ patient's full name and other details notification of death cards ⎭ as requested Mortuary sheet or clean white sheet Gauze bandage Trolley for equipment Receptacle for patient's clothing Patient clothing list book Patient valuables list book Receptacle for patient's valuables Receptacle for soiled linen Receptacle for soiled disposable items.

Guidelines and rationale for this nursing practice

- inform the medical practitioner when a patient is thought to have died *to confirm the diagnosis of death and comply with the legal requirements before the issue of a death certificate* (Births and Deaths Registration Act 1953)
- *to prevent further distress to those persons present*, ensure the patient's privacy and the privacy of the relatives
- ensure that the patient's relatives, if they are not present, are notified of the death. *This will allow the expressed wishes of the deceased to be implemented and funeral arrangements to be initiated*
- assist and support bereaved relatives *as the professional carer is in a key position at this time* (Roper et al 2000)
- inform the nursing officer or deputy and portering staff, or in the patient's home assist the carer, to contact the undertaker *to make the initial arrangements for the transfer of the body to the mortuary or undertaker's premises*
- collect and prepare the equipment *to ensure all the equipment is available*
- wash the hands, apply an apron and gloves *for general hygiene and to prevent cross-infection*
- remove all the upper bed linen, leaving a sheet to cover the patient *to give easy access to the body*
- lay the patient flat, face up, with limbs in a natural position and arms by his or her side. *Rigor mortis occurs 2–4 hours following death; positioning the body after this time is very difficult*
- remove any mechanical aids, for example heel pads or rubber rings, *as they may cause marking of the tissues*
- gently close the eyelids *to protect the tissues should the deceased or relatives give permission for corneal donation and also to improve the facial appearance* (Green & Green 1992)
- clean the patient's mouth and replace any dentures *to enhance the aesthetic appearance of the deceased and maintain hygiene*
- support the mandible in a closed position using a light pillow. An hour may elapse prior to the continuation of the practice, but this interval is not essential. *This will allow rigor mortis to develop prior to the completion of the practice*
- using the disposable bowl, manually express the urinary bladder *as any body fluid leakage will act as a health hazard to staff who come in contact with the deceased*
- remove all tubes and drains, unless otherwise instructed, *to reduce the health hazard*
- re-dress all wounds with a waterproof dressing, *thereby reducing the potential problem of the leakage of body fluids*. Any drains or tubes left in position should also be covered with a padded waterproof dressing
- wash the patient as for 'Bed bath' (*see* p. 31), *for general hygiene purposes*
- a male patient should be shaved *for aesthetic reasons*
- all jewellery, once removed, should be listed in the patient valuables book in the presence of two nurses, *to maintain the security of the deceased's belongings*. In the community, personal belongings should not be removed by the nurse unless a witness is present. Any action should be documented and signed

- apply identification bands and cards to the appropriate limbs and parts of the body as per health authority policy *to ensure continued identification of the deceased*
- apply an incontinence pad or disposable napkin, *which will reduce the health hazard from further body fluid leakage for staff who are in contact with the body*
- place the shroud, or at home fresh bedclothes, in position *to enhance the appearance should relatives wish to view the deceased.*

Institution

- wrap the body in the sheet, ensuring complete coverage, and secure the sheet with adhesive tape or the gauze bandage *to prevent exposure of the deceased during transfer to the mortuary*
- fix an identification card or notification of death card to the sheet using adhesive tape, *for ease of future identification*
- list the patient's clothing, *thus creating a receipt for future use.* Place this clothing and the patient's valuables in a secure place *to ensure safe keeping until removal by the relatives*
- dispose of equipment safely *to reduce any health hazard*
- inform portering staff that the body is ready for collection; *this will permit the body to be cooled as soon as possible after death, thus slowing the decomposition process*
- on the arrival of portering staff with the mortuary trolley, ensure the privacy of the other patients *in an attempt to prevent further distress*
- document the nursing practice appropriately *to provide a written record of the care given*
- in undertaking this practice, nurses are accountable for their actions, the quality of care delivered and record-keeping according to the *Code of Professional Conduct* (UKCC 1992), *Guidelines for Professional Practice* (UKCC 1996) and *Guidelines for Records and Record Keeping* (UKCC 1998).

Community

- cover the patient with a sheet *for aesthetic purposes.* Unless requested otherwise by the carer, leave the face uncovered
- remove any portable nursing material or equipment in order *to reduce the 'clinical' appearance of the room*
- following the removal of the body, arrange for the collection of any residual equipment, *thereby returning the home environment to 'normal'*
- document the nursing practice appropriately *to provide a written record of the care given*
- in undertaking this practice, nurses are accountable for their actions, the quality of care delivered and record-keeping according to the *Code of Professional Conduct* (UKCC 1992), *Guidelines for Professional Practice* (UKCC 1996) and *Guidelines for Records and Record Keeping* (UKCC 1998).

Relevance to the activities of living

Although the patient is deceased, a consideration of the activities of living is important in relation to the family and for the protection of staff.

Maintaining a safe environment

Some health authorities have agreed a policy permitting a senior nurse to confirm the expected death of a patient or resident. The death certificate will be issued by the medical practitioner who was responsible for the patient's care, stating the date and time the patient was last seen.

All equipment should be clean or disposable and all precautions be taken to prevent cross-infection. Nurses should wash their hands before commencing and on completion of the practice. Disposable gloves and apron should be worn when the nurse is handling soiled pads or body fluids from the deceased. On the death of a patient with a contagious disease, such as hepatitis B or HIV/AIDS, isolation techniques should be maintained. The body is placed in a large polythene body bag and sealed, usually with adhesive tape, prior to being wrapped in a sheet. These practices reduce the health hazard to staff who come into contact with the body.

If a patient dies unexpectedly, within 24 hours of surgery or receiving an anaesthetic, or within 24 hours of involvement in some form of trauma, the nurse may be requested to leave in position all drains, tubes and dressings during the practice (Green & Green 1992) as this may help to establish the cause of death. A patient who dies suddenly and unexpectedly will require a post mortem examination.

Communicating

Communication with bereaved relatives can be stressful (Smith 1995). Nurses should not hide their own feelings of loss and sadness from the deceased's relatives as the feeling of sharing may be of great support to them. Informing relations adequately and kindly about immediate practicalities is also crucial. It is, for example, important that the next of kin understand what is written on the death certificate and know that it has to be registered locally as only then can funeral arrangements be made.

Following the death of a patient, other patients may question the nurse about the deceased. The nurse should inform the patients kindly and honestly that the patient has died and give support when needed (Orzel 2000). The nurse may also need to assist and support his or her colleagues prior to, during and after the nursing practice.

Dying

The details of the practice can vary according to the patient's cultural background and religious practices (Nearney 1998, Roper et al 2000) so the nurse must be aware of specific requirements prior to, during or after death. For the body of the Orthodox Jew, for example, there is a ritual purification, no post mortem is permitted, and no organs may be removed for transplantation.

The bereaved relatives will require sensitive and compassionate care. Morris (1988) suggests that nurses shy away from death as it acts as a reminder of our own mortality. Little can be done to ease the relatives' distress, but the nurse should be aware of the many reactions that may be demonstrated and remain calm and supportive (Neuberger 1994). Any request to see the deceased should be arranged as soon as possible as this may assist the relatives during the grieving process; care should be taken to ensure that the patient looks as peaceful as possible, that the environment is cleared of equipment and that a chair is available.

The deceased person's clothing and valuables should be returned to the next of kin in a sympathetic manner. If these can not be returned to the next of kin, they should be transferred to the appropriate administrative department.

In the community, the nurse may make a more gradual withdrawal from the family of the deceased by visiting after the funeral. Referral to other professionals or voluntary agencies who specialise in caring for the bereaved may be required.

References

Green J, Green M 1992 Dealing with death. Chapman & Hall, London

Morris E 1988 A pain of separation. Nursing Times 84(42): 54–56

Nearney L 1998 Practical procedures for nurses: last offices. Nursing Times 94(26): 1–2 (pullout section)

Neuberger J 1994 Caring for dying people of different faiths. 2nd edn. CV Mosby, London

Orzel M 2000 The patient who experiences trauma. In: Alexander M, Fawcett J, Runciman P (eds) Nursing practice – hospital and home: the adult. 2nd edn. Churchill Livingstone, Edinburgh

Roper N, Logan W, Tierney A 2000 The Roper–Logan–Tierney model of nursing. Churchill Livingstone, Edinburgh

Smith C 1995 Bereavement care in A&E departments. British Journal of Nursing 4(9): 485–486

United Kingdom Central Council for Nursing, Midwifery and Health Visiting 1992 Code of professional conduct. UKCC, London

United Kingdom Central Council for Nursing, Midwifery and Health Visiting 1996 Guidelines for professional practice. UKCC, London

United Kingdom Central Council for Nursing, Midwifery and Health Visiting 1998 Guidelines for records and record keeping. UKCC, London

13 Catheterisation: Urinary

There are four parts to this section:

1 Catheterisation
2 Catheter care
3 Bladder irrigation
4 Bladder lavage/washout.

The concluding subsection, 'Relevance to the activities of living', refers to the four practices collectively.

Learning outcomes

By the end of this section, you should know how to:

- prepare the patient for any of these four nursing practices
- collect and prepare the equipment
- carry out catheterisation, catheter care, bladder irrigation and bladder lavage.

Background knowledge required

Revision of the anatomy and physiology of the urinary system and external genitalia
Revision of 'Wound care' technique (*see* p. 407)
Revision of local health authority policy regarding catheter selection, catheter bags and bladder washout solutions.

1 Catheterisation

Indications and rationale for urethral catheterisation

Urethral catheterisation is the passing of a catheter through the urethral orifice to the bladder:

- *to re-establish a flow of urine in urinary retention*
- *to provide a channel for drainage when micturition is impaired*
- *to empty the bladder preoperatively*
- *to allow the monitoring of fluid balance in a seriously ill patient*
- *to facilitate bladder irrigation procedures*
- *to maintain a dry environment in urinary incontinence when all other forms of nursing intervention have failed.*

Equipment

Good light source, such as spotlight or torch
Sterile gloves
Sterile catheterisation or dressings pack
Sterile water-based solution for cleansing the genitalia
Sterile anaesthetic gel if required, or water-soluble lubricant
Sterile receiver
Sterile catheter of the type and size required
Appropriate equipment for catheter balloon inflation for non pre-filled
   catheters only, e.g. syringe, needles and sterile water
Sterile closed drainage system if required, or catheter valve
Hypoallergenic tape
Sterile specimen container appropriately labelled with a completed laboratory
   form and plastic specimen bag for transportation
Trolley or adequate surface for equipment
Receptacle for soiled disposable items.

Catheters and catheter bags

Catheter type   The reason for urinary catheterisation can dictate the type and
size of catheter (Fig. 13.1) to be used:

- a round-ended catheter can be used when a retained catheter is not
  required
- a Foley double-lumen, self-retaining catheter can be used when a short-term
  retained catheter is required
- a Foley triple-lumen, self-retaining catheter can be used when continuous
  bladder irrigation is required
- a Tiemann catheter can be used when the urethral canal is narrowed, for
  example when a male patient has an enlarged prostate gland; the shape
  of the catheter tip aids the passage of the catheter
- a whistle-tipped catheter can be used postoperatively to allow the
  passage of blood clots, particularly when bladder irrigation is
  not being utilised
- a silastic catheter can be used when a retained catheter is required for
  long-term use, as silastic is less irritant to the body tissue.

Sizes   The smallest Charrière size that will drain urine should be used.

- 12–14 FG is a suitable size of catheter for female and male patients
  (Lowthian 1995). Intermittent self-catheterisation catheters are
  usually 10–12 FG in size
- larger-diameter catheters may be used when the urine has an excess of
  sediment and/or blood
- catheters are manufactured in female and male catheter lengths, male
  catheters being approximately 42 cm long and female ones about 26 cm
- for routine use, select a catheter with a 10 ml balloon. A 30 ml balloon may be
  used postoperatively.

Materials   A variety of catheter materials is available, the choice being geared to the needs of the individual patient:

- a latex catheter for use up to 2 weeks
- a PTFE-coated, latex Foley catheter for use up to 2 weeks
- a hydrogel-coated, latex catheter for use up to 12 weeks
- a silicone-coated, latex catheter for use up to 12 weeks

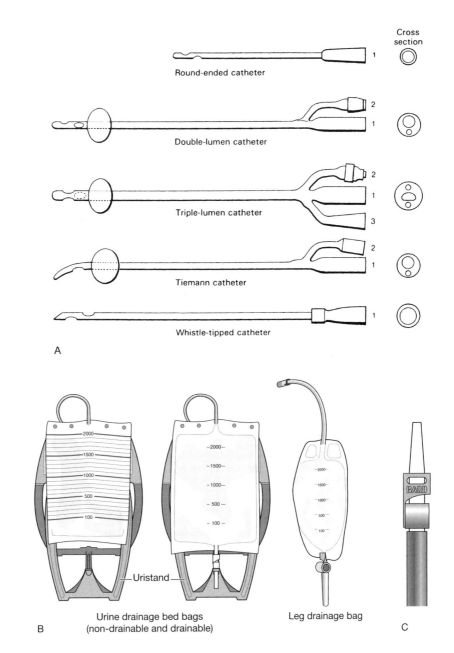

Figure 13.1

Catheterisation

A *Examples of catheters (1, channel for urine flow; 2, channel for balloon inflation; 3, channel for irrigating fluid flow)*

B *Types of drainage bag*

C *Catheter valve*

- a 100% silicone catheter for use up to 12 weeks
- a plastic nelaton catheter for intermittent self-catheterisation (Getliffe & Dolman 1997, Winn 1997)

Only PVC and 100% silicone catheters contain no latex and may be used in patients with a latex allergy.

Catheter bags   There are three elements to be considered when choosing an appropriate catheter bag: the capacity, the length of the inlet tube and the type of outlet tap for emptying (Colley 1998a, b). The selection depends on the rationale for catheter use, patient preference and the patient's manual dexterity. The leg bag can be supported by leg straps or by a variety of garments such as net sleeves.

A catheter valve may be preferable to a catheter bag for patients with bladder sensation and a stable bladder (Pettersson 1997, Woods et al 1999). The valve is released several times a day as sensation indicates.

Guidelines and rationale for this nursing practice

Female patient

- explain the nursing practice to the patient *to obtain consent and co-operation*
- collect and prepare the equipment *to ensure that all equipment is available and ready for use*
- ensure the patient's privacy *to reduce anxiety*
- observe the patient throughout this activity *to note any signs of distress*
- prepare and help the patient into a supine position with the knees bent, the hips flexed and the feet resting on the bed approximately 70 cm apart. *This position provides good access to and visualisation of the genitalia*
- place an incontinence pad or similar waterproof sheet under the patient's buttocks *to prevent any spillage of fluids onto the patient's bed linen*
- arrange the lighting *to assist with good visualisation of the genitalia* (Selfe 2000)
- wash the hands and put on the gloves, *which will act as a barrier between the nurse's skin and the patient's tissues, thus reducing the incidence of contamination* (Horton 1995)
- open and arrange the equipment, maintaining sterility *to reduce contamination*
- cleanse the labia minora, swabbing from above downwards *to reduce the danger of cross-infection from the anal region*
- using the non-dominant hand, separate the labia minora to reveal the urethral meatus. Hold this position until catheter insertion has been completed in order *to prevent recontamination of the urethral meatus by the labia minora after cleansing*
- insert anaesthetic gel or water-soluble lubricant into the urethral meatus *to ease the passage of the catheter*

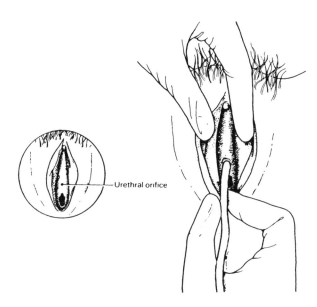

Urethral orifice

Figure 13.2
*Catheterisation: inserting
a catheter into the
female urethra. From
Roper et al (1985), with
permission*

- with the dominant hand, cleanse the urethral meatus *to prevent the introduction of micro-organisms into the urethra and/or bladder* and position the sterile receiver *to collect the urine from the catheter*
- insert the lubricated catheter into the urethra in an upward and backward direction, *which follows the anatomical route of the female urethra* (Marieb 1998) (Fig. 13.2)
- avoid contamination of the surface of the catheter until a flow of urine has been established, *to prevent the introduction of micro-organisms* (Gould 1994)
- if it is not intended that the catheter should be left in situ, gently remove the catheter when the urine flow ceases
- if for retention, gently advance the catheter 4–5 cm and slowly inflate the balloon according to the manufacturer's directions. *The inflated balloon will maintain the catheter's position*
- a complaint of pain may suggest that the inflating balloon is still within the patient's urethra. Stop the inflation and withdraw the fluid inserted into the balloon. Advance the catheter another 4–5 cm and repeat the inflation process. *The length of a patient's urethra can vary so it is important to adjust practice to meet the individual patient's needs and prevent complications*
- attach a drainage system and properly manage all potential entry points of infection *to prevent the development of ascending infection* (Swaffield 2000) (Fig. 13.3).
- anchor the catheter when appropriate by supporting the catheter and drainage tubing *to reduce trauma to the bladder neck and urethra, which could lead to pressure sore development* (Lowthian 1994)
- ensure that the patient is left feeling as comfortable as possible, thus *maintaining the quality of this nursing practice*

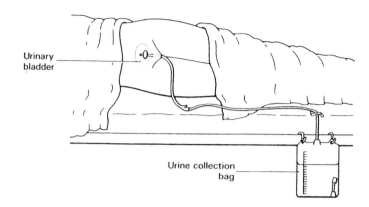

Urinary bladder

Urine collection bag

Figure 13.3 *Closed bladder drainage system showing the drainage bag below the level of the bladder*

- dispose of the equipment safely *to reduce any health hazard*
- document the nursing practice appropriately, monitor the after-effects and report any abnormal findings immediately, *providing a written record and assisting in the implementation of any action should an abnormality or adverse reaction to the practice be noted*
- in undertaking this practice, nurses are accountable for their actions, the quality of care delivered and record-keeping according to the *Code of Professional Conduct* (UKCC 1992a), *Guidelines for Professional Practice* (UKCC 1996) and *Guidelines for Records and Record Keeping* (UKCC 1998).

Male patient

This practice is usually carried out by a medical practitioner, a male nurse or a female nurse who has achieved the required level of competence (UKCC 1992b, Winn 1997).

- explain the nursing practice to the patient *to obtain consent and co-operation*
- collect and prepare the equipment *to ensure that all equipment is available and ready for use*
- ensure the patient's privacy *to reduce anxiety*
- observe the patient throughout this activity *to note any signs of distress*
- prepare and help the patient into a supine position. *This position provides good access to and visualisation of the genitalia*
- place an incontinence pad or similar waterproof sheet under the patient's buttocks *to prevent any spillage of fluids onto the patient's bed linen*
- arrange the lighting *to assist with good visualisation of the genitalia* (Selfe 2000)
- wash the hands and put on gloves, *which will act as a barrier between the nurse's skin and the patient's tissues, thus reducing the incidence of contamination* (Horton 1995)
- open and arrange the equipment, maintaining sterility *to reduce contamination*

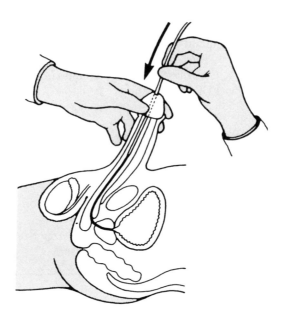

Figure 13.4
*Catheterisation: inserting
a catheter into the male
urethra*

- withdraw the patient's foreskin with the non-dominant hand. Maintain this position until catheter insertion has been completed in order *to prevent recontamination of the urethral meatus by the foreskin after cleansing*
- with the dominant hand, cleanse the glans penis and urethral meatus *to prevent the introduction of micro-organisms into the urethra and/or bladder*
- insert the lignocaine gel and leave for 2 minutes *to allow the local anaesthetic to act*
- position the sterile receiver and, with the non-dominant hand, gently grasp the shaft of the penis, raising it straight up *as this will aid the passage of the catheter along the length of the urethra*
- *as the male urethra is longer than the female* (Marieb 1998), insert the lubricated catheter into the urethral meatus for approximately 20–25 cm until a flow of urine is established (Fig. 13.4)
- continue as for the female patient until the anchoring of the catheter
- replace the patient's foreskin over the glans penis or *a paraphimosis may develop*
- anchor the catheter by taping it laterally to the thigh or abdomen, or use a supportive waist-belt, *to reduce trauma to the urethra and bladder neck, which could cause the development of a pressure sore* (Lowthian 1994)
- ensure that the patient is left feeling as comfortable as possible, *maintaining the quality of this nursing practice*
- dispose of the equipment safely *to reduce any health hazard*
- document the nursing practice appropriately, monitor the after-effects and report any abnormal findings immediately, *providing a written record and assisting in the implementation of any action should an abnormality or adverse reaction to the practice be noted*

- in undertaking this practice, nurses are accountable for their actions, the quality of care delivered and record-keeping according to the *Code of Professional Conduct* (UKCC 1992a), *Guidelines for Professional Practice* (UKCC 1996) and *Guidelines for Records and Record Keeping* (UKCC 1998).

2 Catheter care

Indications and rationale for catheter care

Catheter care is the cleansing of the exposed part of a catheter; this may:

- *help to reduce the risk of infection ascending via the catheter to other parts of the urinary system*
- *remove any crusts or discharge from the catheter as these can harbour pathogenic micro-organisms.*

Equipment

Disposable gloves
Disposable wipes
Mild soap and water
Tray for equipment
Receptacle for soiled disposable items.

Guidelines and rationale for this nursing practice

- explain the nursing practice to the patient *to obtain consent and co-operation*
- collect and prepare the equipment *to ensure that all equipment is available and ready for use*
- ensure the patient's privacy *to reduce anxiety*
- observe the patient throughout this activity *to note any signs of distress*
- help the patient into a suitable position *allowing the nurse easy, comfortable access to the patient*
- wash the hands *to reduce cross-infection* (Horton 1995), apply gloves, and arrange the equipment, *allowing easy access during the practice*
- gently cleanse the external urethral meatus, using the swab only once and in only one direction, swabbing from above downwards in the female patient and away from the catheter–meatus junction *to reduce the risk of cross-infection* (Crow et al 1986)
- in a male patient, retract the foreskin before cleansing, *allowing clear access to the meatus*
- replace the foreskin following the completion of this nursing practice, *preventing the development of a paraphimosis*
- gently swab the shaft of the catheter away from the catheter–meatus junction, *to remove any discharge away from the urethral orifice* (Crow et al 1986)
- ensure that the patient is left feeling as comfortable as possible, *maintaining the quality of this nursing practice*
- dispose of the equipment safely *to reduce any health hazard*

- document the nursing practice appropriately, monitor the after-effects and report any abnormal findings immediately, *providing a written record and assisting in the implementation of any action should an abnormality or adverse reaction to the practice be noted*
- in undertaking this practice, nurses are accountable for their actions, the quality of care delivered and record-keeping according to the *Code of Professional Conduct* (UKCC 1992a), *Guidelines for Professional Practice* (UKCC 1996) and *Guidelines for Records and Record Keeping* (UKCC 1998).

3   Bladder irrigation

Indications and rationale for bladder irrigation

Bladder irrigation is the continuous washing out of the bladder using sterile fluid. Continuous bladder irrigation can be carried out through a three-way urethral catheter or via a suprapubic and a urethral catheter:

- *to prevent the formation of blood clots after surgery to the urinary tract*
- *to aid the removal of blood clots and/or sediment in the bladder*
- *to clear an obstructed catheter.*

Equipment

Sterile disposable gloves
Sterile dressings pack
Sterile normal saline
Sterile irrigating solution at 37.8°C, usually normal saline solution 0.9%
Sterile irrigation set
Sterile drainage bag with outlet tap
Trolley/adequate surface for equipment
Receptacle for soiled disposable items.

Guidelines and rationale for this nursing practice

- explain the nursing practice to the patient *to gain consent and co-operation*
- collect and prepare the equipment *to ensure that all equipment is available and ready for use*
- ensure the patient's privacy *to reduce anxiety*
- observe the patient throughout this activity *to note any signs of distress*
- help the patient into a comfortable position *allowing the nurse easy, comfortable access to the patient*
- wash the hands *to reduce cross-infection* (Horton 1995), apply gloves, and arrange the equipment, *allowing easy access during the practice*
- cleanse the irrigation inlet arm of the catheter with the antiseptic solution *to reduce cross-infection*
- insert the irrigation set connector into the cleansed inlet arm of the catheter *to permit the introduction of the irrigating fluid*
- attach the urine drainage bag if a drainage bag is not already in use. *This will act as a collection container for the returned irrigating fluid*

- empty the drainage bag *to allow accurate monitoring of the volume of returned irrigating fluid and urine output*
- open the valve of the irrigation set and regulate the flow to the prescribed rate, *complying with the medical practitioner's prescription*
- renew the irrigating fluid as stated on the patient's prescription and empty the drainage bag as required *to maintain the bladder irrigation*
- ensure that the patient is left feeling as comfortable as possible, *maintaining the quality of this nursing practice*
- dispose of the equipment safely *to reduce any health hazard*
- document the nursing practice, monitor the after-effects and report any abnormal findings immediately, *providing a written record and assisting in the implementation of any action should an abnormality or adverse reaction to the practice be noted*
- in undertaking this practice, nurses are accountable for their actions, the quality of care delivered and record-keeping according to the *Code of Professional Conduct* (UKCC 1992a), *Guidelines for Professional Practice* (UKCC 1996) and *Guidelines for Records and Record Keeping* (UKCC 1998).

4 . Bladder lavage/washout

Indications and rationale for bladder lavage/ washout

Bladder lavage/washout is the intermittent washing out of the bladder using sterile fluid:

- *to aid the removal of sediment and/or blood clots*
- *to clear an obstructed catheter*
- *to allow the administration of medicine into the bladder.*

Approximately 50% of catheterised patients are susceptible to recurrent catheter encrustation (Getliffe 1994), which can cause blockage of the catheter lumen, the bypassing or retention of urine, pain and unnecessary catheter changes (Rew 1999). The use of bladder washouts for patients with long-term catheters is questionable (Winn 1996) and may lead to an increased risk of infection as a result of breaking the closed drainage system. Washouts have been advocated for recurrent catheter encrustation and blockage (Getliffe & Dolman 1997), particularly when using Suby G or mandelic acid solutions (Button et al 1999), although further evidence for this is required.

Equipment

Sterile disposable gloves
Sterile dressings pack
Sterile normal saline solution
Sterile lavage fluid at 37.8°C, e.g. normal saline
Sterile 50 ml bladder syringe
Two sterile receivers
Sterile drainage bag
Large clean receiver for the returned lavage fluid

Trolley/adequate surface for equipment
Receptacle for soiled disposable items.

Guidelines and rationale for this nursing practice

- explain the nursing practice to the patient *to gain consent and co-operation*
- collect and prepare the equipment required *to ensure that all equipment is available and ready for use*
- ensure the patient's privacy *to reduce any anxiety*
- observe the patient throughout this activity *to note any signs of distress*
- help the patient into a comfortable position *allowing the nurse easy, comfortable access to the patient*
- wash the hands *to reduce cross-infection* (Horton 1995), and arrange the equipment, *allowing easy access during the practice*
- disconnect the drainage bag and discard *to prevent ascending infection should this bag be reconnected*
- cleanse the end of the catheter with the antiseptic solution using the dressing forceps or a gloved hand. *This will reduce the number of micro-organisms present on the end of the catheter and lessen the risk of cross-infection*
- place one sterile receiver under the catheter *to act as a collecting container for the returned lavage fluid*
- *to permit commencement of the lavage,* charge the bladder syringe with the lavage solution, which has been poured into the second receiver
- release the clamp on the catheter and slowly introduce all the solution into the bladder. *A sudden, fast introduction of the lavage fluid may cause the patient extreme discomfort*
- allow this fluid to flow into the sterile receiver *to permit the lavage fluid and any debris to be returned prior to the introduction of the next volume of fluid.* Repeat until the prescribed volume of fluid has been used
- attach the sterile drainage bag *to act as a collection container for any residual lavage fluid and to return the patient's catheter to the former drainage system*
- ensure that the patient is left feeling as comfortable as possible, *maintaining the quality of this nursing practice*
- dispose of the equipment safely *to reduce any health hazard*
- compare the volume, colour and consistency of the fluid injected with that of the fluid returned *to assist in the assessment of the effectiveness of the bladder lavage;* discrepancies should be documented *as this suggests that some lavage fluid has been retained*
- document the nursing practice appropriately, monitor the after-effects and report any abnormal findings immediately, *providing a written record and assisting in the implementation of any action should an abnormality or adverse reaction to the practice be noted*
- in undertaking this practice, nurses are accountable for their actions, the quality of care delivered and record-keeping according to the *Code of Professional Conduct* (UKCC 1992a), *Guidelines for Professional Practice* (UKCC 1996) and *Guidelines for Records and Record Keeping* (UKCC 1998).

Relevance to the activities of living

Maintaining a safe environment

Introducing a catheter into the bladder has the potential to allow pathogenic micro-organisms to enter a sterile environment in a healthy individual, so the nurse must be vigilant in maintaining an aseptic technique throughout the practice (Roper et al 1996). Anchoring the catheter reduces the potential problem of trauma to the internal and external urethral sphincters and bladder tissue (Brunner & Suddarth 1992, Lowthian 1994), and a self-retaining catheter with a small balloon may help to lessen trauma to the bladder epithelium (Lowthian 1989).

The maintenance of a 'closed' drainage system and the use of appropriate infection control measures when emptying a drainage bag will help to reduce the potential problem of ascending infection in the urinary system (Gould 1994) (Fig. 13.5), but the risk of catheter-associated infection has been reported to increase by 5–8% per day (Laurent 1998). Lanara (1987) has suggested that the concept of the 'closed' drainage system as a method of preventing ascending infection is flawed as the system is open to the air when being emptied. It is

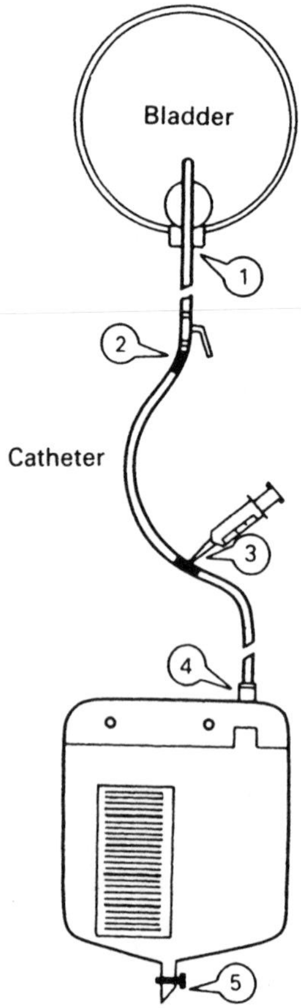

Figure 13.5 *Points at which pathogens can enter a closed urinary drainage system:*
1 the urethral orifice
2 the connection between the catheter and drainage tube
3 where the sample of urine is taken
4 at the connection between the drainage tube and collecting bag
5 at the drainage bag outlet. From Roper et al (1985), with permission

generally agreed that the addition of a disinfectant to the urine drainage bag does not significantly reduce the incidence of infection in catheterised patients (Getliffe & Dolman 1997), and the benefit of catheter care in reducing the risk of ascending infection remain unclear. However, catheter care with mild soap and water and a clean disposable cloth has been found to be as effective as cleansing with other solutions (Button et al 1999, Laurent 1998).

During bladder lavage, the connection between the catheter and drainage bag is broken, with the risk that pathogens may be introduced into the urinary tract. Because of this danger, some health agencies do not advocate bladder lavage (Swaffield 2000).

To prevent blockage by blood clots and/or sediment, a catheter may require regular 'milking' of the tubing. Maintaining a clear flow of urine helps to prevent urinary stagnation, which can be a precursor to the development of infection, and therefore prevents infection of the bladder and urinary tract.

Any patient with an indwelling catheter must know whom to contact if a problem arises with the catheter or/and drainage system (Wright 1989).

A patient who uses intermittent self-catheterisation as a method of bladder control will undertake the catheterisation using a clean technique (Winder 1995).

Catheter leg bags should be changed every 5–7 days (Colley 1998).

Communicating

The patient must be given an easily understood explanation about the reason behind the commencement of any of the nursing practices listed. If these practices are to be used as part of a patient's postoperative care, the explanation should be given preoperatively and will help to reduce patient anxiety. The patient's anxiety must be further lessened by explaining the reason for the appearance and colour of the drainage fluid during a bladder irrigation or lavage.

During bladder irrigation, the patient may experience pain resulting from irritation of the raw areas of the bladder by the irrigating solution. Analgesia should be given as prescribed by the medical practitioner.

The patient with a long-term catheter, and his or her carers, will require an appropriate teaching programme, but this is unfortunately not always seen as a priority in nursing practice. A programme of teaching has been recommended by Wright (1989).

The nurse who is to teach a patient self-catheterisation must have a good understanding of normal bladder function and dysfunction (Winder 1995).

Eliminating

The drainage of urine via a catheter is a deviation from the normal method of micturition but does not interfere with normal defaecation.

Before cleansing the urethra, the nurse should look for any urethral discharge. Any resistance felt during the passage of the catheter, and any bleeding from the urethra following insertion of the catheter, should be noted.

The nurse should also note and record the quantity of urine drained from the patient's bladder. If the catheter has been inserted to re-establish urine flow in urinary retention, only 500 ml of urine should be drained in the first hour; the catheter should then be clamped and 200–300 ml of urine be drained every hour until the patient's bladder is empty. This will help to prevent a loss of bladder muscle tone following the acute retention of urine.

The colour of the urine should be noted. Pale pink or red through to brown is suggestive of blood in the urine (haematuria). Blood or sediment in the urine is suggestive of a malfunction of the renal or urinary system as a result of disease or trauma and should therefore be noted. It should be remembered that certain medicines and foods such as rifampicin (an anti-tuberculosis medication) and beetroot can colour the urine, here reddish-brown and orange respectively; this is not a cause for alarm.

Following the commencement of bladder irrigation, the rate of infusion of the irrigating solution will usually be dependent on the appearance of the fluid returned into the urine drainage bag. After surgery such as a prostatectomy, the patient may require an irrigating volume of 5–10 L in the first 12 hours, but this can usually be reduced to 3–5 L during the following 12–18 hour period. The amount and appearance of the fluid removed from the drainage bag should be recorded and, following surgery, fluid that appears to be rose in colour indicates an adequate irrigation rate (Selfe 2000). The patient's urinary output is calculated by subtracting the amount of drained fluid from the volume of irrigating solution infused. Any resistance or inability to introduce the irrigating or lavage fluid should be reported and documented appropriately.

Eating and drinking

Assistance should be given to patients to increase their oral fluid intake. This will promote an increase in the volume of fluid passing through the urinary system and bladder, which will help to prevent a urinary tract infection developing as a result of urinary stagnation. There is, however, no evidence that increasing the fluid intake has any significant effect on the development of biofilm and the potential for catheter blockage (Getliffe & Dolman 1997). An accurate fluid balance chart must be maintained at all times. Should the patient have both an intravenous infusion and a bladder irrigation system in position, care must be taken not to confuse the urinary irrigation set and solution with the intravenous giving set and fluid.

A patient who practises intermittent self-catheterisation may benefit from a reduction in oral intake during the evening, reducing the necessity for catheterisation during the night.

There is some evidence that cranberry juice may have beneficial effects (Rew 1999), and it has been reported to inhibit bacterial adherence (Avorn et al 1994).

Personal cleansing and dressing

When a catheter is retained over a long period, it is important to ensure that perineal hygiene is maintained; this may involve some education of the patient and carers. The patient should be advised to wear loose underwear, which is less likely to compress the catheter tubing. Showering rather than immersion bathing is preferable to reduce the incidence of ascending infection from the dirty water of a bath. The use of a leg drainage bag in conjunction with trousers or a longer-length skirt can benefit the patient's appearance.

Mobilising

If a catheter is retained, it and the drainage tubing may impede mobilising. Interference may be reduced by using leg drainage bags or catheter valves, which can be easily anchored to the patient's leg.

Catheter movement, which could lead to trauma of the urethra and/or bladder neck when mobilising, can be reduced by supporting the catheter (Lowthian 1994).

Expressing sexuality

The introduction of a catheter can be perceived by the patient as an 'assault' on body image. The adequate provision of privacy during catheterisation and catheter care is conducive to reducing the patient's anxiety and embarrassment.

The appearance of a retained catheter and urine drainage bag can cause a patient a great deal of embarrassment and anxiety. For the bed-bound patient, the discreet placement of the urine drainage bag out of the obvious sight of visitors will be greatly appreciated. Leg drainage bags are less visible and more comfortable for the chair-bound or ambulant patient.

The use of a urinary catheter is a deviation from the normal mechanism of micturition and can thus have an effect on the patient's self-esteem and body image. The nurse and carer must be sensitive to the needs of the patient and assist and support the patient during the period of adaptation to this change. Full sexual activity is not precluded by the presence of a catheter, and patients and their partners should be given leaflets and practical advice (McKnight & Ripley 1995), ideally prior to catheter insertion. It is recognised that this is an area in which many nurses have a knowledge deficit or feel too embarassed to discuss the issue (Atkinson 1997).

Sleeping

A retained catheter may interfere with a patient's usual sleep pattern. As the patient moves during sleep, the catheter and/or tubing may become trapped, causing the patient to awaken from the discomfort caused by tension on the catheter; this possibility should be discussed with the patient in order to reduce alarm should it occur.

A patient at home will require information and education on when to renew and how to keep clean a night drainage bag.

Patient/carer education: key points

In partnership with the patient and/or carer, ensure that they are competent to carry out any practices required. Information should be given on an appropriate point of contact for any concerns that may arise.

Provide verbal and written information on the reason for the use and care of the catheter while it is in situ, for the patient, carer and relatives. When possible, give the patient an indication of the length of time the catheter will be in use, and ensure that the patient knows what to do should a problem develop with the catheter.

A patient who has a catheter on a long-term basis will require extra information and education on the continued care and effect of the catheter on his or her activities of living.

The technique of self-catheterisation may be taught to some patients as a method of coping with their particular urinary problem.

References

Atkinson A 1997 Incorporating sexual health into catheter care. Professional Nurse 13(3): 146–148

Avorn J, Monane M, Gurwitz J, Glynn R, Choodnovsky I, Lipsitz L 1994 Reduction in bacteruria and pyuria after ingestion of cranberry juice. Journal of the American Medical Association 271: 751–754

Brunner L, Suddarth LD 1992 The textbook of adult nursing. Chapman & Hall, London

Button D, Roe B, Webb C, Frith T, Colin-Thome D, Gardner L 1999 Continence promotion and the management by the primary health care team. Consensus guidelines. Whurr, London

Colley W 1998a Catheter care. 1. Nursing Times 94(24 suppl): 1–2

Colley W 1998b Catheter care. 2. Nursing Times 94(25 suppl): 1–2

Crow R, Chapman R, Roe B, Wilson J 1986 A study of patients with an indwelling urethral catheter and related nursing practice. Nursing Practice Research Unit, University of Surrey, Guildford

Getliffe K 1994 The use of bladder washouts to reduce urinary catheter encrustation. British Journal of Urology 73: 696–700

Getliffe K, Dolman M (eds) 1997 Promoting continence: a clinical and research resource. Baillière Tindall/RCN, London

Gould D 1994 Keeping on tract. Nursing Times 90(40): 58–64

Horton R 1995 Handwashing: the fundamental infection control principle. British Journal of Nursing 4(16): 926–933

Lanara V 1987 Catching infection from catheters. Nursing Standard 1(1): 6

Laurent C 1998 Preventing infection from indwelling catheters. Nursing Times 94(25): 60–64

Lowthian P 1989 Catheters – preventing trauma. Nursing Times 85(21): 73–75

Lowthian P 1994 The 'WISSC' – a device to prevent pressure sores in the urethra and bladder neck. Journal of Tissue Viability 4(4): 133

Lowthian P 1995 An investigation of the uncurling forces of indwelling catheters. British Journal of Nursing 4(6): 328–334

McKnight K, Ripley D 1995 Management and care of catheters and collection systems: a guide for nurses. Bard, Crawley

Marieb E 1998 Human anatomy and physiology. 4th edn. Benjamin Cummings, Redwood City, California

Pettersson L 1997 Choosing a catheter valve that suits the patient. Community Nurse 3(4): 9

Rew M 1999 Use of catheter maintenance solutions for long term catheter. British Journal of Nursing 8(11): 708–715

Roper N, Logan W, Tierney A 1985 The elements of nursing. 2nd edn. Churchill Livingstone, Edinburgh

Roper N, Logan W, Tierney A 1996 The elements of nursing. 4th edn. Churchill Livingstone, Edinburgh

Selfe L 2000 The urinary system. In: Alexander M, Fawcett J, Runciman P (eds) Nursing practice – hospital and home: the adult. 2nd edn. Churchill Livingstone, Edinburgh

Swaffield J 2000 Continence. In: Alexander M, Fawcett J, Runciman P (eds) Nursing practice – hospital and home: the adult. 2nd edn. Churchill Livingstone, Edinburgh

United Kingdom Central Council for Nursing, Midwifery and Health Visiting 1992a Code of professional conduct. UKCC, London

United Kingdom Central Council for Nursing, Midwifery and Health Visiting 1992b Scope of professional practice. UKCC, London

United Kingdom Central Council for Nursing, Midwifery and Health Visiting 1996 Guidelines for professional practice. UKCC, London

United Kingdom Central Council for Nursing, Midwifery and Health Visiting 1998 Guidelines for records and record keeping. UKCC, London

Winder A 1995 Intermittent self catheterisation. Journal of Community Nursing 9(2): 24–28

Winn C 1996 Basing catheter care on research principles. Nursing Standard 10(18): 38–40

Winn C 1997 Catheterisation: the scope of professional practice. Nursing Standard 12(13): 57–61

Woods M, McCreanor J, Aitchison M 1999 An assessment of urethral catheter valves. Professional Nurse 14(7): 472–474

Wright E 1989 Teaching patients to cope with catheters at home. Professional Nurse 4(4): 191–194

14   Central Venous Pressure

There are two parts to this section:

1 Insertion of a central venous catheter
2 Measuring and recording central venous pressure.

The concluding subsection, 'Relevance to the activities of living', refers to both practices.

Learning outcomes

By the end of this section, you should know how to:

- prepare and support the patient for this nursing practice
- collect and prepare the equipment
- assist the medical practitioner with safe insertion of the central venous catheter
- monitor and record the central venous pressure (CVP)
- care for the central venous catheter.

Background knowledge required

Revision of the anatomy and physiology of the cardiovascular system, especially the heart, main vessels and veins of the neck and upper thorax

Revision of 'Intravenous therapy', especially part 4, the Hickman catheter (*see* p. 191)

Revision of 'Aseptic technique' (*see* p. 407)

Review of health authority policy in relation to CVP.

Indications and rationale for monitoring central venous pressure

A central venous line may be required for three main reasons:

- *to enable the rapid or high-volume fluid infusion of irritant substances* (e.g. cytotoxic drugs or total parenteral nutrition)
- *to allow frequent venous blood monitoring*
- *to monitor the venous pressure.*

The CVP recording is the measurement of the pressure in the right atrium of the heart and is quantified in cmH_2O. Sixty per cent of the circulating blood volume is held within the venous system, the CVP being the product of blood volume and venous tone. The pressure recorded reflects the circulating fluid volume; *this may need to be assessed in seriously ill patients in whom a close monitoring of fluid balance is needed.* It may be indicated:

- for the preoperative monitoring of patients who have suffered haemorrhage or trauma *to monitor fluid balance closely*
- for postoperative monitoring following major surgery, especially when intravenous therapy or parenteral nutrition is being administered, *to monitor fluid balance* (Daffurn et al 1994)
- for patients who have severe dehydration, for example after vomiting, diarrhoea or haemorrhage, *to monitor fluid replacement therapy*
- for patients who have cardiogenic, bacteraemic or hypovolaemic shock, *as this will adversely affect the circulatory system as the cardiac output falls* (Hayes 2000)
- for patients who have cardiac disease, *to monitor fluid overload*
- for patients who have renal disease, *to monitor fluid overload*
- for patients who have acute renal failure during haemodialysis or ultrafiltration procedures *to monitor fluid balance.*

1   Insertion of a central venous catheter

Outline of the procedure

This procedure is carried out by a medical practitioner using an aseptic technique. The procedure involves the passage of a catheter through the veins to the superior vena cava or the right atrium of the heart (Fig. 14.1). The catheter is then connected to the manometer and giving set, and an intravenous infusion is commenced (*see* 'Parenteral nutrition', p. 263).

The position of the patient

The position of the patient is important during this procedure and is dependent on the choice of the entry site for catheterisation. *Veins on the right side are usually selected because they provide easier access to the heart than do those on the left* (Springhouse Corporation 1999). There are three main entry sites (the first two being more frequently used) (Dougherty 2000).

The subclavian vein   The patient lies supine with the arms by his or her side. The head of the bed is lowered by 10° *to lessen the danger of an embolus occurring.*

The internal jugular vein   The patient lies supine, with no pillow, and with the neck extended. The head is rotated away from the site of entry and well

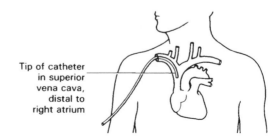

Figure 14.1   *Central venous pressure: position of the catheter in relation to the heart*

Tip of catheter in superior vena cava, distal to right atrium supported in position. The head of the bed is lowered by 10°. *This position is important to prevent an air embolus occurring.*

The median cephalic vein   The patient lies supine. The chosen arm is extended with the palm upwards and the elbow supported *to ensure easy access to the entry site.*

This procedure should ideally be performed in theatre, although it is increasingly being performed on the ward.

Equipment

As for intravenous infusion (*see* p. 181).

Additional equipment

Sterile gown
Sterile gloves
Minor operation sterile pack or sterile drape and towels
Waterproof protection for the bed
Alcohol-based antiseptic for cleansing the skin, evidence suggesting that alcohol-based chlorhexidene is more effective than iodine solution (Pratt 2001)
Venous pressure manometer set
Non-viscous sterile intravenous fluid, e.g. normal saline or dextrose 5% (which will be prescribed by the medical practitioner)
Appropriate sterile catheter depending on the site of entry used, e.g. a single-, double- or triple-lumen catheter (Fig. 14.2)
Sterile needles and black silk sutures
ECG monitoring equipment if required
Local anaesthetic and equipment for its administration.

Guidelines and rationale for this nursing practice

Refer to the section on 'Intravenous therapy' (*see* p. 181) for detailed guidelines.

- help to explain the procedure to the patient *to gain consent and co-operation, and to encourage participation in care*
- check whether the patient has an allergy to the skin-cleansing solution
- ensure the patient's privacy, *respecting his or her individuality*
- prepare the equipment and prime the administration set with the prescribed infusion fluid *in preparation for commencement of the infusion*

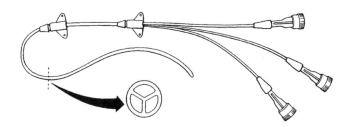

Figure 14.2
Triple-lumen catheter

- help the patient into the correct position depending on the site of entry used *to ensure that access is safely achieved*
- observe the patient throughout this activity *to monitor any adverse effects*
- adjust the angle of the bed so that the patient's head is lowered if required *to increase venous engorgement and prevent an air embolus*
- protect the bed with waterproof material *as some fluid or blood may spill*
- assist the medical practitioner as required, *ensuring safe practice*
- remain with the patient *to help to maintain his or her position and reduce anxiety as far as possible*
- commence the infusion of the prescribed fluid once the catheter is in position and connected to the manometer and administration set. If a double- or triple-lumen catheter is used, the line designated for CVP recording is connected to the appropriate administration set and manometer, and labelled accordingly, *ensuring that all personnel have accurate information*
- ensure that the patient is left feeling as comfortable as possible *so that he or she will tolerate the catheter in situ as long as necessary* (RCN 1992)
- dispose of the equipment safely *to prevent the transmission of infection*
- document the procedure appropriately, monitor the after-effects and report any abnormal findings immediately *to ensure safe practice and enable prompt appropriate medical and nursing care to be initiated as soon as possible*
- monitor and adjust the flow rate *to maintain the infusion at the rate prescribed* (*see* 'Intravenous therapy', p. 181).

A portable chest X-ray image is taken as soon as possible after catheter insertion *to check that the catheter is in the correct position*. A temporary sterile dressing may be applied until this has been performed. The catheter is usually held in place with skin sutures *once it is judged to be correctly positioned*, and a sterile transparent dressing is applied over the site *to maintain asepsis* (Pratt 2001).

Arrhythmias occasionally occur *as a result of irritation of the heart by the passage of the catheter*, and observations may be supplemented by ECG monitoring. The rhythm usually returns to normal *once the catheter is in the correct position*.

---

2 Measuring and recording central venous pressure

The CVP is measured in cmH_2O, the range of normal being 3–10 cmH_2O. The CVP will be measured as advised by the medical practitioner.

Equipment

A central venous catheter, intravenous fluid and associated lines in situ (Fig. 14.3)
A venous pressure manometer (Fig. 14.3)
A spirit level.

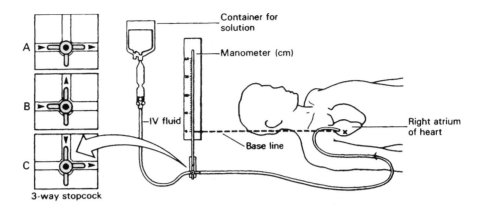

Figure 14.3 *Central venous pressure: position of the patient showing the catheter, manometer and three-way stopcock when reading a central venous pressure*

Guidelines and rationale for this nursing practice

- explain the nursing practice to the patient *to gain consent and co-operation, and to encourage participation in care*
- ensure the patient's privacy *to respect individuality and maintain self-esteem*
- help the patient into the correct position (Fig. 14.3). It is preferable for the patient to lie flat *for absolute accuracy, as this position will stop any upward pressure of the abdominal organs affecting the reading. If lying flat causes the patient any distress,* an acceptable reading can, however, be obtained with the patient sitting comfortably at an angle of about 45°. His or her body should be straight, with the shoulders flat against the back of the bed; *the thorax must not be turned or twisted, or a false reading may result* (Woodrow 1992). The position chosen should be documented and used at each subsequent reading
- position the manometer. It should be supported on a pole *so that it is easily read,* while still allowing the patient freedom of movement in bed between readings. *To prevent disconnection,* there should be no strain on the lines or the catheter
- observe the patient throughout this activity *to monitor any adverse effects*
- assess the baseline. *The baseline is the pressure level above which the measurement of CVP is made.* This is level with the patient's right atrium, where the tip of the catheter is lying. The medical practitioner will note the level at an imaginary 90° angle between the sternal notch and the midline from the axilla. In some areas, it is the practice to use the sternal notch as a proxy for this point. With the patient's consent, this can be marked on his or her skin *to ensure consistency of baseline measurement*
- read the baseline. A spirit level is used to record the level on the manometer gauge that corresponds to the baseline level, which may be marked on the side of the patient's chest; *this ensures that measurement is as accurate as possible*
- turn off all other infusions. Ideally, only the CVP fluid should be infused through the CVP line, but other fluids are on occasion infused through the same line. *As the CVP is measured in centimetres of water, only fluids of similar specific gravity, for example normal saline, should be used.* The use

of multiple-lumen lines overcomes this problem. The tap of the three-way stopcock should be at position A between recordings and before commencing the reading (*see* Fig. 14.3 above)

- flush the line *to ensure patency and to clear all other infusions* (Leighton 1994)
- turn the tap on the three-way stopcock away from the patient and towards the infusion fluid, to position B (*see* Fig. 14.3 above); *this allows the manometer tube to refill with fluid*
- turn the tap towards the patient to position C (*see* Fig. 14.3 above); *this allows the establishment of a free flow of fluid between the manometer tube and the catheter*. The fluid in the manometer tube will fall to a level that *corresponds to the pressure in the right atrium or superior vena cava*. The fluid fluctuates *in relation to the patient's respiration* once it falls to the level for recording
- read the level of the lower fluctuation on the manometer gauge once the fluid in the tube is maintaining a steady level with a fluctuation of 0.2–1.0 cm. *This relates to the pressure in the right atrium*
- subtract the baseline reading from this figure, *the resultant figure being the measurement of CVP*
- if using an electronic monitor, ensure that it is zeroed according to the manufacturer's instructions, align the transducer with the right atrium and continue as before
- turn the tap on the stopcock back to position A (*see* Fig. 14.3 above) *to occlude the manometer and recommence the infusion fluid at the prescribed rate*
- ensure that the patient is left feeling as comfortable as possible *to help to reduce anxiety and promote the healing process*
- document the nursing practice appropriately, monitor the after-effects and report any abnormal findings immediately. *This ensures safe practice and enables prompt appropriate medical and nursing intervention to be initiated.* A single reading is not as valuable as monitoring a series of recordings. *These will show whether the CVP is rising, falling or remaining steady and give some indication of the patient's response to treatment*
- in undertaking this practice, nurses are accountable for their actions, the quality of care delivered and record-keeping according to the *Code of Professional Conduct* (UKCC 1992), *Guidelines for Professional Practice* (UKCC 1996) and *Guidelines for Records and Record Keeping* (UKCC 1998).

Pressure transducers

Pressure transducers are increasingly being used to monitor CVP. The principles of the practice, the care of the patient and the care of the lines are exactly the same. The pressure transducer and the appropriate lines are substituted for the manometer set, and the measurement is recorded on a bedside monitor screen. When a reading is taken, the height of the transducer, which is supported on a pole, is adjusted to be level with the assessed baseline, as previously described.

The monitor may be programmed to assess the reading in mmHg. The normal recording parameters may have to be adjusted (see the manufacturer's instructions).

Relevance to the activities of living	Observations on and further rationale for this nursing practice will be included within each activity of living as appropriate. These are as for intravenous infusion, with the addition of the following.

Maintaining a safe environment

A central venous catheter gives direct access to the heart so the danger of infection is increased, and meticulous care to prevent it must be maintained at all times. An aseptic technique should be used whenever dressings, infusions or lines are changed and a good handwashing technique employed before touching the equipment used for measuring the CVP.

The nurse should ensure that the lines do not become disconnected; otherwise, air may enter and create an air embolus. The lines should be observed for air bubbles and appropriate action taken. The danger from an air embolus is increased because of the direct access to the heart.

The nurse should ensure that the line remains patent and that the infusion is maintained at the required rate to help to prevent clotting or occlusion of the line (*see* 'Intravenous therapy', p. 181).

Breathing

The CVP value is at the lower level of normal in young healthy adults, increasing slightly with age. It is raised in patients who have respiratory disease because of the increased intrapulmonary pressure, and significantly raised in patients with bronchospasm, for example asthma, as this increases the intrathoracic pressure and may mask any change in circulatory fluid volume. The CVP also increases in patients with congestive cardiac failure as a result of the increase in circulatory fluid volume.

A rare complication is the development of a pneumothorax, this being more likely to occur at the time of insertion of the catheter. Any sudden change in the patient's general condition or respiratory function should be reported immediately.

Eating and drinking

The CVP reflects the volume of circulating fluid and any fluid imbalance; it is lower in patients who are dehydrated and raised in patients with fluid overload. An accurate recording of fluid intake should be maintained during the period of monitoring CVP.

Eliminating

Accurate recordings of fluid output should be maintained during the period of monitoring, for the assessment of the patient's fluid balance.

The CVP is raised in patients who have renal disease; it will show a temporary fall during a period of treatment with diuretic medication.

Personal cleansing and dressing

The patient may need appropriate help with personal cleansing while attached to the manometer. The need to wear light clothing to allow unrestricted access to the site of catheterisation should be explained to the patient. Patients are able to bathe or shower with the transparent dressing.

Controlling body temperature

The danger of infection is increased during this procedure as the central line has direct access to the heart, so the patient's temperature should be recorded 2 or 4 hourly during the period of CVP monitoring in order to observe for any signs of developing infection. The temperature should be monitored 4 hourly for 48 hours after the central line has been removed.

Mobilising

The CVP will not be affected by the patient moving around the bed between readings. He or she may be helped into a chair with the manometer and lines adequately supported, as his or her condition allows.

Patient/carer education: key points

In partnership with the patient and/or carer, ensure that they are competent to carry out any practices required. Information should be given on an appropriate point of contact for any concerns that may arise.

The reason for CVP monitoring and its importance for treatment and care should be explained to the patient. This practice will normally only take place in an institutional setting.

The importance of maintaining the catheter in situ should be emphasised, and the dangers of disconnection explained, so that the patient does not pull the lines or dislodge the dressing.

All patients should understand the importance of reporting to the nursing staff any redness, swelling or pain at the infusion site, even after the line has been removed, as this may indicate a developing infection.

References

Daffurn K, Hillman K, Baumn A et al 1994 Fluid balance charts: do they measure up? British Journal of Nursing 3(16): 816–820

Dougherty L 2000 Central venous access devices. Nursing Standard 14(43): 45–50

Gourlay D 1996 Central venous cannulation. British Journal of Nursing 5(1): 8–15

Hayes E 2000 Shock (monitoring haemodynamic state). In: Alexander M, Fawcett J, Runciman P (eds) Nursing practice – hospital and home: the adult. 2nd edn. Churchill Livingstone, Edinburgh

Henderson N 1997 Central venous lines. Nursing Standard 11(42): 49–56

Leighton H 1994 Maintaining patency of transduced arterial and venous lines using 0.9% sodium chloride. Intensive and Critical Care Nursing 10(1): 23–25

Pratt R 2001 Preventing infections associated with central venous catheters. Nursing Times 97(15): 36–39

Royal College of Nursing 1992 Skin tunnelled catheters. Guidelines for care. RCN, London

Sheppard M 2000 Reading central venous pressure. Nursing Times 96(18): 43–44

Springhouse Corporation 1999 Handbook of infusion therapy. Springhouse Corporation, Pennsylvania

United Kingdom Central Council for Nursing, Midwifery and Health Visiting 1992 Code of professional conduct. UKCC, London

United Kingdom Central Council for Nursing, Midwifery and Health Visiting 1996 Guidelines for professional practice. UKCC, London

United Kingdom Central Council for Nursing, Midwifery and Health Visiting 1998 Guidelines for records and record keeping. UKCC, London

Woodrow P 1992 Monitoring CVP. Nursing Standard 6(33): 25–29

15 Chest Drainage: Underwater Seal

There are three parts to this section:

1 Insertion of an underwater seal chest drain
2 Changing a chest drainage bottle
3 Removal of an underwater seal chest drain.

The concluding subsection, 'Relevance to the activities of living', refers to the three practices collectively.

Learning outcomes

By the end of this section, you should know how to:

- support and prepare the patient for these three nursing practices
- collect and prepare the equipment necessary to insert a chest drain and connect it to underwater seal drainage, change a chest drainage bottle and remove an underwater seal chest drain
- assist the competent practitioner in parts 1 and 3
- care for the patient who has a chest drain connected to underwater seal drainage.

Background knowledge required

Revision of the anatomy, physiology and pathology of the respiratory system, including the structures of the chest wall
Revision of 'Aseptic technique' (*see* p. 407).

1 Insertion of an underwater seal chest drain

Indications and rationale for insertion of an underwater seal chest drain

Underwater seal chest drainage is a closed system of drainage that allows air or fluid to pass in one direction only, from the pleural space to the collecting bottle. It may be established in the following circumstance:

- *to bring about re-expansion of the lung* when there is air or fluid, such as blood or pus, in the pleural space as a result of injury, surgery or a respiratory disease or dysfunction (Alexander et al 2000).

Outline of the procedure

Using an aseptic technique, the medical practitioner washes and dries his or her hands, cleanses the patient's skin over the selected site of entry for the drain, injects a local anaesthetic and waits for it to take effect. The doctor then makes a small incision with the scalpel, inserts the drain and introducer, removes the introducer and connects the drain to the equipment already prepared by the nurse. A purse-string suture is inserted round the entry site of the drain to seal the site off when the drain is eventually removed. A dressing is usually placed over the site to help to prevent infection of the small wound (Fig. 15.1).

If there is air in the pleural space, the drain is usually inserted at the level of the 3rd or 4th intercostal space. The insertion site is lower here to promote maximum drainage if fluid has gathered in the pleural space.

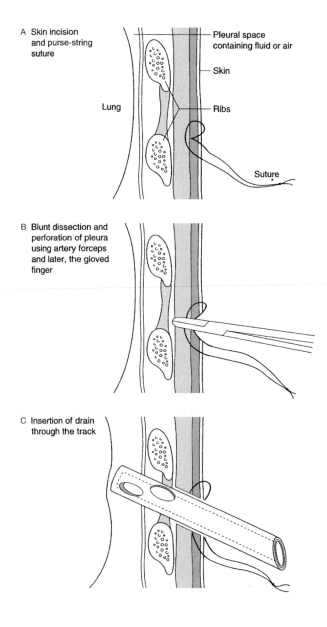

Figure 15.1 *Insertion of a chest drain*
A *Skin incision and purse-string suture*
B *Blunt dissection and perforation of the pleura using artery forceps and, later, the gloved finger*
C *Insertion of the drain through the track*

Equipment 	Trolley Sterile dressings pack Alcohol-based antiseptic for skin cleansing Local anaesthetic and equipment for its administration Sterile scalpel and blade Sterile black silk suture Sterile chest drain and introducer Sterile drainage equipment, e.g. Pleurovac or Argyle double-seal system Two pairs of tubing clamps Receptacle for soiled disposable items.

Guidelines and rationale for this nursing practice

- help to explain the procedure to the patient *to gain consent and co-operation. Patients should be encouraged to be active partners in care*
- ensure the patient's privacy *to help maintain dignity and a sense of self*
- administer a sedative if prescribed by the medical staff. *This may help to reduce the patient's anxiety*
- collect the equipment, *for efficiency of practice*
- help the patient into the position suggested by the medical staff *to allow best access to the site for insertion of the drain*
- observe the patient throughout this activity *to detect signs of discomfort or distress*
- ensure that the drainage equipment is assembled correctly and ready for connection to the drain when required, *for efficient practice*
- open the sterile equipment and help the medical practitioner as requested
- seal all connections *to ensure that they are airtight as this is necessary for maximum functioning of the drain*
- ensure that the collection equipment is always below the level of the patient's chest *so that there is no reflux into the pleural space* (Fig. 15.2)

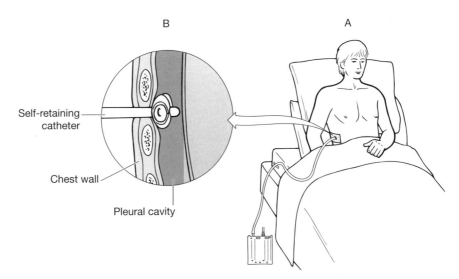

B   A

Self-retaining catheter

Chest wall

Pleural cavity

Figure 15.2
Underwater seal chest drainage
A *Drainage system in position*
B *Detail of the position of the catheter*

- *to allow the apparatus to start functioning*, release the clamps when the drain is connected and the nurse is satisfied that there are no air leaks at the connections
- check that the apparatus is functioning; the fluid should be oscillating in the long underwater tube in time with the patient's respiration. If positive suction is required, connect the short rod of the drainage bottle to the long rod of a second drainage bottle using tubing. The short rod of this second drainage bottle is then connected by tubing to a suction machine, the pressure of which has been decided by the medical practitioner
- apply a sterile dressing to the wound site *to help to prevent infection*
- ensure that the patient is left feeling as comfortable as possible, *to maintain the quality of this practice*
- dispose of the equipment safely *for the protection of others*
- document the procedure appropriately, monitor the after-effects and report any abnormal findings immediately *to ensure safe practice and enable prompt, appropriate medical and nursing intervention to be initiated*
- in undertaking this practice, nurses are accountable for their actions, the quality of care delivered and record-keeping according to the *Code of Professional Conduct* (UKCC 1992), *Guidelines for Professional Practice* (UKCC 1996) and *Guidelines for Records and Record Keeping* (UKCC 1998).

2   Changing a chest drainage bottle

Indications and rationale for changing a drainage bottle

As drainage from the pleural space accumulates and approaches the three-quarters full level, the drainage bottle has to be changed:

- *to enable the equipment to continue functioning efficiently.*

Equipment

Sterile drainage bottle, cap, glass or plastic rods and tubing or a disposable set
500 ml of sterile water or normal saline
Receptacle for soiled disposable items.

Guidelines and rationale for this nursing practice

- collect and prepare the equipment *for efficiency of practice*
- explain this practice to the patient *to encourage active participation in care*
- observe the patient throughout this activity *to detect signs of discomfort or distress*
- clamp off the intercostal drain securely with the two pairs of clamps *to prevent any backflow of air or fluid*
- disconnect the tubing
- connect the fresh tubing and apparatus
- ensure that all the connections are airtight and that the drainage bottle is below chest level *so that it will function correctly*

- release the clamps and check the oscillation of the fluid in the underwater tube *to confirm that the apparatus is functioning correctly*
- ensure that the patient is left feeling as comfortable as possible *to maintain the quality of this practice*
- dispose of the equipment safely *for the protection of others*
- document this nursing practice and report abnormal findings immediately *so that action can be taken to relieve any problems*
- in undertaking this practice, nurses are accountable for their actions, the quality of care delivered and record-keeping according to the *Code of Professional Conduct* (UKCC 1992), *Guidelines for Professional Practice* (UKCC 1996) and *Guidelines for Records and Record Keeping* (UKCC 1998).

3 Removal of an underwater seal chest drain

Indications and rationale for removal of an underwater seal chest drain

Underwater seal drainage is a temporary measure and is removed:

- *when radiological examination demonstrates that the patient's lung has fully reinflated.*

Equipment

Trolley
Sterile dressings pack
Sterile stitch-cutter
Sterile normal saline for wound cleansing
Waterproof tape and scissors
Sterile artery forceps
Receptacle for soiled disposable items.

Guidelines and rationale for this nursing practice

Two nurses, one of whom must be qualified, or the nurse and a medical practitioner are required to carry out this practice.

- explain the nursing practice to the patient *to gain consent and co-operation. Patients should be encouraged to be active partners in their care*
- ensure the patient's privacy *to maintain dignity and a sense of self*
- administer a sedative if it is prescribed by the medical practitioner. *This will help to reduce the patient's anxiety*
- collect the equipment *for efficiency of practice*
- prepare and assist the patient into a suitable position that is as comfortable as possible. *It is necessary to have clear access to the drain site*
- observe the patient throughout this activity *to detect any signs of discomfort and distress*
- remove the dressing from the drain site
- clean the drain site with the normal saline *to cleanse the skin*
- clamp the ends of the purse-string suture with the artery forceps to facilitate tightening the suture *so that the wound is sealed off as quickly as possible*

- raise the drain slightly (this is performed by the assistant) while the qualified practitioner cuts and removes the retaining suture
- request the patient to breathe in; while he or she is breathing out the qualified practitioner holds folded swabs over the puncture site with the non-dominant hand, and with the dominant hand pulls the drain out quickly and smoothly. The assistant tightens the purse-string suture as the drain is removed
- remove the artery forceps from the end of the purse-string suture and knot the suture
- apply a sterile dressing and waterproof tape *to stop as much air as possible accessing the drain site*
- order a chest X-ray *to ensure that the lung is functioning normally*
- ensure that the patient is left feeling as comfortable as possible, *to maintain the quality of this practice*
- dispose of the equipment safely *for the protection of others*
- document the nursing practice, monitor the after-effects and report any abnormal findings immediately *to provide a written record and assist in the implementation of any action should an abnormality or adverse reaction to the practice be noted*
- in undertaking this practice, nurses are accountable for their actions, the quality of care delivered and record-keeping according to the *Code of Professional Conduct* (UKCC 1992), *Guidelines for Professional Practice* (UKCC 1996) and *Guidelines for Records and Record Keeping* (UKCC 1998).

Relevance to the activities of living

Maintaining a safe environment

A meticulous technique must be used for the prevention of infection. Thorough handwashing should be carried out, preferably using an antiseptic detergent.

Ensure that the tubing is not being compressed or kinked by the patient lying on it, as this will cause the equipment to function inefficiently. It is imperative that the drainage bottle is kept below the level of the patient's chest, unless double-clamped, or there may be a backflow of fluid into the pleural cavity.

When the drain is being removed, care must be taken to prevent a pneumothorax (i.e. the entry of air into the pleural space).

Communicating

Because of breathlessness, the patient may have difficulty in talking. A pencil and paper may help communication with staff and visitors, and a bell should always be to hand to summon assistance if necessary. Analgesics may be prescribed to help relieve any pain or discomfort.

Breathing

If the equipment is functioning correctly, the patient's respiratory rate should gradually return to the normal range after the drain has been inserted.

The patient's respiration should be closely monitored after the removal of the drain so that the potential complication of pneumothorax can be quickly detected.

Personal cleansing and dressing

Some assistance with washing and dressing may have to be given to those who are attached to underwater seal drainage equipment as their mobility is reduced. Light, loose clothing should be worn so that breathing is not unduly impaired.

Mobilising

Movement will be restricted by the equipment, but the patient should be encouraged to be as independent as possible.

Sleeping

The patient's normal sleeping pattern may be altered because of difficulty with breathing and because of the presence of the equipment, so the nurse should take measures that help to induce sleep.

Patient/carer education: key points

In partnership with the patient and/or carer, ensure that they are competent to carry out any practices required. Information should be given on an appropriate point of contact for any concerns that may arise.

Continuing information should be given to the patient in order to relieve anxiety. Education on mobility when a chest drain is in situ should also be given.

References

Alexander M, Fawcett J, Runciman P 2000 Nursing care – hospital and home: the adult. 2nd edn. Churchill Livingstone, Edinburgh

Gray E 2000 Pain management for patients with chest drains Nursing Standard 14(23): 34–36

United Kingdom Central Council for Nursing, Midwifery and Health Visiting 1992 Code of professional conduct. UKCC, London

United Kingdom Central Council for Nursing, Midwifery and Health Visiting 1996 Guidelines for professional practice. UKCC, London

United Kingdom Central Council for Nursing, Midwifery and Health Visiting 1998 Guidelines for records and record keeping. UKCC, London

16　Eardrops: Instillation of

Learning outcomes

By the end of this section, you should know how to:

- prepare the patient for this nursing practice
- collect and prepare the equipment
- instil drops safely and effectively into the patient's ear.

Background knowledge required

Revision of the anatomy of the ear
Revision of 'Administration of medicines', especially checking the medication against the prescription (*see* p. 1).

Indications and rationale for instilling eardrops

The instillation of eardrops involves dropping a prescribed solution into the external auditory canal from a dropper. This may be required:

- *to soften wax before syringing*. If the wax has become impacted, syringing the external canal with solution will be ineffective unless the wax has first been softened (Zeitoun 1997)
- *to reduce inflammation and relieve discomfort*
- *to combat infection*.

Equipment

Prescribed eardrops
Cotton wool balls
Receptacle for soiled disposable items.

Guidelines and rationale for this nursing practice

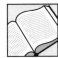

- explain the practice to the patient *to ensure understanding and gain consent and co-operation*
- collect and prepare the equipment *for efficiency of practice*
- ensure the patient's privacy *to preserve dignity and a sense of self*
- assist the patient to sit in an upright position with the head tilted slightly away from the affected ear *so that the drops inserted will run the length of the canal*
- observe the patient throughout this activity *to detect any signs of discomfort*
- check the drug prescription with the label on the eardrops *to ensure that the correct drops are administered*

- check the expiry date on the bottle of eardrops *as expired medication may be ineffective*
- verify which ear should receive the drops, *to avoid errors*
- pull the pinna of the ear gently in an upward and backward direction in adults, and a downward and backward direction in children, *to straighten the external canal*
- insert the prescribed number of eardrops into the canal
- release the pinna
- position a piece of cotton wool at the entrance to the canal if this is local policy
- dispose of the equipment safely *for the protection of others*
- document this nursing practice appropriately, monitor the after-effects and report any abnormal findings immediately *to provide a written record and assist in the implementation of any action should an abnormality or adverse reaction to the practice be noted*
- in undertaking this practice, nurses are accountable for their actions, the quality of care delivered and record-keeping according to the *Code of Professional Conduct* (UKCC 1992), *Guidelines for Professional Practice* (UKCC 1996) and *Guidelines for Records and Record Keeping* (UKCC 1998).

Relevance to the activities of living	***Maintaining a safe environment*** To avoid the risk of cross-infection, each patient should have an individual container of prescribed eardrops. Nurses should wash their hands before commencing and on completion of the practice. ***Communicating*** Any patient who is receiving medication by ear may experience difficulty with hearing, which should be explained. If a patient complains of skin irritation, pain or a burning sensation following the instillation of an ear medication, this should be reported as it may be an indication of a drug allergy. ***Mobilising*** It aids the effectiveness of the eardrops if the ear into which the drops are inserted is kept level or tilted upwards for a period of time after insertion to aid absorption.
Patient/carer education: key points	In partnership with the patient and/or carer, ensure that they are competent to carry out any practices required. Information should be given on an appropriate point of contact for any concerns that may arise. If the patient is expected to self-administer the drops, it will be necessary to teach this technique and ensure proficiency.

References

United Kingdom Central Council for Nursing, Midwifery and Health Visiting 1992 Code of professional conduct. UKCC, London

United Kingdom Central Council for Nursing, Midwifery and Health Visiting 1996 Guidelines for professional practice. UKCC, London

United Kingdom Central Council for Nursing, Midwifery and Health Visiting 1998 Guidelines for records and record keeping. UKCC, London

Zeitoun A 1997 Developing a nurse-led aural care clinic. Nursing Times 93(45): 46–47

17 Ear Syringing

Learning outcomes	By the end of this section, you should know how to: • prepare the patient for this procedure • collect and prepare the equipment • syringe a patient's ear.
Background knowledge required	Revision of the anatomy and physiology of the external and middle ear Review of health authority policy for this procedure.
Indications and rationale for syringing an ear	Syringing an ear is washing out the external auditory canal with a prescribed solution using a special syringe (Booth 1998). This may be required: • *to clear the external canal of an obstruction that may be blocking it* • *to wash out softened wax that may be impeding the transmission of sound waves to the tympanic membrane.*
Outline of the procedure	Using the auriscope, the external canal and ear drum are examined. If the ear drum is intact and no other abnormalities are detected, the practice of syringing the ear can be carried out. It is sometimes not possible to visualise the tympanic membrane at this stage because of the impacted wax. In this case, if there is no history of a ruptured ear drum, and after preparing the equipment and solution as outlined below, insert some of the solution gently to dislodge some of the wax and then check the membrane. The syringe or tubing is primed with the solution, or the pre-prepared equipment assembled, care being taken to expel all the air. The protective covering is placed over the patient's shoulder and the receiver held in place under the ear. The pinna of the ear is gently pulled in an upward and backward direction to straighten out the canal, the fluid then being introduced through the syringe or tubing, which should point to the roof of the canal so that the solution flows along the roof, down and back out, washing any debris with it (Fig. 17.1). After the qualified

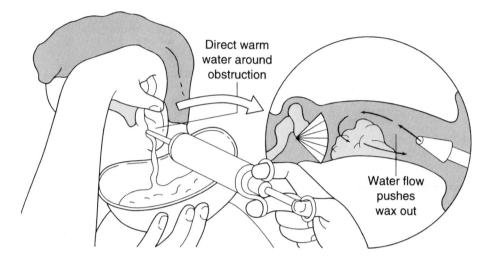

Figure 17.1 *Ear syringing showing fluid being directed towards the roof of the aural canal (the nurse should pull the pinna of the ear gently upwards). From Chilman & Thomas (1987), with permission*

Direct warm water around obstruction

Water flow pushes wax out

practitioner has again examined the canal to assess the result of the syringing, the canal is carefully dried using the dressed applicators (Harkin 2000).

Equipment

Tray
Waterproof protection for the patient
Container with the prescribed amount of solution
Lotion thermometer
Aural (ear) syringe

or

Disposable pre-prepared equipment

or

Electronically operated apparatus with which the operator can control the
   pressure of the fluid
Receiver for return flow
Auriscope
Dressed applicators
Receptacle for soiled disposable items.

Tap water is now commonly used for ear syringing, although sodium chloride 0.9% or a solution of sodium bicarbonate (4 g in 600 ml water) may be ordered. About 500 ml of the solution are usually prepared.

The temperature of the solution should be 38°C. Temperatures other than this are uncomfortable, may injure tissues and may cause the patient to feel dizzy and nauseated. This procedure is normally only carried out if the tympanic membrane is intact, in which case it is a socially clean procedure.

Guidelines and rationale for this nursing practice

- help to explain the procedure to the patient *to ensure that the practice is understood and to gain consent and co-operation*
- assemble and prepare the equipment *to increase the efficiency of the practice*
- ensure the patient's privacy *to help to maintain dignity and a sense of self*
- assist the patient to sit in an upright position with the head tilted slightly to the affected side *to aid the return flow of the solution*
- observe the patient throughout this activity *to detect any signs of discomfort or distress*
- arrange the waterproof protection around the patient's neck and shoulders *to prevent the patient's clothes becoming damp or damaged*
- place the receiver for the return flow under the patient's ear and ask for the patient's assistance in holding it in place
- after examining the external canal, insert the equipment and direct the flow of solution in an upward direction
- continue until the return flow is clear of debris
- dry the patient's ear
- ensure that the patient is left feeling as comfortable as possible and check for improved hearing
- dispose of the equipment safely *for the protection of others*
- document the procedure appropriately, monitor the after-effects and report any abnormal findings immediately *to provide a written record and assist in the implementation of any action should an abnormality or adverse reaction to the practice be noted*
- in undertaking this practice, nurses are accountable for their actions, the quality of care delivered and record-keeping according to the *Code of Professional Conduct* (UKCC 1992), *Guidelines for Professional Practice* (UKCC 1996) and *Guidelines for Records and Record Keeping* (UKCC 1998).

Relevance to the activities of living

Maintaining a safe environment

Although an aseptic technique is not required, the equipment should be clean or disposable, and nurses should wash their hands before commencing and after completing the procedure.

It is important to examine the patient's ear before carrying out this procedure as there is a danger of causing serious damage or introducing infection into the middle ear if the tympanic membrane has been ruptured (Harkin 2000).

The temperature of the solution should be 38°C: colder or hotter solutions may stimulate the labyrinth and cause vertigo or nausea.

Communicating

Eardrops (usually oil) are usually prescribed for a few days prior to syringing to soften hard cerumen (wax).

It is important to explain to the patient that feelings of slight dizziness may be experienced when this procedure is being carried out. If it is being performed to wash away wax that has been impairing the patient's hearing, there should be a marked improvement in hearing afterwards. If the patient wears a hearing aid, the nurse should check that it is working satisfactorily after the practice.

Mobilising

The patient's co-operation in remaining still while the procedure is being carried out is important as the equipment could damage the ear tissue.

If there is any evidence of dizziness, the patient may have to rest for a while following the procedure.

Working and playing

Hearing difficulties may prevent the patient carrying out his or her job efficiently and can also prohibit participation in or limit the enjoyment of hobbies and interests (Bond et al 1995, Roper et al 2000).

Patient/carer education: key points

In partnership with the patient and/or carer, ensure that they are competent to carry out any practices required. Information should be given on an appropriate point of contact for any concerns that may arise.

It should be explained to the patient that nausea or dizziness may be experienced for a short time after the procedure.

If the syringing was carried out to relieve impacted wax and improve hearing, the possibility of the condition recurring must be explained.

References

Bond M, Arthur A, Avis M 1995 Distant voices: hospital care of a woman with sensory impairments highlights the importance of touch in communicating with patients. Nursing Times (19 Jul): 38–40

Booth E 1998 Ear syringing. Practice Nurse 16(9): 580–581

Chilman A, Thomas M (eds) 1987 Understanding nursing care. 3rd edn. Churchill Livingstone, Edinburgh

Harkin H 2000 Evidence based ear care. Primary Health Care 10(8): 25–29

Roper N, Logan W, Tierney A 2000 The elements of nursing. 5th edn. Churchill Livingstone, Edinburgh

United Kingdom Central Council for Nursing, Midwifery and Health Visiting 1992 Code of professional conduct. UKCC, London

United Kingdom Central Council for Nursing, Midwifery and Health Visiting 1996 Guidelines for professional practice. UKCC, London

United Kingdom Central Council for Nursing, Midwifery and Health Visiting 1998 Guidelines for records and record keeping. UKCC, London

18 Enema

Learning outcomes	By the end of this section, you should know how to: ▪ prepare the patient for this nursing practice ▪ collect and prepare the equipment ▪ administer an enema ▪ describe the various enema preparations and their modes of action.
Background knowledge required	Revision of the anatomy and physiology of the colon, rectum and anus Revision of drug administration, particularly checking the drug against the prescription (*see* p. 1).
Indications and rationale for administering an enema	An enema is the introduction of liquid into the rectum by means of a tube. It is used: ▪ *to evacuate the bowel prior to surgery or investigation* ▪ *to administer medication* ▪ *for the treatment of severe constipation.*
Equipment 	Tray Prescribed enema Protective covering for the bed Water-soluble lubricant Disposable gloves Apron Medical wipes/tissues Commode or bedpan if required Receptacle for soiled disposable items.

Types of enema

There are three main kinds of enema (Fig. 18.1):

1 **medication**: enemas containing medication that should be retained as long as possible and should be inserted very slowly over half an hour
2 **evacuant**: stimulant enemas that are usually returned, with faecal matter and flatus, within a few minutes; a solution containing phosphates or sodium citrate is commonly used

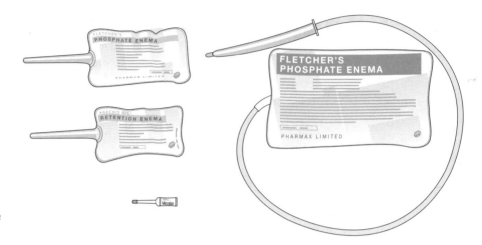

Figure 18.1 *Examples of disposable enemas*

3 **retention**: enemas that soften and lubricate the faeces and should be retained for a specified time; they usually contain arachis or olive oil. They may be inserted, for example, at bedtime to be retained overnight for maximum efficiency of action.

Microenemas are increasingly being used in the community as they cause less discomfort to patients when administered. The other pre-prepared enemas can be obtained with long delivery tubes to facilitate self-insertion by patients.

At one time, a solution containing green soap was prescribed as an evacuant enema, but it has been demonstrated that this can severely damage the mucosa of the bowel so it is no longer in use.

Prior to the administration of any enema, the nurse should check that the patient is not allergic to latex, phosphate or peanuts, arachis oil enema containing peanut oil (Addison 2000).

Guidelines and rationale for this nursing practice

- explain the nursing practice to the patient *to gain consent and co-operation. Patients should be encouraged to be active partners in care*
- assemble and prepare the equipment *for efficiency of practice*
- warm the enema to the required temperature by immersing it in a jug of water (see 'Maintaining a safe environment', below)
- if necessary, allow the patient to empty the bladder first *to reduce discomfort during the procedure* (Mallett & Dougherty 2000)
- ensure the patient's privacy and help the patient into the left lateral position *to allow ease of access to the anal sphincter*
- observe the patient throughout this activity *to detect any signs of discomfort or distress*
- place the protective covering under the patient's buttocks *to contain any soiling or leakage*
- put on disposable gloves and apron

- lubricate the end of the enema tube *to ease entry into the rectum*, and ask the patient to take deep breaths *to encourage relaxation and reduce discomfort on the insertion of the enema*
- squeeze a small amount of fluid down the tube to expel the air, *as air in the rectum will cause discomfort*
- insert the tube into the rectum in an upward and slightly backward direction for about 7.5 cm, *following the natural line of the rectum*
- administer the solution gently and slowly *to minimise any discomfort*, squeezing the bag and rolling it up so that all the contents are administered
- remove the tube when the prescribed amount has been administered. Keeping the enema bag rolled up when removing the nozzle will prevent fluid leaking back into the bag (Nicol et al 2000)
- dry the anal area *to prevent any irritation*
- the protective covering may be left in place *to help prevent soiling of bed linen by leaking faecal matter*
- provide a bedpan or commode when this is required, although access to a toilet is preferable *as it reduces the patient's embarrassment*
- ensure that the patient is left feeling as comfortable as possible, *maintaining the quality of this nursing practice*
- dispose of the equipment safely *for the protection of others*
- document this nursing practice appropriately, monitor the after-effects and report any abnormal findings immediately *to provide a written record and assist in the implementation of any action should an abnormality or adverse reaction to the practice be noted*
- in undertaking this practice, nurses are accountable for their actions, the quality of care delivered and record-keeping according to the *Code of Professional Conduct* (UKCC 1992), *Guidelines for Professional Practice* (UKCC 1996) and *Guidelines for Records and Record Keeping* (UKCC 1998).

Relevance to the activities of living

Maintaining a safe environment

Although an aseptic technique is not required, all the equipment used should be clean or disposable, and nurses should wash their hands before and on completion of the practice. Gloves and aprons are worn for protection.

Some enemas require to be warmed prior to administration (Nicol et al 2000) in order to reduce the risk of bowel spasm and shock (Addison 2000). A temperature of 40.5–43.5°C is recommended, oil retention enemas being warmed to 37.8°C (Mallett & Dougherty 2000).

Care should be taken when there are haemorrhoids or fissures present at the anus (Butler 1998), and to avoid damaging the rectal mucosa when inserting the tube of the enema into the rectum. If the tube meets with resistance, it should be withdrawn slightly and no force used.

Communicating

It is important to explain clearly to the patient the reason for the enema being prescribed so that he or she knows whether it has to be retained for a time or returned quickly. Asking the patient to breathe deeply helps to aid relaxation and minimise discomfort on insertion of the enema (Addison 2000, Nicol et al 2000).

Eating and drinking

If the enema is being administered to relieve constipation, advice should be given on how to avoid this problem in the future. An increased intake of dietary fibre and fluids may be of benefit, as may a review of medication. The long-term use of laxatives, opiates, anticholinergics, iron, antidepressants or anti-Parkinsonian medicines has been implicated in increasing the risk of constipation (Colley 1999a, b, Winney 1998).

An assessment of the patient's mouth is often worthwhile as poor or badly fitting dentition may reduce the ability of the patient to increase the fibre intake (Winney 1998).

Eliminating

Ensure that the patient has ready access to a bedpan, commode or toilet and that assistance is given where necessary.

The foot of the bed may be elevated to an angle of 45° when a retention enema has been administered, in order to facilitate retention (Mallett & Dougherty 2000).

The speed of introduction of the fluid will have an impact on peristalsis: the faster the introduction, the greater being the effect. A retention enema should therefore be administered slowly.

Mobilising

Research has shown that bedfast or immobile patients have a greater tendency to suffer from constipation (Getliffe & Dolman 1997, Winney 1998).

Expressing sexuality

This can be an embarrassing and distasteful practice for the patient, so maximum privacy must be given, together with a clear explanation of the necessity for the practice.

Patient/carer education: key points

In partnership with the patient and/or carer, ensure that they are competent to carry out any practices required. Information should be given on an appropriate point of contact for any concerns that may arise.

If the enema is being administered to treat constipation, a planned programme of increased dietary fibre, fluids and exercise should be explained and encouraged to help to relieve the problem (Hyde et al 1999). A self-completed bowel chart may be helpful in resolving the problem of constipation. Abdominal massage may also be beneficial in the promotion of regular bowel movements (Getliffe & Dolman 1997) and may be taught to the patient and/or carer.

Tell the patient how long the enema requires to be retained for maximum effectiveness.

It may be appropriate to teach patients to administer their own enemas.

References

Addison R 2000 How to administer enema and suppositories. Nursing Times 96(6 suppl): 3–4
Butler M 1998 Laxatives and rectal preparations. Nursing Times 94(3): 56–58
Colley W 1999a Constipation. 1. Causes and assessment. Nursing Times 95(20 suppl): 1–2
Colley W 1999b Constipation. 2. Treatment. Nursing Times 95(21 suppl): 1–2
Getliffe K, Dolman M (eds) 1997 Promoting continence: a clinical and research resource. Baillière Tindall/RCN, London
Hyde V, Tenkinson T, Koch T, Webb C 1999 Constipation and laxative use in older community dwelling adults. Clinical Effectiveness in Nursing 3(4): 170–180
Mallett J, Dougherty L (eds) 2000 Royal Marsden manual of clinical nursing procedures. 5th edn. Blackwell Science, London
Nicol M, Bavin C, Bedford-Turner S, Cronin P, Rawlings-Anderson K 2000 Essential nursing skills. CV Mosby, London
United Kingdom Central Council for Nursing, Midwifery and Health Visiting 1992 Code of professional conduct. UKCC, London
United Kingdom Central Council for Nursing, Midwifery and Health Visiting 1996 Guidelines for professional practice. UKCC, London
United Kingdom Central Council for Nursing, Midwifery and Health Visiting 1998 Guidelines for records and record keeping. UKCC, London
Winney J 1998 Constipation. Nursing Standard 13(11): 49–53

19   Exercises: Active and Passive

Learning outcomes

By the end of this section, you should know how to:

- prepare the patient for this nursing practice
- carry out active and passive exercises.

Background knowledge required

Revision of the anatomy and physiology of the musculoskeletal system.

Indications and rationale for active and passive exercises

Active and passive exercises (Fig. 19.1) are muscle and joint movements carried out *to assist circulation, maintain muscle tone and prevent the development of joint contracture.* These exercises can be performed by the patient (active) or by the nurse or carer helping the patient (passive), and are indicated:

- following an anaesthetic or surgery
- during a period of reduced mobility such as bed-rest
- during prolonged inactivity resulting from the effects of disease or trauma.

Equipment

It may be necessary to include safety equipment, for example bed sides, to prevent a bed-fast patient falling out of bed during passive exercises.

Guidelines and rationale for this nursing practice

These guidelines could be used by the nurse to teach a patient's carer(s) to become involved in this practice.

- explain the nursing practice to the patient *to gain consent and co-operation*
- ensure the patient's privacy *to reduce anxiety and/or embarrassment*
- observe the patient throughout this activity *to note any signs of distress or discomfort*
- wash the hands *to reduce the risk of cross-infection*

- help the patient into a comfortable position. The patient's position may require to be altered during the nursing practice *to permit easy, comfortable access to each limb during the exercise programme*
- assist the patient to move the cervical spine and trunk through their normal range of movement, *preventing damage and strain to any joint or muscle*
- taking each limb separately, assist the patient to move all the joints of the limb through their normal range of movement, *allowing the patient and*

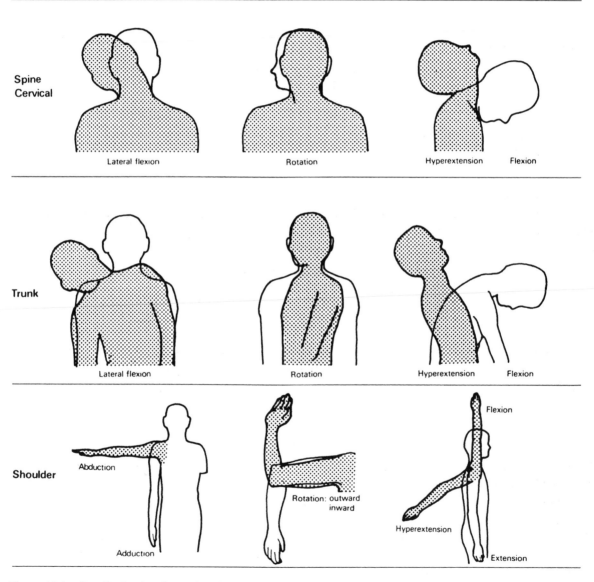

Figure 19.1   *Passive (assisted) exercises for the bed-fast patient. From Roper et al (1985), with permission*
Spine: cervical; Trunk; Shoulder

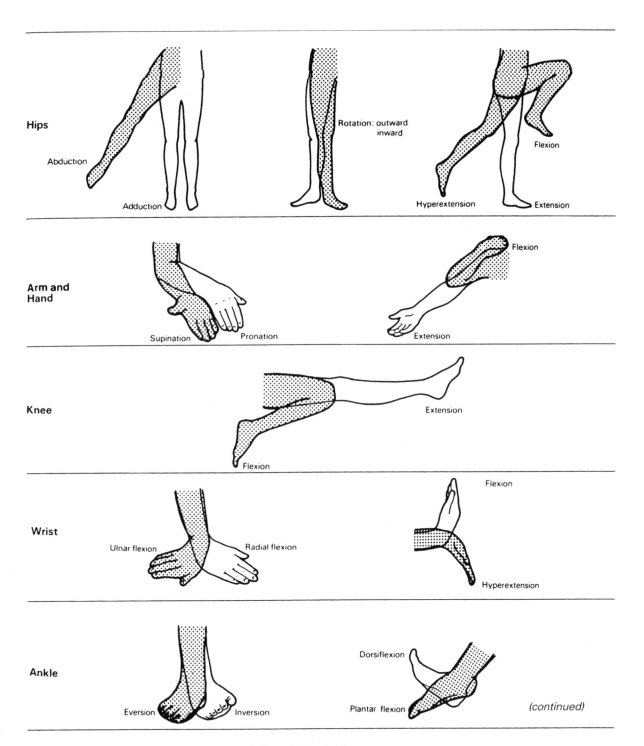

Figure 19.1   (continued) *Hips; Arm and hand; Knee; Wrist; Ankle*

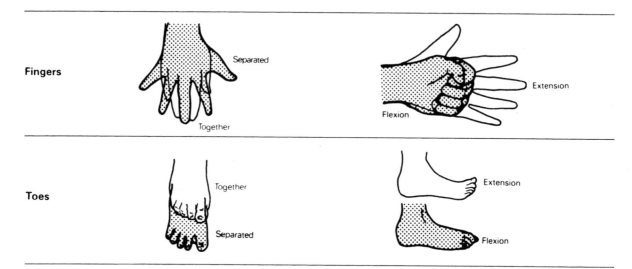

Fingers   Separated   Together   Extension   Flexion

Toes   Together   Separated   Extension   Flexion

Figure 19.1   (continued) *Fingers; Toes*

nurse to concentrate fully on the limb's movement and thus preventing
damage to any tissue
- Maintain open communication with the patient and/or carer during this
  practice *to enable an identification of progress in joint movement*
- ensure that the patient is left feeling as comfortable as possible, *to ensure
  quality of patient care*
- document the nursing practice appropriately, monitor the after-effects and
  report any abnormal findings immediately, *providing a written record and
  assisting in the implementation of any action should an abnormality or
  adverse reaction to the practice be noted*
- in undertaking this practice, nurses are accountable for their actions, the
  quality of care delivered and record-keeping according to the *Code of
  Professional Conduct* (UKCC 1992), *Guidelines for Professional Practice*
  (UKCC 1996) and *Guidelines for Records and Record Keeping*
  (UKCC 1998).

**Relevance to the
activities of living**

Maintaining a safe environment

To prevent cross-infection, nurses should wash their hands before commencing
and on completion of the nursing practice. The patient should not suffer any
discomfort when regularly performing active or passive exercises unless there is
an underlying disease such as rheumatoid arthritis or a developing complication
such as a deep vein thrombosis.

The use of anti-embolic stockings is increasingly being encouraged if there is a
potential risk of a deep vein thrombosis developing. There has been substantial
discussion in the media about the risks of such thromboses developing in

particular in passengers on long-haul air flights, and research is currently ongoing in this area.

Communicating

The nurse should give to the patient an easily understood explanation of the importance of performing the active and/or passive exercises (Roper et al 2000). When appropriate, the nurse should help to teach the patient to perform the exercises independently (Alexander et al 2000). Relatives or informal carers can be involved in the implementation of a regular exercise programme, which can result in psychological benefit to all.

Breathing

Active and passive exercises have the benefit of increasing the patient's depth and rate of respiration, which may help to prevent the development of a chest infection during the period of reduced mobility.

The exercises can assist venous circulation, thus preventing venous stasis, which can cause a deep vein thrombosis. Pulmonary embolism is a serious, occasionally fatal, complication of the development of a deep vein thrombosis, so the exercises should be performed regularly. The benefit of exercise in the prevention of deep vein thrombosis may also be enhanced by the use of anti-embolic stockings and/or the administration of subcutaneous heparin.

Mobilising

In institutional settings, assisting the patient with active and passive exercises is usually the dual responsibility of the physiotherapist and the nurse; at home, the carer may be responsible for implementing the exercise programme.

Exercise helps to maintain muscle tone and movement so that when the patient's normal range of mobility can be resumed, no joint stiffness or muscle weakness will hinder mobilisation. Joints or muscle tissue should never be forced through any movement as this can cause injury, with a resulting effect on the range of mobility.

When the nurse performs passive exercises, the joints and muscles not being exercised must be well supported or injury will occur.

Exercising a paralysed limb may help to prevent joint and/or muscle contracture, which will interfere with the patient's limited remaining mobility and create a problem in positioning the limb.

Patient/carer education: key points

In partnership with the patient and/or carer, ensure that they are competent to carry out any practices required. Information should be given on an appropriate point of contact for any concerns that may arise.

Discuss with the patient and relatives the necessity and benefit of implementing this practice on a regular basis. A plan should be jointly agreed by the patient, carer and nurse for the most appropriate time for these exercises to be carried out. This plan may continue after the patient's discharge from hospital. Responsibility for this practice can help to empower patients in their own care.

Should an abnormality or adverse reaction be noted, inform the patient of the action taken and any subsequent treatment.

References

Alexander M, Fawcett J, Runciman P (eds) 2000 Nursing practice – hospital and home: the adult. 2nd edn. Churchill Livingstone, Edinburgh

Roper N, Logan W, Tierney A 1985 The elements of nursing. 2nd edn. Churchill Livingstone, Edinburgh

Roper N, Logan W, Tierney A 2000 The Roper–Logan–Tierney model of nursing. Churchill Livingstone, Edinburgh

United Kingdom Central Council for Nursing, Midwifery and Health Visiting 1992 Code of professional conduct. UKCC, London

United Kingdom Central Council for Nursing, Midwifery and Health Visiting 1996 Guidelines for professional practice. UKCC, London

United Kingdom Central Council for Nursing, Midwifery and Health Visiting 1998 Guidelines for records and record keeping. UKCC, London

20   Eye Care

There are four parts to this section:

1 Eye swabbing
2 Eye irrigation
3 Instillation of eyedrops
4 Instillation of eye ointment.

The concluding subsection, 'Relevance to the activities of living', refers to the four practices collectively.

Learning outcomes

By the end of this section, you should know how to:

- prepare the patient for these four nursing practices
- collect and prepare the equipment
- carry out eye swabbing, eye irrigation, the instillation of eyedrops and the instillation of eye ointment.

Background knowledge required

Revision of the anatomy and physiology of the eye.
Revision of 'Administration of medicines' (*see* p. 1) and 'Aseptic technique' (*see* p. 407).

1   Eye swabbing

Indications and rationale for eye swabbing

- *to soothe the eye when a patient is suffering from an insensitive or diseased eye*
- *to precede the instillation of an eyedrop or the application of an eye ointment*
- *to remove eye discharge and/or crusts.*

Equipment

Sterile eye dressings pack containing a gallipot, small and other gauze swabs, or gauze swabs and a disposable towel
Sterile swabbing solution, usually normal saline solution, to soften any crusted discharge
Good light source
Trolley or tray for equipment
Receptacle for soiled disposable items.

Guidelines and rationale for this nursing practice

- explain the practice to the patient *to gain consent and co-operation*
- wash the hands *to reduce cross-infection* (Horton 1995)
- collect and prepare the equipment *to ensure that all the equipment is available and ready for use*
- ensure the patient's privacy *to reduce anxiety*
- prepare the patient by helping him into a comfortable position, either lying down or seated with his head inclined backwards, *to allow the patient to maintain the position during the practice and permit easy access to the patient's eyes*
- observe the patient throughout this activity *to note any signs of distress*
- position the light source *to allow maximum observation of the patient's eyes without the beam shining directly into them*
- open and arrange the equipment *in preparation for the practice*
- wash and dry the hands *to reduce the risk of cross-infection* (Horton 1995)
- place the disposable towel around the patient's neck *to catch any spillages and protect the patient's clothing*
- lightly moisten a cotton wool or gauze swab in the prescribed solution. *Excess moisture will cause the patient's face to be soaked with the cleansing solution*
- ask the patient to close his or her eyes in order *to reduce the risk of corneal damage* (Watts 1998)
- gently swab from the inner canthus to the outer canthus of the eye, using each swab only once. *This decreases the risk of cross-infection from one eye to the other or infection of the lacrimal punctum. (If both eyes are being swabbed, the healthy eye should be treated first as this again reduces the risk of cross-infection)*
- gently dry the patient's eyelids *to remove excess moisture*
- ensure that the patient is left feeling as comfortable as possible, *maintaining the quality of this nursing practice*
- dispose of the equipment safely *to reduce any health hazard*
- document the nursing practice appropriately, monitor the after-effects and report any abnormal findings immediately, *providing a written record and assisting in the implementation of any action should an abnormality or adverse reaction to the practice be noted*
- in undertaking this practice, nurses are accountable for their actions, the quality of care delivered and record-keeping according to the *Code of Professional Conduct* (UKCC 1992), *Guidelines for Professional Practice* (UKCC 1996) and *Guidelines for Records and Record Keeping* (UKCC 1998).

2 Eye irrigation

Indications and rationale for eye irrigation

Irrigation involves the continuous washing of the eye surface with fluid:

- *to aid the removal of a corrosive substance from the eye.*

Equipment

Waterproof sheet
Cotton towel
Sterile eye dressings pack containing a gallipot, small and other gauze
    swabs and a disposable towel
Irrigation fluid, e.g. sterile water or sterile normal saline
Lotion thermometer
Irrigating utensil, e.g. undine or intravenous giving set
Receiver for the irrigating fluid
Trolley or adequate surface for equipment
Receptacle for soiled disposable items.

**Guidelines and
rationale for this
nursing practice**

- explain the nursing practice to the patient *to gain consent and co-operation*
- wash the hands *to reduce cross-infection* (Horton 1995)
- collect and prepare the equipment *to ensure that all the equipment is
  available and ready for use*
- ensure the patient's privacy *to reduce anxiety*
- observe the patient throughout this activity *to note any signs of distress*
- warm the irrigating fluid to 37.8°C, *ensuring the comfort of the patient when
  the irrigating fluid is applied*
- help the patient into a suitable position, either sitting or lying with the head
  and neck well supported, *to allow the patient to maintain the position
  throughout the practice and permit easy access to the eyes*
- apply the waterproof sheet and towel around the patient's neck *to absorb
  any spillage*
- help the patient to turn his or her head to the side of the affected eye *to
  prevent any (or further) damage to the other eye by the corrosive substance
  when irrigation is commenced*
- wash and dry the hands *to reduce cross-infection* (Horton 1995)
- position the receiver below the affected eye against the patient's cheek *to
  collect the used irrigating fluid*
- remove any discharge from the eye with a gauze swab *to prevent
  contamination of the eye when the irrigation commences*
- explain to the patient that the flow of fluid is about to begin, *allowing the
  patient to prepare for the introduction of the fluid*
- hold the eyelids apart with the first and second fingers *as the natural defence
  mechanism of closing the eyes when an object approaches closely will
  interfere with the practice*
- direct the flow from the irrigator onto the patient's cheek *to check that the
  temperature is comfortable for the patient*
- hold the irrigator 2.5 cm above the eye *to allow the easy direction of the
  flow of fluid over the eye and prevent further damage to the eye*
- direct a steady flow of irrigating fluid from the inner canthus to the outer
  canthus of the eye, *allowing the fluid to cover the whole of the eye surface*
- ask the patient to move the eye up, down and all around *to ensure that the
  whole eye is irrigated*

- remove the equipment from the patient and ensure that the patient is left feeling as comfortable as possible, *maintaining the quality of this practice*
- dispose of the equipment safely *to reduce any health hazard*
- document the nursing practice appropriately, monitor the after-effects and report any abnormal findings immediately, *providing a written record and assisting in the implementation of any action should an abnormality or adverse reaction to the practice be noted*
- in undertaking this practice, nurses are accountable for their actions, the quality of care delivered and record-keeping according to the *Code of Professional Conduct* (UKCC 1992), *Guidelines for Professional Practice* (UKCC 1996) and *Guidelines for Records and Record Keeping* (UKCC 1998).

3 Instillation of eyedrops

Indications and rationale for the instillation of eyedrops

Instillation involves the introduction of a liquid into a cavity drop by drop. In certain disease conditions and following injury, eyedrops are prescribed:

- *to apply a local anaesthetic topically prior to diagnostic investigations, e.g. tonometry, the removal of a foreign body or minor surgery*
- *to apply topically an antibiotic or anti-inflammatory medicine*
- *to apply topically a muscle constrictor or dilator to the eye*
- *to apply topically an artificial lubricant for the eye.*

Equipment

Sterile eye dressings pack containing a gallipot, small and other gauze swabs and a disposable towel
Sterile solution, usually normal saline, for swabbing
⎫ institutional settings ⎬

Eyedrops to be administered
Automatic dropper for self-administration
Light source
Trolley or tray for equipment
Receptacle for soiled disposable items.

Guidelines and rationale for this nursing practice

- explain the nursing practice to the patient *to gain consent and co-operation*
- wash the hands *to reduce cross-infection* (Horton 1995)
- collect and prepare the equipment *to ensure that all the equipment is available and ready for use*
- ensure the patient's privacy *to reduce anxiety*
- observe the patient throughout this activity *to note any signs of distress*
- help the patient into a comfortable position *to allow easy access to the patient's eye and permit the patient to maintain the position throughout the practice*
- position the light source *to provide good visualisation of the eye*
- check the medicine prescription against the label on the eyedrops *to ensure that the correct medication will be administered*
- check the expiry date on the bottle of eyedrops, *ensuring the administration of stable medication*

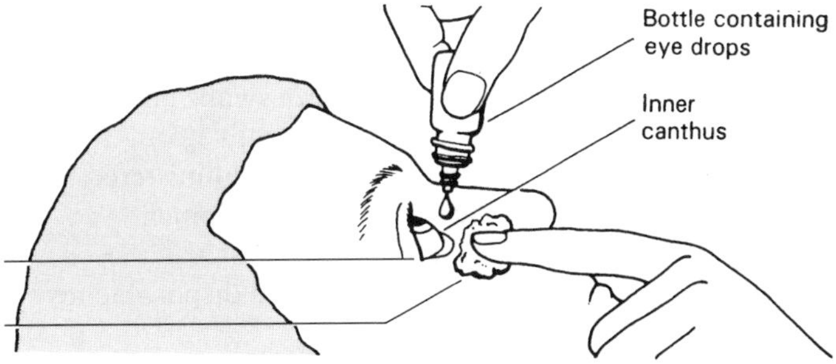

Figure 20.1 *Instillation of eyedrops: the lower lid is pulled gently downwards to create a pouch into which the drop is placed*

- verify which eye should receive the drops *to ensure that the correct eye receives the medication*
- wash and dry the hands *to reduce cross-infection* (Horton 1995)
- swab the eye clean if a discharge is present in order *to remove contaminated debris*
- hold a swab in the non-dominant hand under the lower lid margin *to remove excess moisture after instillation of the drops*
- ask the patient to look up and evert the lower lid, *preventing the patient being aware of the approaching dropper*
- hold the dropper in the dominant hand *to provide controlled application*, about 2 cm above the eye, and allow one drop to fall into the lower conjunctival sac (Fig. 20.1)
- ask the patient to close the eye *to remove excess moisture*
- ensure that the patient is left feeling as comfortable as possible, *maintaining the quality of this practice*
- dispose of the equipment safely *to reduce any health hazard*
- document the nursing practice appropriately, monitor the after-effects and report any abnormal findings immediately, *providing a written record and assisting in the implementation of any action should an abnormality or adverse reaction to the practice be noted*
- in undertaking this practice, nurses are accountable for their actions, the quality of care delivered and record-keeping according to the *Code of Professional Conduct* (UKCC 1992), *Guidelines for Professional Practice* (UKCC 1996) and *Guidelines for Records and Record Keeping* (UKCC 1998).

4   Instillation of eye ointment

Indications and rationale for the instillation of eye ointment

In certain disease conditions, and following injury, eye ointment is prescribed:

- *to instill a medicine topically in place of eyedrops when a prolonged action of the medicine is required*
- *to form a protective film over the corneal surface of the eye*
- *to act as a soothing agent for the patient suffering from an inflamed eye or lid margin.*

Equipment

Sterile eye dressings pack containing a gallipot, small and other gauze swabs and a disposable towel ⎫ institutional
Sterile solution, usually normal saline, for swabbing ⎬ settings
Eye ointment to be administered
Trolley or tray for equipment
Light source
Receptacle for soiled disposable items.

Guidelines and rationale for this nursing practice

- explain the nursing practice to the patient *to gain consent and co-operation*
- wash the hands *to reduce cross-infection* (Horton 1995)
- collect and prepare the equipment *to ensure that all the equipment is available and ready for use*
- ensure the patient's privacy *to reduce anxiety*
- observe the patient throughout this activity *to note any signs of distress*
- help the patient into a comfortable position *to allow easy access to the patient's eye and permit the patient to maintain the position throughout the practice*
- position the light source *to provide good visualisation of the eye*
- check the medicine prescription against the label on the tube of eye ointment *to ensure that the correct medication will be administered*
- check the expiry date on the tube of ointment *to ensure the administration of stable medication*
- verify which eye should receive the ointment, *ensuring that the ointment is inserted into the correct eye*
- wash and dry the hands *to reduce cross-infection* (Horton 1995)
- swab the eye clean *to remove all traces of the previously instilled ointment and/or discharge*
- hold a swab in the non-dominant hand under the lower lid margin *to remove excess ointment after instillation*
- ask the patient to look up and evert the lower lid *to prevent the patient seeing the approaching nozzle, which may cause the eyelid to close*
- hold the tube of ointment in the dominant hand *to permit good control of the insertion of the ointment*
- with the nozzle of the tube 2.5 cm above the lower lid, squeeze the tube *to allow a ribbon of ointment to run into the lower conjunctival sac from the inner to the outer canthus* (Fig. 20.2)
- ask the patient to close the eye *to remove excess ointment*
- inform the patient that he or she may experience blurred vision for a few minutes following the instillation of the ointment *until the oily/greasy base disperses over the eye*
- ensure that the patient is left feeling as comfortable as possible, *maintaining the quality of this practice*
- dispose of the equipment safely *to reduce any health hazard*
- document the nursing practice appropriately, monitor the after-effects and report any abnormal findings immediately, *providing a written record*

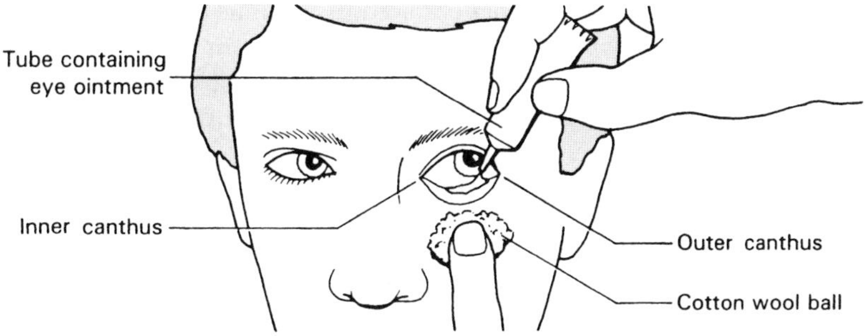

Figure 20.2 *Instillation of eye ointment: the lower lid is pulled gently downwards to create a pouch into which the ointment is placed*

and assisting in the implementation of any action should an abnormality or adverse reaction to the practice be noted

- in undertaking this practice, nurses are accountable for their actions, the quality of care delivered and record-keeping according to the *Code of Professional Conduct* (UKCC 1992), *Guidelines for Professional Practice* (UKCC 1996) and *Guidelines for Records and Record Keeping* (UKCC 1998).

Relevance to the activities of living

Maintaining a safe environment

To reduce the potential risk of cross-infection when caring for a patient's eye, nurses must wash their hands thoroughly (Horton 1995). Only swab the eyes if debris or discharge is present; to reduce cross-infection, swab the cleaner eye first from the inner to the outer canthus. Use sterile swabbing solutions where possible, or at home boiled cooled water; in an emergency, tap water may be used. To reduce the risk of cross-infection, multiple-dose containers of eye medication should be changed regularly, and each patient should have eyedrops or a tube of ointment reserved for his or her use alone (Heywood-Jones 1994). Low-lint swabs, or dental rolls as an alternative, should be used to swab the eye, preventing fibres of swab material being shed into the eye.

When an eyedrop or ointment is to be instilled, care must be taken not to touch the eye surface with the applicator as this could cause injury to the eye and contamination of the applicator (Gardner & Studley 1994). If an eyedrop and eye ointment are to be instilled at the same time, the eyedrop should be instilled first as the greasy/oily base of an ointment would, once applied, prevent the absorption of the medicine within the eyedrop.

The nurse is responsible for instilling the correct medicine into the correct eye, and any discrepancy must be reported immediately. Unconscious or sedated patients are at particular risk of eye damage (Pemberton 2000); care should be taken to avoid damaging the cornea during eye care as the protective blink reflex is inactive (Watts 1998).

If the patient's vision is impaired, the nurse should assist the patient in maintaining a safe environment during his or her stay in hospital and help to identify problems that may occur at home.

Should a patient need to continue eye medication following discharge, the nurse will assess and teach the patient or a relative to become competent in the practice. The self-administration of eyedrops can be assisted with the use of an automatic dropper that clips onto the bottle of eyedrop solution (Heywood-Jones 1994).

Communicating

The nurse should explain the procedure simply to patients and inform them of his or her intended actions. When an emergency eye irrigation is to be performed, the nurse must be quick and precise with the explanation so that the time during which the corrosive substance remains in the patient's eye is minimised. When a patient is extremely anxious or in severe pain, the medical practitioner may prescribe local anaesthetic drops.

Should a patient complain of skin irritation, pain or a burning sensation following the instillation of an eye medication, this should be reported as it may indicate a drug allergy. Following the instillation of an eye ointment, the nurse must warn the patient that the vision will be blurred for 5–6 minutes because of the greasy/oily base of the ointment.

As a result of the injury, disease or the effect of the topical medicine, the patient's previous range of vision may be temporarily or permanently impaired. The nurse will need to assist the patient to adapt to this change.

When a patient wears spectacles, the nurse should assist the patient in the application and care of the spectacles according to the patient's wishes.

Expressing sexuality

The visual appearance of some eye diseases or the effect of trauma to the eye may lead a patient to develop a negative body image, with resultant effects on self-esteem. The patient should be helped to come to terms with this altered body image, whether short-lived or permanent.

If the vision in both eyes is suddenly impaired for any reason, many other activities of living will be affected, and the patient will require help to adapt to this sudden loss of independence.

Patient/carer education: key points

In partnership with the patient and/or carer, ensure that they are competent to carry out any practices required. Information should be given on an appropriate point of contact for any concerns that may arise.

The patient/carer may require to be taught one or all parts of this nursing practice. A patient who requires to use the automatic dropper will need adequate information and practice to ensure the skilled use of the equipment.

The nurse should ensure that the patient at home stores the medication safely and correctly.

The nurse has a responsibility to provide and encourage the education of the general population in the first aid measures needed following contamination of the eye by a corrosive substance.

References

Gardner R, Studley M 1994 Disorders of the eye. In: Alexander M, Fawcett J, Runciman P (eds) Nursing practice – hospital and home: the adult. Churchill Livingstone, Edinburgh

Heywood-Jones I 1994 Eye care. Community Outlook 4(1): 18–19

Horton R 1995 Handwashing: the fundamental infection control principle. British Journal of Nursing 4(16): 926–933

Pemberton L 2000 The unconscious patient. In: Alexander M, Fawcett J, Runciman P (eds) Nursing practice – hospital and home: the adult. 2nd edn. Churchill Livingstone, Edinburgh, p 853

United Kingdom Central Council for Nursing, Midwifery and Health Visiting 1992 Code of professional conduct. UKCC, London

United Kingdom Central Council for Nursing, Midwifery and Health Visiting 1996 Guidelines for professional practice. UKCC, London

United Kingdom Central Council for Nursing, Midwifery and Health Visiting 1998 Guidelines for records and record keeping. UKCC, London

Watts A 1998 Cleaning the eyelids. Nursing Times 94(38 suppl): 1–2

21 Gastric Aspiration

Learning outcomes	By the end of this section, you should know how to: ▪ prepare and support the patient for this nursing practice ▪ collect and prepare the equipment ▪ pass a nasogastric tube ▪ aspirate the stomach contents.
Background knowledge required	Revision of the anatomy and physiology of the nose, pharynx, oesophagus and stomach.
Indications and rationale for gastric aspiration	Gastric aspiration is used *to keep the stomach empty of contents* by passing a tube into it and applying some form of suction (Alexander et al 2000). It is usually performed in the following circumstances: ▪ obstruction of the bowel ▪ paralytic ileus ▪ preoperatively for gastric or some abdominal surgery, e.g. perforated gastric ulcer or oesophageal and gastric varices ▪ postoperatively, e.g. partial gastrectomy or cholecystectomy.
Equipment 	Trolley Disposable gloves Protective covering for the patient Denture dish Equipment for cleaning nostrils, if required Nasogastric tube Lubricant, e.g. iced water or water-soluble jelly Water to sip Catheter-tipped syringe Litmus paper Receiver for aspirated fluid Receptacle for soiled disposable items Hypoallergenic tape Stethoscope Suction pump. The size of tube selected depends on the size and age of the patient, the most commonly used sizes for the average adult are 14 and 16 FG.

Guidelines and rationale for this nursing practice

- explain the nursing practice to the patient *to gain consent and co-operation. Patients should be encouraged to be active partners in their care*
- collect and prepare the equipment *for efficiency of practice*
- ensure the patient's privacy *to maintain dignity and a sense of self*
- help the patient into as comfortable and relaxed a position as possible, sitting upright and leaning forwards either in bed or on a chair *for ease of insertion of the tube*
- observe the patient throughout this activity *to detect any signs of discomfort or distress*
- measure the approximate distance from the patient's nose to his or her stomach and mark it on the nasogastric tube *so that you will have an indication of when the tube is in the region of the stomach*
- put on gloves
- remove the patient's dentures, if present, and place them in a labelled container
- ask the patient to blow the nose and sniff each nostril in turn, or clean the nostrils if necessary *to facilitate the passage of the tube*
- ascertain whether the patient has any nasal defect or tenderness and change to the other nostril if the first nostril appears to be blocked. *Do not use great force as this may damage the nasal mucosa*
- ask the patient to relax as much as possible while the tube is being passed. *This eases the passing of the tube*
- insert the tube and slide it gently but firmly inwards and backwards along the floor of the nose to the nasopharynx
- encourage the patient to swallow and breathe through his or her mouth when the tube reaches the pharynx, keeping the chin down and the head forward in order to assist the passage of the tube. *This is to try to overcome the gag reflex, which is present in the pharynx. Swallowing helps the tube to pass down by peristalsis*
- when the tube has reached the measured distance, confirm, by testing (see below), that it is in the stomach
- secure the tube with tape when there is confirmation that it is in the stomach
- aspirate the stomach contents. Either continuous or intermittent aspiration will be ordered by the medical practitioner
- ensure that the patient is left feeling as comfortable as possible, *to maintain the quality of this practice*
- dispose of the equipment safely *for the protection of others*
- document this nursing practice appropriately, monitor the after-effects and report any abnormal findings immediately *to provide a written record and assist in the implementation of any action should an abnormality or adverse reaction to the procedure be noted*
- in undertaking this practice, nurses are accountable for their actions, the quality of care delivered and record-keeping according to the *Code of Professional Conduct* (UKCC 1992), *Guidelines for Professional Practice* (UKCC 1996) and *Guidelines for Records and Record Keeping* (UKCC 1998).

The recommended test to confirm the presence of the tube in the stomach is the aspiration of some of the stomach contents using a catheter-tipped syringe and their testing for acidity with litmus paper. If the aspirate is from the stomach, the acidity will turn blue litmus paper pink. If it is not possible to aspirate sufficient stomach contents for testing, some air can be blown into the stomach through the syringe, while a second nurse listens with a stethoscope for the noise of the bubbles of air entering the stomach.

Continuous aspiration can be carried out by some form of pump, the recommended suction pressure being 20–25 mmHg. A lower pressure is ineffective and a greater pressure can damage the lining of the stomach. Sometimes, usually postoperatively, a drainage bag and tubing may be attached to the end of the nasogastric tube. If the drainage bag is placed lower than the patient's stomach, the stomach contents will siphon into the bag.

Intermittent aspiration can be performed by pump or catheter-tipped syringe. Between aspirations, a clean spigot should be inserted in the end of the tube.

Relevance to the activities of living

Maintaining a safe environment

Although an aseptic technique is not required, all the equipment should be clean or disposable, and nurses should wash their hands before commencing and after completing this practice. Disposable gloves should be worn for the nurse's protection.

In order to prevent damage to the respiratory and alimentary mucosa, it is the nurse's duty to ensure that the tube is in the correct position and that the correct pressure of suction is applied.

Communicating

Communication, especially verbal, may be restricted so a pad of paper and a pen may be helpful to the patient.

Breathing

The presence of a nasogastric tube may affect the rate and quality of respiration. It may also cause dryness and irritation of the patient's nose; a lubricant placed at, and just beyond, the nasal orifice may reduce discomfort.

Mouth breathing often occurs because of the size of the tube, so oral hygiene should be maintained.

Eating and drinking

When nasogastric aspiration is in progress, the patient will not be permitted any solid food by mouth, but restricted fluids may be allowed.

Personal cleansing and dressing

The presence of the tube may predispose to dry mucous membranes in the nose and mouth, so frequent oral and nasal hygiene will be necessary.

Mobilising

Mobility may be limited because of the presence of the nasogastric tube and a possible connection to suction apparatus.

Expressing sexuality

When a nasogastric tube is in position, the patient may be concerned about his or her appearance; if the tube remains in position for a length of time, body image may be affected.

Sleeping

Sleep may be affected by the presence of the tube. The patient's sleeping pattern may also be interrupted if intermittent suction is being performed.

Patient/carer education: key points

In partnership with the patient and/or carer, ensure that they are competent to carry out any practices required. Information should be given on an appropriate point of contact for any concerns that may arise.

Explaining why the tube is needed will help the patient to cope with discomfort it causes.

The importance of not interfering with the tube should be explained to the patient, but if pain or extreme discomfort is experienced, he or she should tell someone. It should also be explained that, because the patient is unable to eat or drink, he or she may experience a dry mouth but that staff will help by giving mouthwashes, ice to suck, etc.

References

Alexander M, Fawcett J, Runciman P 2000 Nursing care – hospital and home: the adult. 2nd edn. Churchill Livingstone, Edinburgh

United Kingdom Central Council for Nursing, Midwifery and Health Visiting 1992 Code of professional conduct. UKCC, London

United Kingdom Central Council for Nursing, Midwifery and Health Visiting 1996 Guidelines for professional practice. UKCC, London

United Kingdom Central Council for Nursing, Midwifery and Health Visiting 1998 Guidelines for records and record keeping. UKCC, London

22 Gastric Lavage

Learning outcomes	By the end of this section, you should know how to: ■ prepare and support the patient for this procedure ■ collect and prepare the equipment ■ assist with the procedure of gastric lavage.
Background knowledge required	Revision of the anatomy and physiology of the upper alimentary tract Review of health authority policy on gastric lavage.
Indications and rationale for gastric lavage	Gastric lavage involves the introduction of a wide-bore tube into the stomach and the washing out of the contents by pouring in and siphoning off a prescribed solution. It is sometimes necessary: ■ *to obtain a specimen of gastric contents* ■ *to remove harmful substances swallowed either accidentally or deliberately.* Gastric lavage is now rarely used except when substances have been swallowed that cannot be absorbed by activated charcoal (Jones & Volans 1999).
Outline of the procedure	Health authority policies vary on who is qualified to perform a gastric lavage. As a general rule, medical practitioners or experienced nurses who have received specific training carry it out on unconscious patients after the assessment and securing of the airway by an anaesthetist, and experienced nursing staff in accident and emergency units can carry it out on conscious patients. The tube will be passed through the patient's mouth; if the patient is conscious, he or she will be asked to swallow it. Once the marked length on the tube has been reached, one of the tests to check that the tube is in the stomach, described in Chapter 21, will be performed. Some of the stomach contents may then be aspirated to obtain specimens for analysis. The tubing and funnel are attached to the stomach tube and approximately 300 ml of warmed tap water are poured into the stomach. Care should be taken because if the stomach is overfilled, some of the contents may be forced through the pylorus. The funnel is then lowered and the gastric contents siphoned into the bucket. The lavage is repeated until the return flow is relatively clear. Activated charcoal and an osmotic laxative such as sorbitol will usually be introduced into the stomach via the tube before it is removed. The tube is

pinched when it is being withdrawn to maintain suction and prevent stimulation of the vomiting reflex.

Equipment

As for 'Gastric aspiration' (*see* p. 161), but the tube should have a much larger lumen (e.g. a 30 FG stomach tube)

and

Apron, gloves and goggles
Funnel and connecting tubing
Bucket for the aspirate
Tap water or water at body temperature
Sterile containers appropriately labelled for specimens of aspirate
Laboratory form
Plastic specimen bag for transportation
Airway
Lubricating gel.

Guidelines and rationale for this nursing practice

- collect and prepare the required equipment *for efficiency of practice*
- explain the procedure to the patient if possible, *to gain consent and co-operation*
- ensure the patient's privacy *to maintain dignity and a sense of self*
- remove dentures if appropriate and place in a labelled container
- insert an airway if it is usual practice. *This helps to prevent airway obstruction. On some occasions, an anaesthetist will be standing by in case it is necessary to insert an endotracheal tube to maintain the patient's airway*
- measure the approximate distance between mouth and stomach, and mark the tube. *This is helpful in indicating when the end of the tube has reached the stomach*
- help the patient into the position requested by the practitioner passing the tube. The patient is often requested to lie on his or her side, but because of the unpleasant nature of the procedure, may need to have the hands firmly held to prevent him or her reflexly pulling out the tube
- observe the patient throughout this activity *to detect any signs of discomfort or distress, although, as already indicated, this is an unpleasant procedure*
- lubricate the end of the tube *to ease its passing to the stomach*
- aspirate some stomach contents if required for examination
- connect the funnel to the tube and pour approximately 300 ml fluid into it
- pinch the tube and invert it into the bucket so that the contents will be siphoned out of the stomach
- repeat the above two stages as often as necessary
- ensure that the patient is left feeling as comfortable as possible, *to maintain the quality of this practice.* Patients who have intentionally ingested poisonous substances should be offered additional psychological and emotional support until they can be seen by a mental health practitioner
- dispose of the equipment safely *for the safety of others*

- document this procedure appropriately, monitor the after-effects, and report any abnormal findings immediately *to provide a written record and assist in the implementation of any action should an abnormality or adverse reaction to the procedure be noted*
- dispatch the labelled specimens and completed forms to the laboratory
- in undertaking this practice, nurses are accountable for their actions, the quality of care delivered and record-keeping according to the *Code of Professional Conduct* (UKCC 1992), *Guidelines for Professional Practice* (UKCC 1996) and *Guidelines for Records and Record Keeping* (UKCC 1998).

Relevance to the activities of living

Maintaining a safe environment

Although an aseptic technique is not required, all the equipment should be clean or disposable, and nurses should wash their hands before commencing and on completion of the procedure. Gloves should be worn.

The safety of the patient is a prime consideration; because of the obvious risks, only a medical practitioner or a suitably qualified member of the nursing staff will carry out this practice. If the patient is unconscious, a medical practitioner will undertake the procedure. For the safe transport of specimens, *see* 'Specimen collection' (p. 317). The nurse should also ensure that he or she is adequately protected from any spray of gastric contents.

Breathing

If the patient is unconscious, a nasotracheal tube will be passed before the stomach tube to ensure the maintenance of a clear airway. The patient should be positioned in a way that will prevent aspiration of the stomach contents.

Eating and drinking

The tube used for this procedure has a large lumen and cannot be left in position for a long period as it will cause tissue irritation and damage.

Sleeping

As above mentioned, this procedure may be carried out on an unconscious patient, so all reasonable precautions must be taken for the patient's safety. He or she should be placed in the recovery position and constantly observed, and the vital signs should be monitored.

Patient/carer education: key points

In partnership with the patient and/or carer, ensure that they are competent to carry out any practices required. Information should be given on an appropriate point of contact for any concerns that may arise.

A clear explanation of the procedure and the reasons for performing it needs to be given to the patient to gain co-operation.

References

Jones A, Volans G 1999 Management of self poisoning. British Medical Journal 319: 1414–1417

United Kingdom Central Council for Nursing, Midwifery and Health Visiting 1992 Code of professional conduct. UKCC, London

United Kingdom Central Council for Nursing, Midwifery and Health Visiting 1996 Guidelines for professional practice. UKCC, London

United Kingdom Central Council for Nursing, Midwifery and Health Visiting 1998 Guidelines for records and record keeping. UKCC, London

23 Hair Care

There are two parts to this section:

1 Washing the hair
2 Care of the infested head.

The concluding subsection, 'Relevance to the activities of living', refers to both practices collectively.

Learning outcomes

By the end of this section, you should know how to:

- prepare the patient for these nursing practices
- collect and prepare the equipment
- carry out washing the hair and care of the infested head.

Background knowledge required

Revision of the anatomy and physiology of the skin, with special reference to the hair follicles of the scalp
Revision of the life cycle of the head louse (*Pediculus capitis*)
Review of the health authority policy on the use and type of insecticide.

1 Washing the hair

Indications and rationale for washing the hair

The hair covers the skin of the scalp so sweat, sebum, dust and dead epithelial cells become trapped between the hair strands. The patient's hair, if left unwashed, may appear greasy and limp, and generally makes him or her feel unkempt. The patient may be unable to maintain hair hygiene due to the effect of disease or injury, following surgery or because of age (being either a young child or a frail elderly person). The hair may therefore need to be washed:

- *to maintain hygiene*
- *to improve the patient's self-esteem.*

Equipment

Basin
Large container of warm water ⎫
Container for used water, or a bed-fast rinser ⎬ for a bed-fast patient
Small jug or hair spray tap attachment
Cotton towels
Polythene sheeting

Patient's shampoo/conditioner
Patient's own brush and/or comb
Flannel or disposable cloth
Disposable plastic apron
Hair dryer
Trolley or adequate surface for equipment
Receptacle for soiled disposable items.

Guidelines and rationale for this nursing practice

- explain the nursing practice to the patient *and gain consent and co-operation*
- collect and prepare the equipment *to ensure that all the equipment is available and ready for use*
- wash the hands and apply an apron *to reduce cross-infection* (Horton 1995)
- ensure the patient's privacy *to reduce anxiety*
- observe the patient throughout this activity *to note any signs of distress.*

The bed-fast patient

- help the patient into a comfortable position, e.g. with the head overhanging the edge of the bed or on the bed-fast rinser (Baker et al 1999), *to promote comfort and allow the patient to maintain the position during the practice*
- protect the patient's clothing, pillows and bedclothes using the polythene sheeting *to reduce water penetration*
- place a towel around the patient's shoulders *to absorb any water spillage*
- position the basin under the patient's head *to catch the water as it drains from the head*
- protect the patient's eyes with the flannel or disposable cloth, *preventing irritation from the shampoo*
- using the basin to catch the water, wet the hair, and apply the shampoo *to commence washing the patient's hair*
- rinse off the lather *to remove the shampoo and leave the patient's hair clean.* Repeat if the patient wishes
- apply the patient's hair conditioner if used, and leave for the manufacturer's recommended time before rinsing. *This helps to detangle the hair and may improve the hair's overall hair condition*
- towel the hair dry, *removing excess moisture*
- assist the patient to comb his or her hair into its usual style and dry using the hair dryer *to allow a positive body image to be reinstated*
- ensure that the patient is left feeling as comfortable as possible, *confirming the quality of care delivered*
- dispose of the equipment safely *to reduce any health hazard*
- document the nursing appropriately, monitor the after-effects and report any abnormal findings immediately, *providing a written record and assisting in the implementation of any action should an abnormality or adverse reaction to the practice be noted*
- in undertaking this practice, nurses are accountable for their actions, the quality of care delivered and record-keeping according to the *Code of*

Professional Conduct (UKCC 1992), *Guidelines for Professional Practice* (UKCC 1996) and *Guidelines for Records and Record Keeping* (UKCC 1998).

The ambulant patient

- help the patient to the bathroom and ensure that he or she is sitting comfortably, *to promote comfort and allow the patient to maintain the position during the practice*
- protect the clothing using the polythene sheeting *to reduce water penetration*
- drape a towel around the shoulders *to absorb any water spillage*
- protect the patient's eyes with the flannel or disposable cloth, *preventing irritation from the shampoo*
- using the small jug or the hair spray tap attachment, wet the hair, and apply the shampoo *to commence washing the patient's hair*
- rinse off the lather *to remove the shampoo and leave the patient's hair clean.* Repeat if the patient wishes
- apply the patient's hair conditioner if used, and leave for the manufacturer's recommended time before rinsing. *This helps to detangle the hair and may improve the hair's overall hair condition*
- towel the hair dry, *removing excess moisture*
- assist the patient to comb his or her hair into its usual style and dry using the hair dryer, *to allow a positive body image to be reinstated*
- ensure that the patient is left feeling as *comfortable as possible, confirming the quality of care delivered*
- dispose of the equipment safely *to reduce any health hazard*
- document the nursing practice appropriately, monitor the after-effects and report any abnormal findings immediately, *providing a written record and assisting in the implementation of any action should an abnormality or adverse reaction to the practice be noted*
- in undertaking this practice, nurses are accountable for their actions, the quality of care delivered and record-keeping according to the *Code of Professional Conduct* (UKCC 1992), *Guidelines for Professional Practice* (UKCC 1996) and *Guidelines for Records and Record Keeping* (UKCC 1998).

Patients can also have their hair washed during a shower or an immersion bath, using a hair spray tap attachment.

Patient/carer education: key points	In partnership with the patient and/or carer, ensure that they are competent to carry out any practices required. Information should be given on an appropriate point of contact for any concerns that may arise.

Emphasise the importance of an adequate nutritional intake and daily grooming to maintain the health of the hair.

Patients who are undergoing specialised treatment regimes involving the head and neck will require individualised information and education regarding the care of their hair. Patients receiving radiotherapy to the scalp may, for example, not be permitted to wash their hair during and immediately after the course of treatment.

2   Care of the infested head

Indications and rationale for care of the infested head

Scalp infestation is the parasitic infestation of the scalp by the head louse. The louse and its pre-louse stage, the nit, cause irritation, which may lead to scratching and potential infection of the abrasions. An insecticide is used:

- *to remove the parasites*
- *to prevent the infestation spreading to family members, other patients and staff.*

Equipment

Shampoo or lotion containing an insecticide.

Medicated shampoo treatment

Shampoo containing an insecticide, e.g. phenothrin, permethrin or malathion
Disposable cap, gown and gloves
Fine-tooth comb
Equipment as for hair washing (*see* above).

Medicated lotion treatment

Head lotion containing an insecticide, e.g. phenothrin, permethrin or malathion
Polythene sheeting
Disposable paper towel, cap and gown
Fine-tooth comb.

12 Hours later, equipment for hair washing (see above)

Trolley or tray for equipment
Receptacle for soiled disposable items.

Guidelines and rationale for this nursing practice

- explain the nursing practice to the patient *to gain consent and co-operation*, and explain that you will wear a cap, gown and gloves *for your protection*
- collect and prepare the equipment *to ensure that the equipment is available and ready for use*
- wash the hands and apply gloves *to reduce cross-infection and the possible absorption of insecticide*
- apply a disposable cap and gown *for personal protection*
- ensure the patient's privacy *to reduce anxiety*
- observe the patient throughout this activity *to note any signs of distress*
- assist the patient into a comfortable position *to promote comfort and allow the patient to maintain the position during the practice.*

Medicated shampoo method

- follow the guidelines for washing the hair (*see* above)
- protect the patient's eyes *as the medication can be irritant to the eyes*
- use the medicated shampoo as recommended by the manufacturer. *Non-compliance may cause the medication to be ineffective*
- rinse the hair thoroughly *to remove any excess insecticide, which could act as a skin irritant*
- comb the hair with the fine-tooth comb *to remove the nits and lice*, collecting them on a disposable paper towel with each stroke of the comb
- allow the patient's hair to dry, *for the comfort and appearance of the patient*
- ensure that the patient is left feeling as comfortable as possible, *confirming the quality of care delivered*
- disinfect the patient's comb and/or hair brush using the shampoo *to prevent reinfestation of the patient's hair*
- dispose of the equipment safely *to reduce any health hazard*
- remove the protective cap and gown and dispose of them safely *to prevent any cross-infestation*
- document the nursing practice appropriately, monitor the after-effects and report any abnormal findings immediately, *providing a written record and assisting in the implementation of any action should an abnormality or adverse reaction to the practice be noted*
- in undertaking this practice, nurses are accountable for their actions, the quality of care delivered and record-keeping according to the *Code of Professional Conduct* (UKCC 1992), *Guidelines for Professional Practice* (UKCC 1996) and *Guidelines for Records and Record Keeping* (UKCC 1998).

Medicated head lotion method

- protect the patient's clothing using the polythene sheeting *to prevent staining by the medicated lotion*
- protect the patient's eyes *to prevent accidental spillage into them*
- apply the head lotion as recommended by the manufacturer *to ensure effectiveness*, paying particular attention to the area above the ears and the nape of the neck *as the nits and lice tend to gather in these areas*
- leave the hair to dry naturally *as drying with a hair dryer can alter the effectiveness of the insecticide and cause a health hazard*
- disinfect the patient's comb and/or hair brush *to prevent reinfestation of the hair*
- 12 hours later, or as suggested by the manufacturer, wash the hair with a normal shampoo *to remove the insecticide*
- comb the hair with the fine-tooth comb *to remove the nits and lice*, collecting them on a disposable paper towel with each stroke of the comb
- allow the patient's hair to dry naturally
- ensure that the patient is left feeling as comfortable as possible, *confirming the quality of care delivered*
- disinfect the fine-tooth comb with the head lotion *to prevent reinfestation of the hair*

- dispose of the equipment safely *to reduce any health hazard*
- remove the cap and gown and dispose of them safely *to prevent any cross-infestation*
- document the nursing practice appropriately, monitor the after-effects and report any abnormal findings immediately, *providing a written record and assisting in the implementation of any action should an abnormality or adverse reaction to the practice be noted*
- in undertaking this practice, nurses are accountable for their actions, the quality of care delivered and record-keeping according to the *Code of Professional Conduct* (UKCC 1992), *Guidelines for Professional Practice* (UKCC 1996) and *Guidelines for Records and Record Keeping* (UKCC 1998).

Either of the two forms of treatment should be repeated as recommended by the manufacturer and according to the success of the treatment.

Patient/carer education: key points

In partnership with the patient and/or carer, ensure that they are competent to carry out any practices required. Information should be given on an appropriate point of contact for any concerns that may arise.

The patient and carer or parents require to be given information and education regarding the care and future prevention of infestation of the head. Myths such as lice can fly or lice prefer clean to dirty heads or long to short hair should be dispelled (Cook 1998, McKay 1999).

At home, advice and information regarding the treatment of potentially infested bed linen should be given.

Relevance to the activities of living

Maintaining a safe environment

Although hair care does not require an aseptic technique, all equipment should be clean or disposable and all precautions be taken to prevent cross-infection. Nurses should wash their hands before commencing and on completion of hair care.

The nurse should test the temperature of the water prior to washing a patient's hair and be aware of any temperature change during the nursing practice, so that the patient's comfort is maintained. Protecting the patient's eyes reduces the potential problem of the accidental introduction of shampoo or medicated head lotion into the eyes, acting as an irritant. Once an infestation has been noted, treatment should start immediately as the condition spreads rapidly. Transmission of the louse is by direct physical contact or by contact with an infested comb, hair brush, wig, hat or bedding (McKay 1999). All family members and close contacts must be treated at the same time as the patient or reinfestation of the patient can occur. For the nurse's own safety, he or she should wear a disposable cap, gown and gloves during the treatment of an infested scalp.

If left untreated, the sufferer may develop a variety of complications such as impetigo, dermatitis or undefined general malaise.

The louse can develop resistance to an insecticide (Burgess 1999). Many health authorities now use insecticides on a rotational basis to reduce resistance; advice on the locally recommended preparation should be obtained from the pharmacy department (Burgess 1999). In the community, the treatment regime is often the responsibility of the parent or carer, with some input from the school or community nurse. Alternative methods of treatment that do not use insecticides are receiving positive recognition from children and parents (Ibarra 1995).

Communicating

The patient with an infested scalp must be given a tactful, easily understood explanation of the reason for and the form of treatment. The patient's relatives and/or close contacts will also need to be told about the infestation and given the necessary information about their own treatment. Some education of the patient and family about the head louse may be necessary.

Personal cleansing and dressing

For normal hair cleanliness, the use of a dry shampoo can be of benefit to the patient who is unable to have his or her hair washed using shampoo and water. Wide-handled brushes or combs can assist patients with hand grip problems or limited shoulder movement to remain independent in their hair care (Roper et al 1996).

Patients who experience a chronic disease or a prolonged period of immobility will benefit both physically and psychologically from a visit by a hairdresser to cut and style their hair either in hospital or at home.

Consideration must be given to cultural and religious beliefs when dealing with hair care (Mallett & Dougherty 2000). Some patients' beliefs do not allow hair washing, whereas others place a restriction on hair cutting. Sensitivity is also required where a patient may be experiencing hair loss as a result of chemotherapy.

As far as the infested head in concerned, the nits remain firmly attached to the hair even following insecticide treatment, so the fine-tooth comb must be used to remove them. The patient's hair should be left to dry naturally after insecticide application as most of the lotions have an inflammable alcoholic base.

Expressing sexuality

A patient's hair should be kept in good condition as this helps to create a positive body image and maintain self-esteem.

The nurse should style the patient's hair in the usual manner or as the patient wishes as this helps to maintain individuality.

Most people are embarrassed if it is discovered that their hair is infested with lice, and although the nurse should wear a disposable cap and gown while assisting the patient to remove the infestation, the explanation for doing so should be tactful and should not detract from the patient's dignity and self-esteem.

References

Baker F, Smith L, Stead L 1999 Washing a patient's hair in bed. Nursing Times 95(5 suppl): 1–2

Burgess I 1999 Headlice. In: Clinical Evidence. BMJ Publishing Group issue 2: pp 650–653

Cook R 1998 The treatment of headlice. Nursing Standard 12(19): 49–52

Docherty C, Hodgson R 2000 Skin disorders. In: Alexander M, Fawcett J, Runciman P (eds) Nursing practice – hospital and home: the adult. 2nd edn. Churchill Livingstone, Edinburgh

Horton R 1995 Handwashing: the fundamental infection control principle. British Journal of Nursing 4(16): 926–933

Ibarra J 1999 Commentary, originating data and references for the bug buster teaching pack. Community Hygiene Concern, London

McKay S 1999 Myths and facts about headlice. Nursing 29(6): 30

Mallett J, Dougherty L 2000 The Royal Marsden manual of clinical nursing procedures. 5th edn. Blackwell Science, Oxford

Roper N, Logan W, Tierney A 1996 The elements of nursing. 4th edn. Churchill Livingstone, Edinburgh

United Kingdom Central Council for Nursing, Midwifery and Health Visiting 1992 Code of professional conduct. UKCC, London

United Kingdom Central Council for Nursing, Midwifery and Health Visiting 1996 Guidelines for professional practice. UKCC, London

United Kingdom Central Council for Nursing, Midwifery and Health Visiting 1998 Guidelines for records and record keeping. UKCC, London

24 Intrapleural Aspiration

Learning outcomes

By the end of this section, you should know how to:

- prepare the patient for this nursing practice
- collect and prepare the equipment
- assist the medical practitioner during chest aspiration.

Background knowledge required

Revision of the anatomy and physiology of the respiratory system
Revision of 'Aseptic technique' (*see* p. 407).

Indications and rationale for aspirating the pleural cavity

The lungs are covered by the visceral pleura, the inner chest wall being lined by the parietal pleura. Between these pleura lies a thin layer of serous fluid whose surface tension holds the two pleural linings together. As a result, the lung follows the movement of the chest wall, the lung volume being determined by the size of the thorax.

An increase in the amount of fluid in the space upsets this mechanism. Chest aspiration involves the introduction of a needle into the pleural cavity between the visceral and parietal pleura. It may be performed for the following reasons:

- *to examine a specimen of the pleural fluid as an aid to the diagnosis of disease, e.g. tuberculosis or carcinoma*
- *to relieve dyspnoea, by removing excess pleural fluid*
- *to introduce medication, e.g. antibiotics, into the pleural cavity.*

Harvey & Prescott (1994) suggest that chest aspiration may be used as an alternative to the insertion of an intercostal drain for the treatment of a spontaneous pneumothorax in a patient with normal lungs.

Outline of the procedure

Using an aseptic technique, the medical practitioner washes and dries his or her hands, cleanses the patient's skin over the selected site of entry of the aspiration needle, injects a local anaesthetic and waits for it to take effect. The aspiration needle is then inserted into the cavity between the visceral and parietal layers of the pleura (Fig. 24.1). After withdrawing the stilette from the needle, specimens of fluid can be obtained from the cavity for laboratory investigation, and the remaining fluid can be allowed to drain out. If the fluid is purulent, it may have to be aspirated by attaching a large syringe to the needle.

At the end of the procedure, the aspirating needle is withdrawn, a sterile plastic spray is applied to the wound puncture, and an adhesive dressing is placed over it.

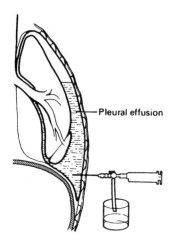

Pleural effusion

Figure 24.1 *Aspiration of pleural fluid. From Chilman & Thomas (1987), with permission*

Equipment

Trolley
Sterile dressings pack
Sterile gloves
Alcohol-based antiseptic for skin cleansing
Local anaesthetic and equipment for its administration
50 ml sterile syringe
Sterile aspiration needles
Sterile two-way tap with a length of sterile tubing
Sterile bowl for collecting fluid
Sterile specimen bottles and an appropriately labelled laboratory form
Plastic specimen bag for transportation
Sterile plastic spray and adhesive dressing
Receptacle for soiled disposable items.

Guidelines and rationale for this nursing practice

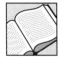

- help to explain the procedure to the patient, *ensuring that he or she has some understanding of the procedure, and obtain consent and co-operation*
- ensure the patient's privacy *to help maintain dignity and a sense of self*
- collect the equipment *for efficiency of practice*
- administer a sedative, if prescribed by the medical staff, *to help to relieve stress and anxiety in the patient*
- help the patient into a back-fastening gown *so that there is ease of access to the site for aspiration*
- assist the patient to sit up with arms extended over a bed table on which a pillow has been placed for the head to rest. If this is not comfortable for the patient, lying in bed on the unaffected side should still allow good access to the needle site. *The medical practitioner requires unobstructed access to the site of needle insertion*
- observe the patient throughout this activity *to detect any signs of discomfort or distress*
- wash the hands and apply an apron *to reduce cross-infection* (Horton 1995)

- open the sterile equipment as it is required by medical staff
- remain with the patient and help to maintain the chosen position as required. *Continuing explanation and support will help the patient through this procedure*
- observe the patient's respirations and attend to any complaints of pain during the procedure. *This may indicate that the needle has penetrated through the pleura and into the lung*
- ensure that the patient is left feeling as comfortable as possible
- dispose of equipment safely *for the protection of others*
- immediately despatch the labelled specimen container, in a plastic specimen bag, to the laboratory, along with the completed form. *Immediate despatch ensures that the specimen arrives in optimal condition for any tests required*
- document this nursing practice appropriately, monitor the after-effects and report any abnormal findings immediately *so that measures to overcome these can be instigated as soon as possible*
- in undertaking this practice, nurses are accountable for their actions, the quality of care delivered and record-keeping according to the *Code of Professional Conduct* (UKCC 1992), *Guidelines for Professional Practice* (UKCC 1996) and *Guidelines for Records and Record Keeping* (UKCC 1998).

| **Relevance to the activities of living** | *Maintaining a safe environment* |

Intrapleural aspiration is an invasive procedure, and all precautions for the prevention of infection must be taken. A meticulous technique should be used and thorough handwashing carried out using an antiseptic detergent and alcohol-based hand cleansing solution as appropriate.

For the safe transport of specimens *see,* 'Specimen collection' (p. 317).

During and after this procedure, there is some risk of a pneumothorax occurring, that is, a collapse of the lung as a result of atmospheric air entering the pleural space and causing the loss of the normally negative intrathoracic pressure. The clinical features are chest pain, rapid respiration and dyspnoea. The patient should be observed closely and a chest X-ray performed in case this complication occurs (McMahon-Parkes 1997).

Breathing

By removing excess fluid from the pleural cavity and allowing the lungs to expand during inspiration, this procedure should help to relieve some of the patient's breathing problems and alleviate any attendant pain. A patient who may have recurring pleural effusions caused by malignant disease may receive sclerotherapy to slow down the rate of development of the effusion (Patz 1998).

Controlling body temperature

If infection is present in the pleural space, the patient may have an elevated temperature and will require the care designated for a pyrexial patient.

Mobilising

Chest aspiration as such will not alter the patient's ability to mobilise, but rest is usually advised for 4–6 hours following the procedure.

Patient/carer education: key points

In partnership with the patient and/or carer, ensure that they are competent to carry out any practices required. Information should be given on an appropriate point of contact for any concerns that may arise.

A detailed explanation and step-by-step guidance through the procedure should help the patient to maintain co-operation.

If medication has been instilled into the cavity, the patient should be helped to turn into different positions over the next couple of hours to facilitate its dispersal.

References

Chilman A, Thomas M (eds) 1987 Understanding nursing care. 3rd edn. Churchill Livingstone, Edinburgh

Harvey J, Prescott R 1994 Simple aspiration vs intercostal tube drainage for spontaneous pneumothorax in patients with normal lungs. British Medical Journal 309(6965): 1338–1339

Horton R 1995 Handwashing: the fundamental infection control principle. British Journal of Nursing 4(16): 926–933

McMahon-Parkes K 1997 Management of pleural drains. Nursing Times 93(52): 48–52

Patz E 1998 Malignant pleural effusions: recent advances in ambulatory sclerotherapy. Chest 113(1) suppl: 74–77

United Kingdom Central Council for Nursing, Midwifery and Health Visiting 1992 Code of professional conduct. UKCC, London

United Kingdom Central Council for Nursing, Midwifery and Health Visiting 1996 Guidelines for professional practice. UKCC, London

United Kingdom Central Council for Nursing, Midwifery and Health Visiting 1998 Guidelines for records and record keeping. UKCC, London

25 Intravenous Therapy

There are four parts to this section:

1 Commencing an intravenous infusion
2 Priming the equipment for intravenous infusion
3 Maintaining the infusion for a period of time
4 Care of a Hickman catheter for long-term intravenous therapy.

The concluding subsection, 'Relevance to the activities of living', refers to all four practices collectively.

Learning outcomes

By the end of this section, you should know how to:

- prepare and support the patient for these nursing practices, both at home and in an institutional setting
- collect and prepare the equipment
- assist the medical practitioner with the safe insertion of an intravenous cannula or catheter
- maintain an intravenous infusion as prescribed.

Background knowledge required

Revision of the anatomy and physiology of the cardiovascular system, with special reference to the circulation of the blood, and body fluids
Revision of 'Aseptic technique' (*see* p. 407)
Review of health authority policy in relation to intravenous therapy in both community and institutional care.

Indications and rationale for intravenous infusion

An intravenous infusion is the introduction of prescribed sterile fluid into the blood circulation; it may be indicated for the following reasons:

- *to maintain a normal fluid, nutrient and electrolyte balance when the patient is unable to maintain adequate intake by mouth and nasogastric feeding is inappropriate*, e.g.:
  — a patient during the preoperative and postoperative periods
  — a patient who has had surgery involving the alimentary system
  — a patient who has malabsorption problems
- *to replace severe fluid loss in emergency situations*, e.g.:
  — a patient who has severe haemorrhage and haemorrhagic shock
  — a patient who has severe burns or scalds

— a patient dehydrated by vomiting or diarrhoea usually associated with enteric infection
- *to administer medication when other routes are not appropriate or when there is a need for a rapid-onset action or accurate titration of the dose*, e.g.:
  — analgesic medication for effective pain relief
  — chemotherapy for the treatment of patients with malignancy.

1   Commencing an intravenous infusion

Outline of the procedure

Intravenous therapy is prescribed by the medical practitioner and initiated by a doctor or a nurse who has undertaken specialist training and is deemed competent to carry out this procedure. The non-specialist nurse may be required to help with the procedure, to maintain the infusion safely for a period of time and to undertake removal of the cannula.

Using an aseptic technique, the competent practitioner chooses a suitable vein site for access, the skin area being shaved as necessary and cleansed with antiseptic lotion, which is allowed to dry fully before the skin is punctured. A topical preparation of local anaesthetic, i.e. EMLA cream, can be applied to the skin surface approximately 1 hour prior to the procedure.

A sterile cannula is inserted into the vein so that the prescribed infusion fluid can enter the patient's blood circulation. The infusion fluid flows into the cannula through an administration set that will have been primed ready for use. The cannula is secured in position and covered by a sterile dressing. The flow of infusion fluid is maintained, and the containers of fluid replaced as prescribed, until the intravenous infusion is discontinued (Lamb 1995).

Sites chosen for intravenous cannulation

Short-term intravenous therapy   The veins at the back of the hand or the superficial veins of the wrist or lower arm are chosen for short-term infusions expected to last for a few hours or days. Cannulation increases the risk of venous thrombosis in the veins used for access; if this occurs in the smaller branches of the peripheral veins following an infusion, it is still possible to use the larger branches of the same vein at a later date if required. The veins of the lower limbs are rarely used because of the increased risk of thrombosis as a result of a slower venous flow. The non-dominant limb should be used if possible to minimise the patient's discomfort.

Long-term intravenous therapy   For long-term intravenous infusions lasting for several days or weeks, a long catheter is inserted into the subclavian or internal jugular vein so that the tip of the catheter lies in the superior vena cava (*see* 'Care of a Hickman catheter', p. 191 and 'Central venous pressure', p. 113) (Gabriel 1994).

Equipment

Trolley or tray
Sterile dressings pack, if required
Sterile cannula
Alcohol-based antiseptic for cleansing the skin (as per local policy)
Gloves
Sterile administration set
Prescribed sterile infusion fluid
Sterile cannula dressing
Infusion stand
Tourniquet
Hypoallergenic tape
Receptacle for soiled disposable items.

Additional equipment if required

Equipment for shaving the skin area
Local anaesthetic and equipment for its administration
Air inlet for glass containers
Holder for glass containers (bottle holder)
Continuous infusion pump and appropriate cassette (*see* 'Parenteral nutrition', p. 263).

Infusion fluids

The most commonly prescribed fluids are:

- normal saline (sodium chloride 0.9%)
- dextrose 5% in water
- Ringer's lactate/Hartmann's solution
- plasma or plasma expanders, e.g. Haemaccel
- blood (*see* 'Blood transfusion', p. 51)
- parenteral nutrients (*see* 'Parenteral nutrition', p. 263).

Most prescribed fluids are commercially prepared in sterile containers, being labelled 'FOR INTRAVENOUS INFUSION'. They may also be prepared by the hospital pharmacy. The containers used for these preparations are frequently soft plastic bags protected by an outer covering (see the manufacturer's instructions), although glass bottles or semi-rigid plastic containers (Polyfusors) continue to be used for some preparations.

Cannulae

Various cannulae (Fig. 25.1) are available and are prepared commercially in sterile packs. Those chosen by the competent practitioner may have an inner needle surrounded by a plastic cannula. The needle is withdrawn once the vein has been punctured, allowing blood to flow back. Once the cannula is safely in situ, the infusion fluid is connected and the cannula secured in position.

Figure 25.1

Intravenous infusion: cannulae in common use A Cannula used when intravenous drugs are to be administered with the infusion or post infusion B Cannula used preoperatively for short-term infusion

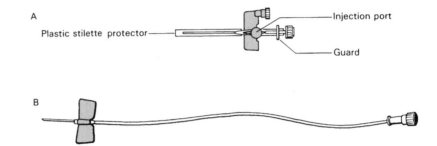

Figure 25.2

Administration set for intravenous infusion

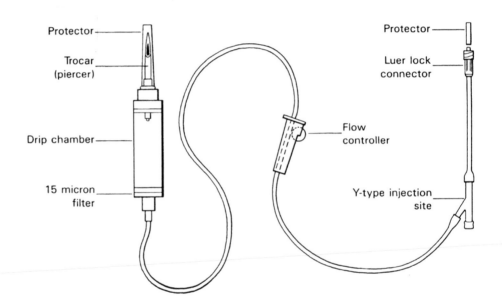

Some cannula packs include an accompanying syringe, for example Medicut. Small winged needles are used for access to scalp veins in babies and young children, and for elderly patients who have fragile veins.

Administration sets

Administration sets are commercially prepared in sterile packs. The set contains specialised sterile tubing with, at one end, a rigid trocar protected by a sterile sheath. At the other end is a similarly protected Luer connector nozzle. Towards the trocar end, the tubing widens into a drip chamber. An adjustable roller clamp surrounds the tubing below the drip chamber, which allows the flow of fluid to be regulated at the prescribed flow rate. Blood administration sets include a filter; simple administration sets are available without a filter, for the infusion of clear fluids (Fig. 25.2).

Specialised administration sets (burette sets)

A specialised administration set is used for infusions when a volumetric infusion pump is not available and a more accurate control of flow rate is needed. This is particularly important to reduce the risk of fluid overload when infusions are prescribed for babies or young children. The burette set has a calibrated drip chamber with one roller clamp above and one roller clamp below. The drip chamber is filled with the amount of fluid prescribed in millilitres per hour, and this amount of fluid is infused during 1 hour. The flow rate will depend on the drop factor and the amount prescribed (see the manufacturer's instructions). For the infusion to continue, the drip chamber has to be refilled as prescribed each time it has emptied.

Volumetric infusion pumps

Some volumetric infusion pumps are used with specific sterile cassettes (e.g. Accuset) as well as a normal administration set so that an accurate flow of fluid can be maintained during the infusion. When primed and connected, these can be set to infuse fluid within a range of 1–999 ml per hour. Other volumetric infusion sets simply use a specifically adapted administration set. The infusion is controlled by a column of electronically controlled rollers that adjust the flow rate as required, constantly monitoring the rate, total volume infused and infusion pressure. This equipment must be mechanically serviced as per the manufacturer's guidelines and local policy.

Guidelines and rationale for this nursing practice 	■ Help to explain the nursing practice to the patient *to gain consent and co-operation and encourage participation in care* (Corbett et al 1993) ■ ensure the patient's privacy, *respecting his or her individuality* ■ help to collect and prepare the equipment. Gloves should be worn *to prevent contamination with body fluids* ■ check the prescribed infusion fluid with a registered nurse or medical practitioner. *This is a legal requirement and part of professional practice* ■ prime the administration set with the infusion fluid, maintaining asepsis, *so that it is ready once the cannula is in position* ■ place the infusion fluid on the stand beside the patient, check that it is running freely,and that all air has been expelled from the system. *This prevents any danger of air embolus.* If not connected immediately, the end should be protected by replacing the sterile cap *to prevent contamination* ■ help the patient into as comfortable a position as possible *so that he or she will tolerate the intravenous therapy without distress* ■ observe the patient throughout this activity *to monitor any adverse effects as well as any improvement in condition* ■ expose and support the area for cannulation *to facilitate access*

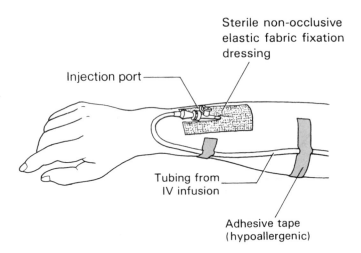

Injection port

Sterile non-occlusive elastic fabric fixation dressing

Tubing from IV infusion

Adhesive tape (hypoallergenic)

Figure 25.3   *Anchoring the tubing with adhesive tape*

- help to prepare the sterile equipment as required, *to maintain a safe environment* (Recker 1992)
- apply pressure around the limb above the cannulation site as directed using a tourniquet. *This will retain more blood in the veins and facilitate cannulation*
- release the pressure as directed once the venous cannula is correctly positioned and the infusion lines are connected, *to commence the flow of fluid to the veins*
- regulate the flow rate as prescribed *to maintain the prescribed fluid intake*
- help the competent practitioner to secure the dressing and tubing *to maintain asepsis and prevent disconnection of the tubing and cannula* (Fig. 25.3)
- apply a splint to the limb *if the site of the infusion requires the limb to be immobilised.* This is not routine practice
- ensure that the patient is left feeling as comfortable as possible *so that he or she will continue to tolerate the intravenous therapy. Comfort helps to reduce stress levels and promotes healing*
- dispose of equipment safely *to prevent the transmission of infection*
- document this nursing practice appropriately, monitor the after-effects and report any abnormal findings immediately, *ensuring safe practice and enabling prompt, appropriate medical and nursing intervention to be initiated as soon as possible*
- maintain the infusion at the prescribed flow rate *for continuation of the treatment.* To reduce the risk of infection, administration sets should be changed as per local policy and immediately following the infusion of blood products (Fox 2000). On-going care involves regular monitoring of the site to identify localised infection, infiltration of fluid into the surrounding tissue or the development of thrombophlebitis. Fox (2000) advocates the formal monitoring of cannulation sites daily using a graded 5-point assessment tool. Similarly, Burke (2000) has created a tool that also includes guidance on appropriate interventions for each grade

■ in undertaking this practice, nurses are accountable for their actions, the quality of care delivered and record-keeping according to the *Code of Professional Conduct* (UKCC 1992), *Guidelines for Professional Practice* (UKCC 1996) and *Guidelines for Records and Record Keeping* (UKCC 1998).

2   Priming the equipment for intravenous infusion

This is the preparation of the prescribed infusion fluid by running it through the administration set. Asepsis should be maintained during this part of the practice *to prevent any internal or exposed areas being contaminated*.

Equipment

Prescribed intravenous infusion fluid
Sterile administration set
Sterile gallipot
Receptacle for soiled disposable items
Infusion stand
Alcohol-saturated swab
Sterile air inlet
Bottle holder for use with glass container
Trolley or tray.

Guidelines and rationale for this nursing practice

■ check the infusion fluid, which is prescribed by the medical practitioner. Each container of fluid is checked by two people, one of whom must be a registered nurse or a medical practitioner (*see* 'Administration of medicines', p. 1), *for safe practice*
■ check the following details against the patient's own documentation and the label on the infusion fluid *to make sure that the correct prescribed infusion is given*:
— the patient's name and unit number
— the date of the prescription
— the type of infusion prescribed
— the amount of infusion prescribed
— the container labelled 'FOR INTRAVENOUS INFUSION'
— the expiry date of the infusion fluid
— the time prescribed for commencement of the infusion
— the time to be taken for completion of the infusion
— the signature of the medical practitioner
■ check the fluid for cloudiness, sediment or discoloration. The container should be checked for flaws, leaks or evidence of contamination. Any suspect fluid or containers must be discarded immediately according to health authority policy *to prevent any introduction of infection or contamination and to maintain a safe environment*
■ include the serial number of the fluid as well as the signature of the nurse or medical practitioner checking the infusion prescription in the documentation.

If the patient suffers any adverse effects, the particular infusion can then be identified (UKCC 1992)

- establish the identity of the patient by appropriate means, e.g. identification bracelet, thus *maintaining safe practice*.

When using a soft plastic container (bag)

- perform the appropriate handwashing technique and wear gloves *to prevent infection*
- remove the outer plastic covering of the container *in preparation for use*
- remove the sheath covering the entry channel without contaminating the inside, thus *maintaining asepsis*
- remove the administration set from its package *in preparation for use*
- close the flow control clamp *to prevent any uncontrolled flow of fluid*
- remove the protective sheath from the trocar of the administration set, maintaining asepsis *in preparation for insertion*
- insert the trocar firmly through the seal of the container's entry channel *so that fluid flows into the first part of the administration set*
- invert the container and hang it on the infusion pole *so that gravity will aid the flow*
- gently squeeze the chamber of the administration set *to allow it partly to fill*
- temporarily remove the protective sheath covering the Luer connector at the end of the administration set and hold it over a sterile container (e.g. gallipot) *to prevent any contamination*
- slowly release the flow control clamp *to allow the fluid to fill the rest of the tubing*
- eliminate any air bubbles from the fluid in the tubing by running some fluid into a sterile container if necessary, *to prevent any danger of air embolus*
- close the flow control clamp *to stop the flow of fluid*
- replace the protective cover on the Luer connector nozzle *to prevent any infection*
- place the free end of the tubing in the notch provided on the flow control clamp *to keep the Luer connector nozzle protected from contamination*
- place the primed equipment on the infusion stand beside the patient's bed *ready for connection to the intravenous cannula.*

The equipment should only be primed immediately prior to the infusion *to minimise the risk of infection. If contamination occurs or the container is punctured while priming the equipment, the infusion and the administration set are discarded and the procedure recommenced.*

When using a glass container (bottle)

- maintain an aseptic technique as before
- remove the seal from the top of the checked infusion fluid bottle *to expose the rubber bung*
- clean the rubber bung with alcohol solution and allow it to dry completely, *to prevent the transmission of infection*
- prepare the administration set as before

- push the trocar firmly through the rubber bung *to access the fluid*
- remove the sterile air inlet from its outer package and remove the protective sheath from the needle
- insert the needle of the air inlet through the rubber bung *to equalise the pressure in the bottle and thus facilitate the flow of fluid*
- hang the inverted bottle on the infusion stand using a bottle holder if required, and if necessary support the end of the air inlet above the level of the fluid in the bottle *to allow the fluid to flow freely*
- proceed to prime the equipment as before.

When using a semi-rigid plastic container (Polyfusor)

- maintain an aseptic technique as before
- remove the outer package of the checked infusion fluid
- snap off the end of the entry channel *to maintain asepsis*
- prepare the administration set as before
- insert the trocar into the entry channel and twist it for a firm fit *to gain access*
- invert the container and hang it on the infusion stand *for gravity to aid the flow*
- proceed to prime the equipment as before (no air inlet being required for this container).

3 Maintaining the infusion for a period of time

The number of drops per minute required for each particular infusion has to be accurately calculated *in order to maintain the flow of infusion at the prescribed rate*. Volumetric pumps are now used routinely.

Guidelines and rationale for this nursing practice

Calculating the flow rate of infusion fluids

All administration sets include details of the number of drops delivered per millilitre for that particular set, this being known as the drop factor. Some sets include within the pack a scale of drops per minute for a given time. Using this information, an accurate assessment of the flow rate needed can be calculated.

Formula used for calculation

$$\frac{\text{Total volume of infusion fluid} \times \text{Drop factor (see administration set)}}{\text{Total time of infusion in minutes}}$$

Example

Total volume of fluid $= 500\,\text{ml}$

Time for completion $= 4$ hours, i.e. 240 minutes (4×60)

Drop factor $= 15$

$$\frac{500 \times 15}{[240]} = 31.2 = 30 \text{ drops (approximately)}$$

Thus the number of drops required to maintain the infusion at the required rate is 30 per minute when the drop factor is 15 drops/ml.

The position of the cannula in the vein and the movement of the patient's limbs may have an effect on the flow rate. *It is therefore important to assess visually the rate of fall of fluid in the infusion container as well as to regulate the number of drops required per minute.* For example, when the time for completion is 4 hours, one-quarter of the fluid should have been infused after 1 hour and half the fluid after 2 hours.

Changing the infusion container

Within 24 hours, the empty container can be replaced with a full container of prescribed infusion fluid without changing the administration set depending on the duration of infusion. The containers should be exchanged before the level of fluid drops below the point of the trocar in the neck of the container. Preparation for changing a container should begin while a small amount of fluid remains in the infusion container; *this prevents the formation of air bubbles in the system and the danger of air embolus.*

Guidelines and rationale for this nursing practice

- explain the nursing practice to the patient *to gain consent and co-operation*
- perform handwashing *and maintain asepsis during this practice as before*
- check the prescribed infusion fluid
- prepare the new container of infusion fluid as for priming the equipment
- temporarily turn off the infusion by closing the roller clamp
- remove the trocar of the administration set from the empty container and insert it into the new infusion fluid, *maintaining asepsis*. A new air inlet should be used when changing glass bottles
- recommence the infusion as soon as possible at the prescribed flow rate
- maintain observations as before
- dispose of the used container safely *to prevent the transmission of infection*
- document the nursing practice appropriately, monitor the after-effects and report any abnormal findings immediately *to ensure safe practice and enable prompt appropriate medical and nursing intervention to be initiated as soon as possible* (Locher 1992)
- in undertaking this practice, nurses are accountable for their actions, the quality of care delivered and record-keeping according to the *Code of Professional Conduct* (UKCC 1992), *Guidelines for Professional Practice* (UKCC 1996) and *Guidelines for Records and Record Keeping* (UKCC 1998).

Removal of the intravenous cannula

This is performed using an aseptic technique when intravenous infusion is discontinued or when a new site for access is needed to continue an infusion.

- explain the procedure to the patient *to obtain consent and co-operation*
- ensure the patient's privacy, *respecting his or her individuality*

- close the flow clamp *to discontinue infusion of the fluid*
- prepare a trolley and sterile dressings as required *to maintain a safe environment*
- apply gloves *to protect against blood-borne infection*
- expose the site of insertion of the cannula, *maintaining asepsis*
- hold a sterile swab lightly over the entry site using the non-dominant hand and slowly withdraw the cannula with the dominant hand, applying pressure once it has been removed *to reduce any bleeding*
- retain pressure on the puncture site as required *until the bleeding stops, maintaining asepsis*
- cover the site with a small sterile dressing, e.g. Airstrip, *to prevent infection*
- dispose of equipment safely *to prevent the transmission of infection*
- resume the observation of the site as appropriate *to monitor the healing process*
- document the nursing practice appropriately, monitor the after-effects and report any abnormal findings immediately, *ensuring safe practice*
- in undertaking this practice, nurses are accountable for their actions, the quality of care delivered and record-keeping according to the *Code of Professional Conduct* (UKCC 1992), *Guidelines for Professional Practice* (UKCC 1996) and *Guidelines for Records and Record Keeping* (UKCC 1998).

The tip of the cannula is occasionally sent to the laboratory for microbiological investigation. If this is ordered, the tip must be cut off with sterile scissors, put into an appropriately labelled sterile specimen container, maintaining asepsis, and sent to the appropriate laboratory with the completed laboratory form (*see* 'Specimen collection', p. 317).

---

4 Care of a Hickman catheter for long-term intravenous therapy

General indications and rationale for use of a Hickman catheter

These are as for 'Intravenous therapy' (*see* p. 181).

Specific indications and rationale for use of a Hickman catheter

The use of a Hickman catheter may be chosen by the medical practitioner for continuous or intermittent intravenous therapy for a period of months or even for as long as 3 years.

The patient may be at home or in an institutional setting (Stillwell 1992). This method is chosen because the radio-opaque silastic catheter, which is usually 'tunnelled', can safely remain in situ for a long period if efficient care of the catheter is maintained. Patient education should help patients to become independent in their own care so that they can be discharged home with a long-term catheter in place, under the supervision of the community team (Sheldon & Bender 1994).

A Hickman catheter may be required for:

- the administration of medicines, for example chemotherapy to give repeated doses of cytotoxic medication for the treatment of malignant disease such as leukaemia, over a period of weeks. Cytotoxic medication can cause damage to the peripheral vessels, but *central venous access allows the irritant medication to be diluted rapidly in the circulating fluid of the large veins and transported safely round the body*
- long-term parenteral nutrition (*see* 'Parenteral nutrition', p. 263). Nutrients in the parenteral feeding regime may also irritate the lining of the peripheral blood vessels; *access via a central line prevents irritation as the nutrients are infused directly into the central veins*
- taking blood samples over a period of time *to monitor the progress of treatment*, for example in children or adults with malignant disease *to prevent repeated venepuncture.*

Skin-tunnelled catheters

A Hickman catheter will remain in situ for a period of time. The distal end of the catheter is usually tunnelled subcutaneously so that the entry site to the vein is separated from the skin exit site, thus reducing the risk of infection entering the circulation from the catheter insertion site. This is particularly important for patients receiving chemotherapy as both the disease and the treatment may cause immunosuppression, further reducing resistance to infection (RCN 1992).

A Hickman catheter has a Dacron cuff at the distal end, around which fibrous tissue will form, anchoring the catheter in position and ensuring safer long-term use (Fig. 25.4).

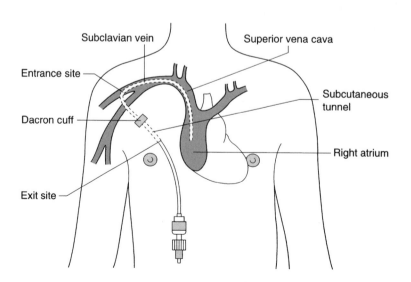

Figure 25.4 *Hickman catheter in situ*

Outline of the procedure	*See* 'Insertion of a central venous catheter' (p. 114) and 'Parenteral nutrition' (p. 263).

Equipment 	***Equipment for insertion of a Hickman catheter*** This is as for 'Intravenous therapy' (p. 181) and 'Insertion of a central venous catheter' (p. 114). Procedure performed in theatre. In addition: Hickman catheter – a flexible, radio-opaque, silicone tube, approximately 90 cm long, incorporating a Dacron cuff at the distal end Injectable cap with a Luer lock for access to the line. ***Equipment for care outside the hospital setting*** Equipment for dressing the entry site if required (semi-permeable polyurethane dressing; Pratt 2001) – *see* 'Wound care' (p. 405). Instruction sheet or booklet to reinforce the patient education commenced prior to transfer Suitable container for storing equipment Spare Luer lock caps. Most Hickman catheters have two ports, blood line and drug line (see the manufacturer's instructions) Sterile 5 ml syringe Sterile 19 G needle for drawing up the heparin Prepared heparinised saline, 50 iu in 5 ml (local policy may vary) Alcohol-impregnated swabs Approved container for the disposal of sharps. All the above should be available in the patient's home and continuously replaced as required for as long as the treatment continues. It is helpful if all the equipment is stored in a suitable container and used only for the care of the catheter so that safe environment can be obtained.

Guidelines and rationale for this nursing practice 	These guidelines are applicable to the nurse and also to the patient or carer as the patient develops confidence in his or her own care. <ul><li>help to explain the procedure to the patient *to obtain consent and co-operation, and encourage participation in care*</li><li>ensure the patient's privacy, *respecting his or her individuality*</li><li>collect and prepare the equipment *so that everything is easily available*</li><li>help the patient into as comfortable a position as possible, *ensuring that there is easy access to the Hickman line and entry port*</li><li>apply sterile gloves after efficient handwashing *to reduce any risk of infection and contamination with body fluids*. If the patient performs this procedure, he or she will usually need to use gloves; a good handwashing technique</li></ul>

should be part of patient education prior to discharge and should be continually reinforced afterwards (Cochrane 1994)

- draw up heparinised saline solution into the syringe, *maintaining asepsis in preparation for flushing the line*
- observe the catheter site for redness, swelling or exudate, *which may indicate infection*. The patient should inform the medical practitioner and the community nurse of any change in condition of the site
- observe the catheter for any damage or cracks, *which may cause infection or an air embolus*. Report any problems immediately and clamp the line above the damage until it has been repaired or replaced
- clamp the line above the Luer lock cap if the cap needs changing. *This will ensure that air does not enter the line to cause an air embolus*
- maintaining asepsis, change the cap. *This may be necessary to ensure the continued efficiency of the valve and to reduce any risk of infection or contamination*. Refer to the health authority policy and manufacturer's instructions
- release the clamp from the line once the cap is safely in position, *to ensure that the line is safely patent again*
- swab the end of the entry port of the cap with alcohol *to prevent the transmission of infection*
- flush the line with heparinised saline, maintaining asepsis, *to prevent a clot forming that would block the patency of the central line and prevent its continued use* (Fig. 25.5). Health authority policy will dictate the frequency of flushing with heparin. If resistance is felt, flushing should not be continued *as a clot may be dislodged*. Resistance to flushing should be reported immediately *as it may indicate a clot blocking the line*
- dress the catheter site as appropriate (*see* 'Wound care', p. 405). The site may initially be covered by a semi-permeable dressing (Keenlyside 1993). There may be no need for a dressing once the site is clean and healed after the stitches have been removed, usually after the first 10 days
- wash the site with prescribed solution and dry thoroughly with low-linting swabs *to keep the site clean and prevent any risk of infection*. Catheter care can be timed to follow a shower or bath *to prevent further any risk of*

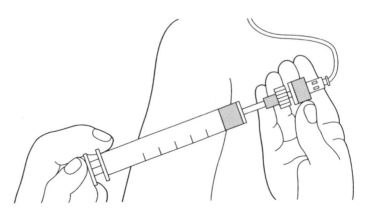

Figure 25.5 *Care of a Hickman catheter: flushing the line with heparinised saline*

infection, but the site itself should still be cleaned separately *to prevent contamination*

- ensure that the patient is left feeling as comfortable as possible *so that he or she can resume the normal activities of living*
- dispose of equipment safely *to prevent the transmission of infection*
- document this nursing practice appropriately, monitor the after-effects and report any abnormal findings immediately *to ensure safe practice and enable prompt, appropriate medical or nursing intervention to be initiated*
- in undertaking this practice, nurses are accountable for their actions, the quality of care delivered and record-keeping according to the *Code of Professional Conduct* (UKCC 1992), *Guidelines for Professional Practice* (UKCC 1996) and *Guidelines for Records and Record Keeping* (UKCC 1998).

Relevance to the activities of living

Observations and further rationale for intravenous therapy will be included within each activity of living as appropriate.

Maintaining a safe environment

Intravenous infusion is an invasive practice so all precautions must be maintained to prevent any infection occurring at the venous access site or any infection entering the blood circulation via the infusion itself (Fig. 25.6).

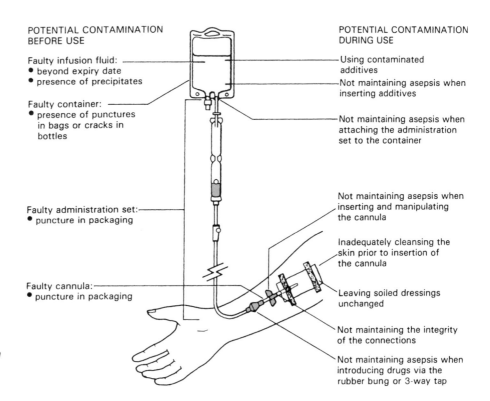

POTENTIAL CONTAMINATION BEFORE USE

Faulty infusion fluid:
- beyond expiry date
- presence of precipitates

Faulty container:
- presence of punctures in bags or cracks in bottles

Faulty administration set:
- puncture in packaging

Faulty cannula:
- puncture in packaging

POTENTIAL CONTAMINATION DURING USE

Using contaminated additives

Not maintaining asepsis when inserting additives

Not maintaining asepsis when attaching the administration set to the container

Not maintaining asepsis when inserting and manipulating the cannula

Inadequately cleansing the skin prior to insertion of the cannula

Leaving soiled dressings unchanged

Not maintaining the integrity of the connections

Not maintaining asepsis when introducing drugs via the rubber bung or 3-way tap

Figure 25.6 *Potential routes for contamination associated with intravenous infusion*

An efficient handwashing technique should be employed when handling equipment.

The drip rate and flow rate should be monitored to check that there is no occlusion in the system and that the prescribed flow is being maintained. Spasm of the vein or movement of the limb may cause a slowing or cessation of the infusion; repositioning the limb may help to relieve the occlusion. If the stoppage is associated with soreness or swelling of the vein site, this may indicate that the cannula is no longer in the vein and that fluid is seeping into the surrounding tissues; alternatively, it may be evidence of developing thrombophlebitis. If this occurs, the medical practitioner should be informed and the infusion discontinued and resumed at another site.

All the equipment connections should be inspected for disconnections, flaws or leakage in order to prevent contamination or an air embolus. The tubing should be inspected to check that there are no air bubbles.

A careful, considerate explanation of what the practice involves will help the patient to co-operate in maintaining a safe environment. He or she should understand why the lines must not be pulled or the dressing touched. Patients who are confused or disorientated may, only if absolutely necessary, require the use of splints and bandages to maintain the infusion safely in position.

The administration set should be changed every 24 hours, maintaining asepsis to minimise the risk of infection, unless long-term (96 hour) filters are used (Johnson 1994). Local policy should be followed as the frequency of changing administration sets is related to the type of fluid used in the system (Pratt 2001).

The dressing should be changed according to local practice. A transparent semi-permeable polyurethane dressing enables the site and the cannula to be observed without disturbing the dressing, thus minimising the risk of infection and enabling the patient to shower or bathe. Gloves should be worn to prevent the risk of blood-borne infection.

Any abnormalities should be reported immediately, and the infusion discontinued or the rate of infusion reduced to a minimum until further instructions are given. Maintaining the minimum flow will prevent clotting in the vein and also reduce the risk of further complications developing until the problem has been dealt with.

The use and complexity of the different types of infusion device has resulted in an increasing number of human errors in relation to such equipment (Quinn 2000). This highlights the need for all practitioners to be competent in the use of any devices they are using in clinical areas.

Communicating

The patient may find this practice very stressful so the nurse should give appropriate support and simple explanations at each stage of the procedure.

It may be difficult for the patient to position spectacles or a hearing aid if one hand is immobilised. By anticipating such needs, the nurse can greatly enhance the patient's ability to communicate. He or she should be reassured that a nurse is always nearby and constantly observant. When leaving the patient, the nurse should ensure that articles likely to be needed are easily accessible and that a bell or other means of communication is available.

Breathing

Intravenous therapy should not in itself affect the patient's breathing, but vital signs should be monitored according to the circumstances so that complications can be identified as soon as possible. For patients undergoing long-term intravenous therapy, for example with a Hickman line in situ at home, monitoring may only be necessary if the site is infected or any associated problems are identified.

- **Pulse rate.** Tachycardia may indicate an infusion reaction or infection. It may also indicate circulatory overload if the rate of infusion is too rapid and the patient's cardiac output has difficulty in responding to the extra fluid in the circulation.
- **Respiration rate.** A rise in respiration rate may indicate infection or circulatory overload. Dyspnoea accompanied by a cough and frothy sputum may indicate pulmonary oedema and should be reported immediately.
- **Blood pressure.** Changes in blood pressure will depend on the reason for the infusion. If the infusion is given to replace fluid loss, the patient may initially be hypotensive, and a gradual rise in blood pressure will be expected. Recordings outside the normal range should be reported.

The prescribed rate of the infusion will depend on the individual patient's requirements and condition. Patients who have congestive cardiac failure and elderly patients will have a lower infusion rate prescribed by the medical practitioner.

The prescribed rate of infusion for babies and young children will be adjusted for their age, weight and height ratio. A volumetric infusion pump or burette set should be used to maintain an accurate flow rate, and observations should frequently be recorded.

For seriously ill patients, a catheter may be inserted to record the central venous pressure, which can accurately monitor changes in circulating fluid volume during the period of intravenous infusion (*see* 'Central venous pressure', p. 113).

Disconnection of the infusion lines may cause a backflow of blood, increasing the risk of haemorrhage. Pressure over the venous site will prevent further blood loss while appropriate action is taken by qualified staff.

An air embolus may occur if a bubble of air enters the blood circulation, but the bubble may remain unnoticed until it reaches the heart. A large air embolus may cause a cardiac arrest, whereas a small one may enter the pulmonary circulation and cause some respiratory distress. Every effort should be made to eliminate air from the tubing when priming the infusion equipment, and observations should be maintained to prevent any risk of air embolus (*see* 'Central venous pressure', p. 113).

Eating and drinking

Fluid intake should be recorded and fluid balance charts accurately maintained (Daffurn et al 1994).

The amount of infusion fluid is normally documented after the completion of each unit. With seriously ill patients, however, both intake and output are recorded hourly. In such cases, the infusion fluid is usually given via continuous infusion pump or a burette set.

The patient may be unable to eat or drink normally during this procedure. Oral hygiene should be performed as appropriate to maintain a healthy oral and oropharyngeal mucosa (*see* 'Mouth care', p. 225).

The infusion may continue while the patient recommences oral feeding. Food should be prepared so that the patient can comfortably use his or her available hand, and the nurse should ensure that prescribed oral fluids are readily accessible if one arm is partly immobilised by the infusion equipment.

Eliminating

An accurate documentation of fluid output should be maintained. This will help to monitor the patient's renal function during the infusion.

When using a commode, the patient may need help to support the administration lines and prevent disconnection of tubing.

Personal cleansing and dressing

The condition of the skin should be noted. Local redness or heat may indicate infection, and swelling may indicate fluid leakage into the surrounding tissues. Sweating, shivering, rigor, pallor or a rash may indicate an adverse systemic reaction (see the pharmaceutical literature). Monitor the infusion site 4–6 hourly.

The patient may need appropriate help with personal cleansing and dressing, and clothing may have to be adapted to maintain access to the infusion site. The need for this and for appropriate light clothing should be explained.

Controlling body temperature

Body temperature should be monitored according to circumstances. A sudden rise in body temperature, or shivering and signs of rigor, may indicate an infusion reaction or the onset of infection and should be reported immediately (*see* 'Blood transfusion', p. 51). For long-term intravenous therapy, the temperature should be monitored at the discretion of the community team if any infection is suspected.

It may be necessary for the area of the infusion site to be exposed for observation. The patient may need help to adjust his or her own clothing, or the bed covers, for any perceived change in temperature.

Mobilising

Patients are increasingly being encouraged to move around and even to take a shower as their condition allows while an intravenous infusion is still in progress, especially during the postoperative period. The nurse should ensure that the lines are supported and that all precautions for the prevention of infection and disconnection are, with the patient's co-operation, maintained during the period of mobilisation.

Working and playing

The nurse should ensure that patients maintain their interests, as their condition allows, while this practice is in progress. Access to newspapers, radio and television should be available if required. Family and friends should be encouraged to visit the patient if there are no contraindications.

Sleeping

The patient's general condition, for example restlessness, drowsiness and level of consciousness, should be noted.

The patient may find it difficult to lie in his or her normal sleeping position because of the infusion. Help in adjusting to a suitably comfortable position may induce sleep. Necessary observations may waken the patient, but an explanation of the need for these and reassurance may reduce the waking period. The observations that cause most disturbance are the recording of temperature and blood pressure; these may be reduced in frequency as the patient's condition allows, while maintaining the frequency of the pulse rate recording and observations of the lines and infusion rate.

Patient/carer education: key points

In partnership with the patient and/or carer, ensure that they are competent to carry out any practices required. Information should be given on an appropriate point of contact for any concerns that may arise.

The reason for the particular intravenous therapy should be explained to the patient. The importance of maintaining the cannula or catheter in situ should be emphasised and the danger of disconnection explained, so that the patient does not pull the lines or dislodge the dressing.

Specific written education for care of the site and lines should be given to the patient discharged home with an intravenous infusion. This may include:

- care of the infusion site and cannula or catheter port
- changing the infusion fluid as prescribed
- flushing the line to maintain patency for intermittent intravenous therapy
- observing the site for any adverse effects.

Patients at home should know what to do if the lines become disconnected. They and their carers should be familiar with the use of a simple clamp and be able to apply a dressing with firm pressure and a tight bandage while waiting for help from the community team.

All patients should understand the importance of immediately reporting any redness, swelling or pain at the infusion site, as well as any disconnection or blockage of the lines and any other adverse symptoms. A telephone help-line gives the patient at home added confidence to be self-caring.

References

Burke K 2000 Combating phlebitis: a peripheral cannula grading scale. Nursing Times 96(29): 38–39

Cochrane S 1994 A mask of approval: patient satisfaction with self infusion teaching programme. Professional Nurse 10(2): 106–111

Cooper C, Hodgson J 1992 A learning experience (district nurses extended role in administering I.V. therapy to an AIDS patient). Journal of Community Nursing 6(2): 18–20

Corbett K, Meehan L, Sackey V 1993 A strategy to enhance skills. Developing intravenous therapy skills for community nursing. Professional Nurse 9(1): 60–63

Daffurn K, Hillman K, Baumn A et al 1994 Fluid balance charts: do they measure up? British Journal of Nursing 3(16): 816–820

Fox 2000 Managing the risks posed by intravenous therapy. Nursing Times 96(30): 37–39

Gabriel J 1994 An intravenous alternative. Nursing Times 90(31): 39–41

Johnson S 1994 A time and money saver. Cost comparison of I.V. therapy with and without Pale 96 filters. Professional Nurse 10(2): 94–96

Keenlyside D 1993 Avoiding an unnecessary outcome. A comparative trial between I.V. 3000 and conventional film dressing to access rates of catheter related sepsis. Professional Nurse 8(5): 288–291

Lamb J 1995 I.V. therapy. Nursing Standard 9(30): 31–35

Locher C 1992 How to make the best of your charting. Journal of Practical Nursing 42(2): 35–43

Pike S 1989 Family participation in the care of central venous lines. Nursing 3(47): 30–31

Pratt R 2001 Preventing infections associated with central venous catheters. Nursing Times 97(15): 36–39

Quinn C 2000 Infusion devices: risks, functions and management. Nursing Standard 14(26): 35–41, 43

Recker D 1992 Catheter related sepsis: an analysis of research (I.V. catheters). Dimension of Critical Care Nursing 11(5): 249–262

Royal College of Nursing 1992 Skin tunnelled catheters. Guidelines for care. RCN, London

Royal College of Nursing 1999 Guidance for nurses giving intravenous therapy. RCN, London

Sheldon P, Bender M 1994 High technology in home care. An overview of intravenous therapy. Nursing Clinics of North America 29(3): 507–519

Stillwell B 1992 Skills update. Central venous lines (using Hickman lines). Community Outlook 2(5): 22–23

United Kingdom Central Council for Nursing, Midwifery and Health Visiting 1992 Code of professional conduct. UKCC, London

United Kingdom Central Council for Nursing, Midwifery and Health Visiting 1996 Guidelines for professional practice. UKCC, London

United Kingdom Central Council for Nursing, Midwifery and Health Visiting 1998 Guidelines for records and record keeping. UKCC, London

Willis J 1995 Infusion devices: volumetric and peristaltic pumps. Professional Nurse 10(7): 433–435

26   Isolation Nursing

There are three parts to this section:

1 Source isolation (barrier nursing)
2 Protective isolation (reverse barrier nursing)
3 Radioactive hazard isolation.

The concluding subsection, 'Relevance to the activities of living', refers to the three practices collectively.

Learning outcomes

By the end of this section you should know how to:

- prevent the spread of infection while nursing a patient with a specific communicable disease (source isolation)
- protect a patient from infection when he or she may be at a greater risk than normal (protective isolation)
- prevent hazard to carers and visitors when radioactive substances are used.

Background knowledge required

Revision of the modes of transmission of infection and related microbiology
Awareness of legislation on infection control (Proudfoot & Whyte 2000)
Review of health authority policy in relation to the control of infection in both institutional and community settings
Knowledge of the role of the infection control officer/nurse in your area
Understanding of universal blood and body fluid precautions (Roberts 2000)
Review of health authority policy in relation to the handling of radioactive substances.

Indications and rationale for isolation nursing

The aim of this nursing practice is to create an effective barrier between an infected area and a non-infected area, *to prevent the occurrence of cross-infection*, or to use appropriate measures *to prevent contamination from radioactive substances*.

This is a constantly changing area of practice so local policy should always be followed. In general, it is advised that all practitioners use the same general prevention strategies with all patients at all times (Loveday 2001). The application of universal precautions (DoH 1998) is the foundation for this and includes:

- an appropriate handwashing technique
- the use of gloves for clinical practices

- the protection of any broken skin
- the prevention and treatment of needle-stick injuries
- the use of protective clothing/equipment (aprons, gowns, eye goggles) when required
- the use and disposal of 'sharps'
- the management of spillages
- the collection and disposal of waste products.

1   Source isolation (barrier nursing)

In this instance, the infected area is the isolation area where the infected patient is being nursed, the non-infected area being that outside the isolation area.

Indications and rationale for source isolation

This is carried out *to prevent the spread of infection from patients who have or are suspected of having a specific communicable infection*, for example:

- a wound infection caused by *Staphylococcus aureus*
- an infection caused by methicillin-resistant *Staphylococcus aureus* (MRSA). This infection, especially if present in sputum, poses the greatest problem for patients who are already immunosuppressed. Guidelines for MRSA vary between care settings and barrier nursing may not be required
- a respiratory infection caused by *Mycobacterium tuberculosis*
- an enteric infection caused by Salmonella.

Equipment

The equipment required will depend on the infection, the patient's condition and the health authority's policies. It may include the following:

Single room with toilet facilities
Handwashing facilities for personnel inside and outside the isolation area
Alcohol-based hand rub (Loveday 2001)
Protective clothing, which may include:
— cap (not routinely used)
— filter-type mask
— gown
— plastic apron
— gloves
— overshoes (not routinely used)
— goggles (not routinely used)
These items should be disposable and a supply of them kept just outside the isolation area
Linen for the bed
Disposable or individual crockery and cutlery
Facilities for the treatment, or disposal, of infected linen and rubbish
All equipment needed for appropriate nursing care should remain within the isolation area *to prevent the transmission of infection*

Thermometer, sphygmomanometer, stethoscope and watch or clock with a second hand as required for recording vital signs

Special containers for the collection of laboratory specimens if required

The patient's documentation should remain outside the isolation area and details of recordings and care be completed by 'uncontaminated' personnel *to maintain a safe environment.*

Guidelines and rationale for this nursing practice

- consult appropriate personnel *to obtain advice and guidance.* All health authorities and hospitals have a member of staff designated to be responsible for the control of infection in that area, for example an infection control nurse (Alderman 1992)
- carry out a risk assessment of infection (Clarkson & McGhee 1999)
- plan the nursing so that everything required is carried out during one period of time in the isolation area: *personnel continually entering and leaving the area greatly increase the risk of cross-infection*
- if possible, choose personnel with known immunity to care for patients with specific infections *as they will be resistant to the infection*
- explain the importance of the precautions to the patient *to gain consent and co-operation, and encourage participation in care*
- wash the hands and apply alcohol solution before entering the isolation area *to maintain a safe environment*
- don protective clothing as required *to create an effective barrier against the infection* (Ayton 1984)
- enter the isolation area
- perform all necessary nursing care. Two nurses may be needed for certain nursing practices (Bowell 1990), for example passing equipment, the patient's meals or prescribed medication in from outside the isolation area. One nurse should remain in protective clothing within the area. The second nurse should remain at the entrance of the area and transfer articles to the nurse within the area without allowing any contamination to occur. *This prevents the transmission of infection*
- observe the patient throughout this activity *to monitor any change in condition*
- ensure that the patient is left feeling as comfortable as possible *to help to promote the healing process*
- ensure that the patient has some means of communication, such as a nurse call system, *as patients can feel very isolated in this situation* (Denton 1986)
- safely dispose of any infected material according to health authority policy *to prevent cross-infection*
- wash the hands within the isolation area *to prevent the infection being transferred out of the area*
- remove protective clothing without touching the outside of the garments and dispose of them safely *to prevent any cross-infection and maintain a safe environment for all*
- leave the isolation area once all the nursing care has been completed

- repeat handwashing outside the isolation area and apply alcohol solution *to further ensure no contamination occurs* (Elliot 1992)
- document the nursing practices appropriately, monitor any after-effects and report abnormal findings immediately *so that care can be evaluated and any nursing or medical interventions altered as required*
- explain the precautions to visitors, who should be restricted to close relatives and friends, *to obtain their co-operation in maintaining isolation for the patient by wearing protective clothing*
- in undertaking this practice, nurses are accountable for their actions, the quality of care delivered and record-keeping according to the *Code of Professional Conduct* (UKCC 1992), *Guidelines for Professional Practice* (UKCC 1996) and *Guidelines for Records and Record Keeping* (UKCC 1998).

Disposal of infected material

Local guidelines should be followed regarding the disposal of contaminated waste. In an institutional setting, two nurses are required: one to remain in protective clothing within the isolation area, the second nurse to remain free from contamination outside it.

Disposal of waste   This should be put in a clinical waste disposal bag and closed as appropriate inside the isolation area by the isolation nurse. The second nurse, who is outside the area, remains at the entrance with an open clinical waste bag into which the isolation nurse places the infected bag without touching the outside of the second bag. The second bag is closed without contaminating its outside and is treated as normal clinical waste. This procedure is known as 'double-bagging' (Fig. 26.1).

Disposal of linen   Infected linen should be 'double-bagged' in clear plastic bags and sent to the laundry in carriers designated for infected linen; disposable linen is sometimes used.

Disposal of 'sharps'   The infected 'sharps' container should be safely closed by the isolation nurse and placed in a clear plastic bag held by the second nurse, keeping the outside uncontaminated. It should then be sealed and disposed of in accordance with health authority policy *to prevent any transmission of infection*.

Domestic cleaning

The domestic manager should be informed whenever isolation procedures are required. Arrangements for cleaning the isolation area will be made in co-operation with the hospital infection control personnel, thus *maintaining a safe environment*.

Decontamination of the isolation area

When a patient leaves an isolation area, the nursing staff should dispose of all the infected equipment. The room or cubicle and its associated furniture

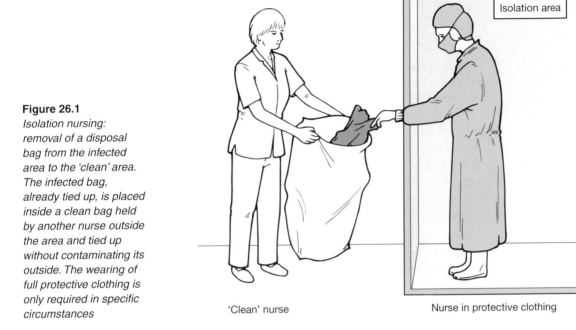

Figure 26.1
Isolation nursing: removal of a disposal bag from the infected area to the 'clean' area. The infected bag, already tied up, is placed inside a clean bag held by another nurse outside the area and tied up without contaminating its outside. The wearing of full protective clothing is only required in specific circumstances

'Clean' nurse   Nurse in protective clothing

should be decontaminated as health authority policy dictates before being used again, *to ensure that it is free from any infection.*

Specific precautions

Different precautions may be needed for specific infections.

Respiratory infections   The patient should be nursed in a single room or cubicle with the door kept closed *to reduce air-borne and/or droplet infection.*

Gloves should be worn during all care procedures; *this prevents contamination with body fluids.* A good handwashing technique along with gloves should give adequate protection, this *preventing contamination with body fluids.*

Urine and faeces do not require special treatment, but should be disposed of immediately; *the use of a separate toilet or commode helps to reduce the risk of cross-infection.*

Wound infections   The patient may need to be nursed in a single room or cubicle. Gloves should be worn, especially when performing dressings or handling potentially infected bed linen or clothing, to *prevent contamination with body fluids* as well as *prevent the transmission of infection* (Thomas 1994).

A plastic apron may be adequate protective clothing depending on the organism causing the infection.

A good handwashing technique is essential *to ensure that there is no transmission of infection.*

Enteric infections   The patient should be nursed in a single room or cubicle with adequate individual toilet facilities *as enteric infections are readily transmitted* (Epton 1990). Gowns, plastic aprons and gloves should be worn, but a mask is not necessary. Individual or disposable crockery and cutlery should be used as required *to prevent infection.*

Vomitus and faeces will be infected and should be disposed of according to local policy. This may include covering the infected matter with disinfectant for a period of time *to destroy the causative organisms.* Toilet utensils should be disposable and treated as infected waste *to maintain a safe environment.*

Before removing protective clothing, the gloved hands should be washed *to reduce contamination*, and further handwashing should be performed as in the guidelines above.

Viral infections   Special precautions are applicable when a patient has a viral infection caused by:

- the hepatitis B or C virus
- human immunodeficiency virus (HIV), which may develop into acquired immune deficiency syndrome (AIDS) (Pratt 1994).

These patients may be suffering from the disease or carrying the virus in their blood and should be treated as having infected blood and body fluids. The caring personnel are most at risk of infection in this situation. Precautions should be maintained for all patients suspected of being 'carriers' until investigations prove negative. According to current knowledge, those most likely to be infected are:

- addicts who take drugs via the intravenous route and use contaminated needles *as the infection is blood borne*
- male homosexuals and heterosexual couples, especially those with numerous partners and practising unprotected sex, *as HIV can be transmitted during sexual intercourse*
- babies born to mothers who are infected *because the virus crosses the placental barrier*
- people who have been transfused with contaminated blood or blood products
- patients from, or who have recently visited, tropical or subtropical countries, *where there is a relatively higher incidence of the disease.*

Every precaution should be taken to prevent personnel in contact with the patient being infected by the virus; it has to enter the blood circulation via a break in the skin or through the mucosa of the non-infected individual. The degree of risk is assessed by the appropriate practitioner and precautions prescribed accordingly.

Low-risk situations   Precautions should be taken when handling blood and body secretions, and gloves should be worn at all times. Special care should be taken when handling and disposing of syringes and needles. Sharps containers should be treated as infected and labelled with special stickers. Blood and other specimens for investigation should be labelled with special 'at risk of infection' stickers.

High-risk situations   Additional precautions may be prescribed, for example when carrying out an invasive procedure for patients known to be infected with HIV or hepatitis B virus. Strict isolation nursing should be maintained, the protective clothing including goggles worn by any attending personnel as well as efficient masks *to prevent any infected secretions or blood splashing the eyes or mouth of the carer*. In some areas where such patients are known to be admitted, a protective 'pack' is available for immediate use. The infection control personnel should be the resource centre for up-to-date requirements.

Health-care personnel should be vaccinated against hepatitis B (refer to health authority policies).

2   Protective isolation (reverse barrier nursing)

In this situation, the infected area is the environment of the ward and the non-infected area is the isolation area. Pathogens are prevented from entering the isolation area by the protective isolation of the patient. The principles and the guidelines are the same as above, but the procedure is reversed.

Indications and rationale for protective isolation

This is carried out *to prevent the spread of infection to patients who have a reduced resistance to infection as a result of their disease condition or prescribed treatment*, for example:

- patients who have leukaemia, which leads to immature and defective white blood cells and decreases resistance to infection
- patients who have reduced autoimmunity as a result of cytotoxic medication used in the treatment of malignant disease, and have a reduced white blood cell count
- patients who are receiving immunosuppressive medication following transplant surgery, which also reduces the number of white blood cells.

The following precautions are emphasised. A filter-type mask may be used by personnel *to protect the prolonged neutropenic patient from droplet infection*.

The form of protective clothing depends on the patient's condition. Gowns should be worn when nursing children, but in most instances a plastic apron will be sufficient *to prevent cross-infection from the nurse's uniform*.

All personnel must be meticulous in their handwashing technique *to maintain a safe environment* (Gould 1994). An alcohol hand rub should be applied frequently to the nurse's hands *to further reduce the risk of cross-infection*.

Special air flow facilities, for example a laminar flow system, may be used to prevent a flow of air from the ward area to the isolation area. This *decreases the risk of infection being transferred from the ward environment.*

The precautions should be explained to visitors, who should be limited to close relatives and friends, thus *reducing the risk of infection.* Appropriate protective clothing should be worn *to maintain a safe environment for the patient* (Curran 1994).

Visitors and other personnel should not be in contact with the patient if they have a cold, sore throat or other infection, however mild, *which might infect the immunosuppressed patient.* The reason for this precaution should be explained. Nursing should be planned so that only one or two staff are caring for the patient during a span of duty, *to reduce the risk of infection from ward personnel.*

3   Radioactive hazard isolation

Patients receiving large doses of radioactive isotopes, either systemically or by implantation, are normally nursed in specially equipped units that have in-built barriers against radioactivity and are equipped with specialised screens. Radioactive isotopes are, however, being used more frequently for diagnostic purposes, and nurses may care for patients undergoing such investigations in general wards. Local policy should always be followed.

Indications and rationale for radioactive hazard isolation

This is carried out *to prevent the radioactive contamination of carers and others when radioactive substances are used*:

- to treat patients who have malignant tumours with radioactive implants or radioactive isotopes
- for diagnostic investigations using radioactive isotopes.

The isolation technique aims *to reduce the risk of radiation for other patients and caring personnel* by limiting the time spent near the patient having radioactive treatment, and enforcing a safe distance at other times. The patient should be nursed in a single room or confined to one particular area of the ward. Lead screens should be used *as a shield from radiation when radioactive implants are inserted*, according to individual requirements. Radioactive material should be transported in lead containers *to prevent any escape of radioactivity.*

Guidelines and rationale for this nursing practice

- consult the radiation protection officer and health authority policy *to ascertain the precautions appropriate for particular radioactive substances used in treatment or investigation*
- explain the precautions and their implications to the patient *and gain consent and co-operation*
- ensure that all staff wear radiation detection badges. This will *monitor individual doses of radiation and ensure that no one is exposed to a dangerous level*

- plan the nursing so that no nurse is in an area of radiation for longer than necessary, and share care *so that each nurse has a reduced exposure time*
- don protective lead aprons or use a lead board if appropriate *to block the passage of radiation*
- wear gloves and apron for all nursing practices and when handling any bedclothes or linen that may be contaminated by radioactive excreta or body fluids, *to prevent contamination* (Thomas 1994)
- dispose of linen and waste according to health authority policy, labelling materials with special radioactive warning stickers, *in order to maintain a safe environment*
- follow local policy when dealing with any spillage of suspected radioactive material
- display radiation hazard notice near to the patient to alert others to the radioactive risk
- in undertaking this practice, nurses are accountable for their actions, the quality of care delivered and record-keeping according to the *Code of Professional Conduct* (UKCC 1992), *Guidelines for Professional Practice* (UKCC 1996) and *Guidelines for Records and Record Keeping* (UKCC 1998).

Radioactive materials have a reducing 'half-life' so that *precautions need only be carried out for a specific, prescribed period of time*. Once the danger of radioactivity is considered negligible, the precautions may be discontinued.

It is advisable that staff who have had close contact with radioactive materials should have a shower and a change of clothing when coming off duty, *as an extra precaution.*

In radiotherapy units, special guidelines may apply, i.e. for pregnant staff, and a Geiger counter may be used to assess the radioactivity level before disposing of radioactive material.

Relevance to the activities of living

Observations and further rationale for this nursing practice will be included within each activity of living as appropriate.

Maintaining a safe environment

The whole concept of isolation nursing is related to maintaining a safe environment for patients and those who come into contact with their fomites.

With infected patients, the emphasis is on maintaining a safe environment for other people by preventing the spread of the infection. The nursing and medical personnel are the key figures here. The safe environment of other hospital staff, for example porters and laundry staff, as well as the general public, is maintained by the safe disposal of infected waste and linen. Bagging and labelling infected blood products for investigation ensures a safe environment for transportation and laboratory staff.

Protective isolation aims to maintain a safe environment for the patient at risk of infection while the treatment for the disease is underway. Once the patient's immune system is able to maintain his or her own safe environment, the isolation procedures can gradually be reduced. Patients may initially be allowed to eat unsterile food, the staff still practising reverse barrier nursing. Patients are then reintroduced to a normal environment over a period of days. During the isolation period, it is important that they are not exposed to any known infection. Staff and visitors with colds or sore throats should thus be excluded at all times and the reason for this explained.

Radiation isolation acts to maintain a safe environment for those in the vicinity of the radiation while giving nursing care to the patient.

An appropriate handwashing technique is a most important means of maintaining a safe environment.

Communicating

This activity of living is most influenced by isolation nursing as isolation immediately affects the normal person-to-person communication process. Patients often become depressed and bored because the number of people in contact with them is greatly reduced: visitors are limited, and staff restrict the number of times they enter and leave the area. The isolation increases when the door to a room needs to be shut and when the door and corridor wall are not made of glass. Nurses need to be perceptive to patients' needs (Ward 2000), discussing with them and their visitors the best way of coping with the isolation problem.

An individual television and video is a great help and should be considered essential equipment. A voice link system will enable staff to chat to the patient, and the patient to call the staff, thus reducing the feeling of isolation while still maintaining the safe environment. A call system must be available so that the patient can summon assistance.

Interests such as reading, crafts, letter-writing and jigsaw puzzles should be encouraged as the patient's condition allows. Most articles can be decontaminated or sterilised as required.

Isolation areas should ideally be glass cubicles from which the patient can see the outside environment, and they should possess a window with an interesting view.

Blood-borne infections such as HIV have a high media profile. Nurses should be responsible communicators to promote health education on the subject, and should also help to minimise intolerant attitudes by using appropriate verbal and non-verbal communication skills.

Eating and drinking

Some patients are prescribed sterile food and drink, available in cans, while in protective isolation, although they may find these boring after a while. It is important that the patient maintains an adequate diet while treatment continues. Microwave ovens can sterilise normal food and utensils so food can be safely prepared in this way. The dietitian should be asked for help as appropriate.

Patients with enteric infections may have an intravenous infusion in situ. When they are able to eat and drink, individualised or disposable crockery and cutlery should be used.

Eliminating

Ideally, all isolation patients should be nursed in a single room with individual toilet and washing facilities. Special precautions are needed for patients who have diarrhoea caused by enteric infection.

Personal cleansing and dressing

Patients undergoing source isolation may have to wear hospital garments or disposable clothes, which may add to the problems of isolation and stigma. Patients in protective isolation should be encouraged to wear their own freshly laundered day and night clothes. This will help to encourage individuality and self-esteem.

Controlling body temperature

Patients isolated because of a specific infection should have their temperature recorded as appropriate to monitor the course of the infection and any associated fever. All equipment necessary for recording should remain within the isolation area. Documentation should remain uncontaminated outside the area.

Expressing sexuality

The whole procedure of isolation may give the patient an impression of having an altered body image arising from the stigma caused by the infection. Perceptive and supportive nursing care and good communication skills will help to alleviate the feeling of rejection.

Patient/carer education: key points

In partnership with the patient and/or carer, ensure that they are competent to carry out any practices required. Information should be given regarding an appropriate point of contact for any concerns that may arise.

- the reason for the specific precautions should be explained to the patient and relatives
- detailed patient education on the specific precautions for each individual infection will be needed throughout this nursing practice
- the specific teaching of self-care skills such as mouth care will be needed for immunosuppressed patients and the importance of these reinforced
- patients with MRSA should understand the importance of reporting that they have had this infection when visiting the outpatient department or on readmission, as recurrence may be a problem
- patients with HIV and AIDS should have a good knowledge of the precautions for the prevention of cross-infection in order to maintain a safe

environment. Good communication skills, both verbal and non-verbal, are required to reinforce the nurse's non-judgemental attitude and to reduce any feeling of stigma on the part of the patient and family

- patients being discharged following recent investigation using radioactive isotopes should be given information sheets concerning any specific precautions. Liaison with the community team will help to reinforce any precautions needed.

References

Alderman C 1992 Never a dull moment. Role of the infection control nurse. Nursing Standard 6(2): 18–19

Ayton M 1984 Protective clothing. What do we use and when? Nursing Times 80(20): 68–69

Bowell E 1990 Assessing infection risks. Nursing 4(12): 19–23

Clarkson J, McGhee C 1999 Assessing the risk of infection. In: National Board for Nursing, Midwifery and Health Visiting for Scotland, Focus on update 4; Issues in infection control. NBS, Scotland

Curran E 1994 Taking down the barriers. Professional Nurse 9(7): 472–478

Denton F 1986 Psychological and physiological effects of isolation. Nursing 3(3): 88–91

Department of Health 1998 Guidance for clinical healthcare workers: protection against infection with blood-borne viruses. Recommendations of the Expert Advisory Group on AIDS and the Advisory Group on Hepatitis. HMSO, London

Elliot P 1992 Hand washing: a process of judgement and effective decision making. Professional Nurse 7(5): 292, 294–296

Epton V 1990 Salmonella. What risk? Nursing 4(20): 14–16

Gould D 1994 Making sense of hand hygiene. Nursing Times 90(30): 63–64

Loveday H 2001 Standard principles for preventing HAI. Nursing Times 97(13): 36–39

Oakley K 1994 Making sense of universal precautions. Nursing Times 90(27): 34–36

Pratt R 1994 Safe practice (HIV and AIDS). Nursing Times 90(27): 64–68

Pratt R 2001 Guidelines for preventing hospital acquired infections. Journal of Hospital Infections 47(suppl): S1–S82

Proudfoot L, Whyte L 2000 Infection control in the community. In: National Board for Nursing, Midwifery and Health Visiting for Scotland, Focus on update 4; Issues in infection control. NBS, Scotland

Roberts C 2000 Universal precautions: improving the knowledge of trained nurses. British Journal of Nursing 9(1): 43–47

Thomas L 1994 Glove story: cost benefit analysis. Nursing Times 90(36): 31–35

United Kingdom Central Council for Nursing, Midwifery and Health Visiting 1992 Code of professional conduct. UKCC, London

United Kingdom Central Council for Nursing, Midwifery and Health Visiting 1996 Guidelines for professional practice. UKCC, London

United Kingdom Central Council for Nursing, Midwifery and Health Visiting 1998 Guidelines for records and record keeping. UKCC, London

Ward D 2000 Infection control; reducing the psychological effects of isolation. British Journal of Nursing 9(3): 162–170

27 Liver Biopsy

Learning outcomes	By the end of this section, you should know how to:

- prepare the patient for this procedure
- collect and prepare the equipment
- assist the medical practitioner during the liver biopsy
- care for the patient prior to, during and after a liver biopsy.

Background knowledge required

Revision of the anatomy and physiology of the liver, with special reference to the position and the functions of the liver
Revision of 'Aseptic technique' (*see* p. 407).

Indications and rationale for a liver biopsy

A liver biopsy is the removal of a small piece of liver tissue, using a specially designed needle

- *to aid in the diagnosis of a liver disease*
- *to assess the effectiveness of treatment*
- *to monitor the course of the liver disease.*

Outline of the procedure

Prior to this investigation, the patient will have blood samples taken for the estimation of bleeding, clotting and prothrombin times (Long et al 1995). A platelet count, grouping and cross-matching will also be requested by the medical practitioner (Topping 1992). A patient who requires a liver biopsy may be suffering from a blood clotting defect that may prevent or defer investigation.

The patient will be given intravenous sedation during the procedure. Hypnosis is increasingly being used as an alternative to sedatives as the metabolism of sedative drugs is impaired in some patients with hepatic disease. The biopsy will normally be preceded by ultrasound imaging to ascertain the anatomy of the area.

A medical practitioner will carry out the biopsy using an aseptic technique. It may be necessary for the biopsy to be obtained under ultrasound imaging if cells from a specific area of the liver are required by the medical practitioner. The patient should lie in a supine position, using one pillow, with the right hand under his or her head. The biopsy is obtained using a biopsy gun, which inserts the biopsy needle into the area and quickly removes a sliver of tissue (Fig. 27.1). Pressure should be applied to the biopsy site for 5 minutes using a sterile swab to prevent bleeding. A sterile dry dressing can then be applied to the puncture site.

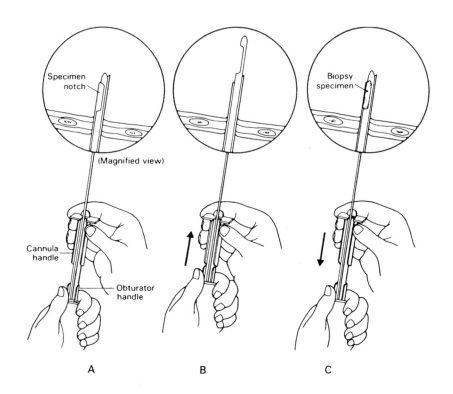

Figure 27.1 *Liver biopsy: method of securing a specimen of tissue*
A *Introducing a biopsy needle: cannula (outer) and obturator (inner)*
B *Obtaining tissue specimen by advancing the obturator handle, and pushing the cutting edge of the obturator's specimen notch into the liver tissue*
C *Withdrawing the obturator handle to enclose the specimen within the cannula, then removing the entire biopsy needle*

Equipment

Sterile gloves and gowns
Sterile dressings pack
Alcohol-based antiseptic for skin cleansing
Sterile disposable biopsy gun
Sterile adhesive dressing
Sterile specimen container with preservative appropriately labelled and with a completed laboratory form and plastic specimen bag for transportation
Trolley for equipment
Receptacle for soiled disposable items
Intravenous cannulae and dressings for the site
Appropriate sedation as prescribed by the medical practitioner, e.g. midazolam
Ultrasound gel.

Guidelines and rationale for this nursing practice

- help the medical practitioner to explain the procedure to the patient *in order to gain consent and co-operation*
- ensure that the patient has fasted for 4–6 hours before the procedure *to reduce the risk of inhalation of aspirate while sedated*
- wash the hands *to reduce cross-infection* (Horton 1995)
- assist the medical practitioner in the siting of the intravenous cannula
- ensure the patient's privacy *to further assist in the reduction of anxiety*

- collect and prepare the equipment and trolley as required *to ensure that all the equipment is available and ready for use*
- help the patient into the supine position with one pillow and the right arm under the head *as this will help to ensure a positive outcome for the procedure*
- ensure that the patient is as comfortable as possible *as this position will need to be maintained throughout the procedure*
- observe the patient throughout this activity *to note any signs of distress*, which should immediately be conveyed to the medical practitioner
- assist the medical practitioner as necessary during the procedure *to permit the procedure to be completed in a safe and competent manner*
- remain with the patient and help to maintain his or her position as required during the biopsy, *providing physical and psychological support during an unfamiliar experience*
- help the patient to reposition herself or himself on the right side for 2 hours after the liver biopsy (Topping 1992) *in order to lessen the escape of blood and bile from the biopsy site*
- ensure that the patient is left feeling as comfortable as possible, *maintaining the quality of this nursing practice*
- monitor the patient's pulse and blood pressure every 15 minutes for 1 hour, every 30 minutes for 3 hours and then hourly for 2 hours *to assess for signs of haemorrhage*
- check the biopsy site hourly for the first 6 hours *to monitor for swelling or staining with blood or bile*
- the patient should continue to fast for 4 hours after the procedure *to allow the effects of the sedative to resolve and in case complications demand intervention*
- the patient should remain in bed for 6 hours *to allow recovery from the procedure*
- dispose of the equipment safely *to reduce any health hazard*
- dispatch the labelled specimen to the laboratory immediately, with the completed laboratory form, *to permit microscopic examination of the tissue of the correct patient*
- document the nursing practice appropriately, monitor any after-effects and report any abnormal findings immediately, *providing a written record and assisting in the implementation of any action should an abnormality or adverse reaction to the practice be noted*
- in undertaking this practice, nurses are accountable for their actions, the quality of care delivered and record-keeping according to the *Code of Professional Conduct* (UKCC 1992), *Guidelines for Professional Practice* (UKCC 1996) and *Guidelines for Records and Record Keeping* (UKCC 1998).

Relevance to the activities of living

Maintaining a safe environment

As this is an invasive procedure, all precautions against, and observations to detect, infection should be implemented. Unless a complication arises, the adhesive dressing can be removed 2–3 days after the biopsy.

For safe transportation of the specimen collection, *see* p. 317.

Some patients who require a liver biopsy may be intravenous drug users and therefore have a high risk of being HIV or hepatitis B or C positive. Universal precautions should be used to reduce or eliminate the cross-infection of staff and other patients prior to, during and after this procedure (Roberts 2000). Local practices for the disposal of contaminated materials must be rigidly adhered to.

Communicating

An easily understood explanation of the procedure and aftercare should be given to the patient. This is primarily undertaken by the medical practitioner, but the nurse may be required to repeat the explanation.

It may be helpful to ask the patient to turn his or her head to the left during the procedure in order to prevent increased anxiety brought about by observing the medical practitioner's actions and the equipment used.

The patient should not experience any discomfort or pain following the biopsy. Any pain must be reported to the medical practitioner immediately as this may be a sign of developing complications such as biliary peritonitis.

Patients requiring a liver biopsy may have altered liver function tests as a result of their infection or disease process. They also have a prolonged clotting time and propensity to haemorrhage, which may be exacerbated by the biopsy because of the highly vascular nature of the liver tissue. Any signs of haemorrhage must be communicated immediately to the medical practitioner.

Breathing

The patient should have frequent recordings of blood pressure, pulse and respiration rate for 24 hours following a liver biopsy, and the biopsy site should be observed for continued bleeding or haematoma formation (Topping 1992).

A sudden change in the patient's cardiovascular status or respiratory function, such as a drop in blood pressure or dyspnoea, must be reported. This may signify injury to other tissues during the biopsy leading to the development of the known complications of haemorrhage or pneumothorax. The risk of tearing the liver and damaging the lung tissue is greatly reduced if the patient holds his or her breath in full expiration as the biopsy needle is advanced into the liver (Long et al 1995).

Mobilising

The patient may remain in bed for 24 hours after the biopsy, the first 2 hours of the period spent quietly lying on the right side to compress the liver against the chest wall. This will help to reduce the possibility of haemorrhage.

Patient/carer education: key points

In partnership with the patient and/or carer, ensure that they are competent to carry out any practices required. Information should be given on an appropriate point of contact for any concerns that may arise.

The medical practitioner and the nurse should provide information on the need for this procedure. The patient and relatives will also need time to ask questions and discuss any aspects of the planned procedure that concern them.

Before the procedure, the nurse should provide information and the rationale for the position the patient should adopt during and after the biopsy, as well as for the aftercare that will be delivered.

References

Horton R 1995 Handwashing: the fundamental infection control principle. British Journal of Nursing 4(16): 926–933

Long B, Phipps W, Cassmeyer V (eds) 1995 Adult nursing: a nursing process approach. Mosby-Times Mirror, London

Roberts C 2000 Universal precautions: improving the knowledge of trained nurses. British Journal of Nursing 9(1): 43–47

Topping A 1992 Caring for patient with disorders of the liver, biliary tract and exocrine pancreas. In: Royle J, Walsh M (eds) Watson's medical–surgical nursing and related physiology. 4th edn. Baillière Tindall, London

United Kingdom Central Council for Nursing, Midwifery and Health Visiting 1992 Code of professional conduct. UKCC, London

United Kingdom Central Council for Nursing, Midwifery and Health Visiting 1996 Guidelines for professional practice. UKCC, London

United Kingdom Central Council for Nursing, Midwifery and Health Visiting 1998 Guidelines for records and record keeping. UKCC, London

28   Lumbar Puncture

Learning outcomes   By the end of this section, you should know how to:

- prepare the patient for this nursing practice
- collect and prepare the equipment
- assist the medical practitioner to perform a lumbar puncture.

Background knowledge required   Revision of the anatomy and physiology of the brain and spinal cord, with special reference to the cerebrospinal fluid and meninges
Revision of the anatomy of the lumbar vertebrae
Revision of 'Aseptic technique' (*see* p. 407).

Indications and rationale for lumbar puncture   Lumbar puncture is the insertion of a specialised needle into the lumbar subarachnoid space to gain access to the cerebrospinal fluid. This may be required:

- *to obtain a sample of cerebrospinal fluid for investigative and diagnostic purposes*, e.g.:
  — bacteriological investigation for patients suspected of having meningitis or encephalitis
  — cytological investigation for patients suspected of having a malignant tumour
- *to identify the presence of blood in the cerebrospinal fluid* following trauma or a suspected subarachnoid haemorrhage
- *to introduce radio-opaque fluid into the subarachnoid space* for radiographic investigation
- *to identify raised intraspinal/intracranial pressure and provide relief*, if appropriate, by removing some of the cerebrospinal fluid
- *to introduce intrathecal medication* such as cytotoxic agents or antibiotics.

Outline of the procedure   A lumbar puncture is performed by a medical practitioner using an aseptic technique. The patient is helped into the correct position. An area of skin above the 3rd, 4th and 5th lumbar vertebrae is prepared and cleansed with antiseptic solution prior to the administration of local anaesthesia. A special lumbar puncture needle is inserted between the 3rd and 4th, or 4th and 5th, lumbar vertebrae in order to gain access to the subarachnoid space below the spinal cord in the region of the cauda equina (Fig. 28.1). Once in position, the stilette

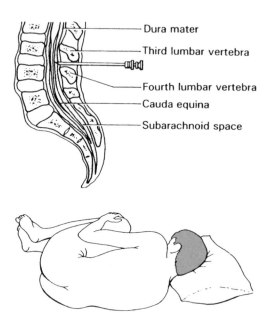

- Dura mater
- Third lumbar vertebra
- Fourth lumbar vertebra
- Cauda equina
- Subarachnoid space

Figure 28.1 *Lumbar puncture: position of the needle in relation to the vertebrae*

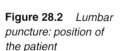

Figure 28.2 *Lumbar puncture: position of the patient*

of the needle is removed. A disposable manometer is attached to the end of the needle via a two-way tap, and the cerebrospinal fluid is allowed to flow into the manometer to record the intraspinal pressure.

When the pressure recording has been completed, the manometer is occluded, and 2–3 ml of cerebrospinal fluid is allowed to flow into three separate sterile specimen containers as required while still maintaining asepsis. The medical practitioner will note the colour, consistency and opacity of the cerebrospinal fluid as well as observing the presence or absence of blood. On completion of this stage, the needle is removed, and the puncture site is covered by a small sterile dressing or plastic sealant spray. The patient remains lying flat in bed for 4–8 hours depending on extent of symptoms following this procedure, appropriate neurological observations, wound site assessment and the monitoring of any pain being maintained during this period (Allan 1989).

The position of the patient

The correct position is important in order to ensure the success and safety of this procedure. Patients should lie on their side on a firm bed with one pillow, stretching their lumbar vertebrae by flexing their head and neck and drawing their knees up to the abdomen, holding them with their hands (Fig. 28.2). The nurse can assist by supporting the patient behind the knees and the neck, and helping to maintain the extension of the lumbar vertebrae, thus widening the intervertebral space. This will help to ensure that the insertion and correct placement of the lumbar puncture needle is safely achieved. Once the needle is in position, the medical practitioner may ask patients to straighten their legs slowly without moving the position of their back. This will reduce the intra-abdominal pressure, which can cause an abnormal reading of intraspinal pressure.

This procedure is occasionally performed with a patient sitting straddled on a chair and facing the back of the chair with his or her head resting on folded arms. This position may be chosen by the medical practitioner when performing a lumbar puncture for an obese patient with dyspnoea who may be distressed when lying flat.

Equipment

Trolley
Sterile dressings pack
Sterile drapes
Sterile surgical gloves for the medical practitioner
Lumbar puncture needles of different sizes
Spinal manometer
Two-way tap
Alcohol-based antiseptic lotion for cleansing the skin
Local anaesthetic and equipment for its administration
Syringe and needles for administering the local anaesthetic
Sterile dressing, e.g. Airstrip or plastic sealant spray
Three sterile specimen containers appropriately labelled, completed laboratory forms, and a plastic specimen bag for transportation. These may be required for three separate samples of cerebrospinal fluid for microbiological, biochemical and cytological investigation
Receptacle for disposable items.

Lumbar puncture needle

This is a rigid stainless steel needle approximately 5 cm in length, complete with its own sharp-pointed stilette; this helps the passage of the needle into the correct position. Once the stilette has been removed, the blunt end of the needle lies within the subarachnoid space and should cause no damage to the tissues during the procedure. Needles are usually supplied with their own metal two-way tap, but a Luer disposable tap may be used.

Guidelines and rationale for this nursing practice

- help to explain the procedure to the patient *to gain consent and co-operation, and to encourage participation in care*
- ensure the patient's privacy *to respect his or her individuality and maintain self-esteem*
- help to collect and prepare the equipment
- help to prepare the sterile field *to maintain asepsis*
- help the patient into the appropriate position, and remain with him or her *to maintain that position and maximise safety during the procedure*
- observe the patient throughout this activity *to monitor any adverse effects*
- help to expose the lumbar region of the patient's back and assist the medical practitioner, as required, *to maintain asepsis and reassure the patient*
- encourage the patient to breathe quietly *in order to prevent hyperventilation, which gives a falsely low pressure reading*

- hold the appropriate sterile containers *to receive the flow of cerebrospinal fluid as directed, maintaining asepsis*
- ensure that the puncture site is covered with a sterile dressing or plastic sealant spray once the needle has been removed *in order to prevent leakage of the cerebrospinal fluid and maintain asepsis*
- help the patient into a comfortable position once the procedure has been completed. In some clinical areas, patients may be requested to lie supine for 4–8 hours after the procedure, *which may stabilise the cerebrospinal fluid pressure and reduce incidence of headache*
- carry out patient observations as detailed under 'Relevance to the activities of living', below
- ensure that the patient is left feeling as comfortable as possible with everything he or she requires at hand *to provide reassurance and help the healing process*. A period of rest should ideally be encouraged after any stressful experience
- dispose of the equipment safely *to maintain a safe environment and prevent the transmission of infection*
- document the procedure appropriately, monitor any after-effects, and report abnormal findings immediately, *ensuring safe practice and enabling prompt appropriate medical and nursing action to be initiated*
- immediately dispatch the labelled cerebrospinal fluid specimens, with their completed forms, to the laboratory *so that investigations may be initiated and decisions about appropriate treatment made as soon as possible*
- in undertaking this practice, nurses are accountable for their actions, the quality of care delivered and record-keeping according to the *Code of Professional Conduct* (UKCC 1992), *Guidelines for Professional Practice* (UKCC 1996) and *Guidelines for Records and Record Keeping* (UKCC 1998).

Relevance to the activities of living

Observations and further rationale for this nursing practice will be included within each activity of living as appropriate.

Maintaining a safe environment

This is an invasive procedure that involves direct access to the spinal and brain tissue via the cerebrospinal fluid. Asepsis should therefore be maintained during and after the procedure, and an adequate handwashing technique should be practised to prevent cross-infection. The puncture site should be observed for evidence of localised infection or leakage; accurate observations of the patient's condition will help to monitor any signs of developing infection. Urgent medical attention must be sought if cerebrospinal fluid leakage occurs.

A lumbar puncture is performed as a neurological investigation. A patient who is confused or disorientated may need cot sides on the bed to prevent falls and maintain the safety of the environment.

A lumbar puncture should not be performed if raised intracranial pressure is suspected as the raised pressure might cause the brain stem tissue to herniate through the foramen magnum. This is known as 'coning' and could be fatal.

The safety of staff transporting specimens should be maintained by enclosing containers in plastic specimen bags (*see* 'Specimen collection', p. 317).

Communicating

After the procedure, the patient should lie horizontally with only one pillow, either supine or on his or her side. This will minimise the effect of changes in intraspinal pressure caused by the removal of 2–3 ml of cerebrospinal fluid during the procedure, and help to prevent headache or dizziness. This position is usually maintained for 4–8 hours, depending on the patient's condition, but there is conflicting evidence on the length of time the patient needs to remain horizontal following this procedure (Carpaat & Vancrevel 1981, Bassett, 1997).

The patient's general condition, for example orientation, restlessness, drowsiness and nausea, should be noted. Any evidence of cerebral irritability should be observed. Fitting, twitching, spasticity or weakness of limb movements should be reported immediately and recorded (Hart et al 1988). The patient's level of consciousness should be recorded as prescribed, depending on his or her condition. Neurological observations should be maintained according to local policy after this investigation (*see* 'Unconscious patient', p. 367).

The patient may complain of a headache following this procedure. Analgesic medication should be administered as prescribed. The nurse should be observant for any non-verbal communication indicating pain, and anticipate the patient's needs as appropriate. The fact that the patient might experience discomfort should be explained to him or her.

Breathing

The pulse, respiration and blood pressure should be recorded 4 hourly or as indicated by the patient's condition. Abnormalities may indicate developing infection or evidence of cerebral changes and should be reported immediately.

Eating and drinking

A normal diet may be ordered as the patient's condition allows, but while he or she is lying flat, some adjustments and help may be needed. An adequate fluid intake should be maintained following the procedure. Drinks should be easily accessible to the patient and specialised cups or straws used as appropriate.

Eliminating

It may be necessary for the patient to use a urinal or bedpan instead of a commode for a period after the procedure because of the bed rest. The reason for this should be explained to the patient.

Controlling body temperature

The temperature should be monitored for as long as necessary after the procedure. Four-hourly recordings should be maintained for 24–48 hours, and any rise in temperature that might indicate a developing infection should be reported.

Mobilising

The patient should have a short period of rest and then mobilise as directed. Mobilisation should commence with the patient sitting up in bed for a period of time before progressing to further activity as the condition allows. This will reduce any further risk of headaches or dizziness, which can occur if the patient changes position too rapidly following this procedure (Bass & Vandervoort 1988).

Patient/carer education: key points	In partnership with the patient and/or carer, ensure that they are competent to carry out any practices required. Information should be given on an appropriate point of contact for any concerns that may arise.

The reason for the investigation and the importance of a lumbar puncture for diagnostic purposes should be explained. This should include the fact that the investigation itself should have no long-term effects. The importance of keeping in the correct position should be carefully explained and reinforced.

Following the lumbar puncture, the patient should be told the importance of remaining flat for a period of time, and the reason for this. The patient should understand the necessity of reporting a headache or any other adverse effects to the nursing staff, who will be monitoring his or her condition following a lumbar puncture.

Any redness, swelling or soreness at the site should be reported. If the patient is discharged home, adverse effects should immediately be reported to the medical practitioner or community nurse.

References

Allan D 1989 Making sense of ... lumbar puncture. Nursing Times 85(49): 39–42
Bass B, Vandervoort MK 1988 Post lumbar puncture headache. Canadian Nurse 84(4): 15–18
Bassett C 1997 Medical investigations 1: lumbar puncture. British Journal of Nursing 6(7): 405–406
Carpaat P, Vancrevel H 1981 Lumbar puncture headache. Controlled study. Lancet 8256(11): 1133–1134
Hart I, Bone I, Hadley D 1988 Development of neurological problems after lumbar puncture. British Medical Journal 296(2): 51–52
United Kingdom Central Council for Nursing, Midwifery and Health Visiting 1992 Code of professional conduct. UKCC, London
United Kingdom Central Council for Nursing, Midwifery and Health Visiting 1996 Guidelines for professional practice. UKCC, London
United Kingdom Central Council for Nursing, Midwifery and Health Visiting 1998 Guidelines for records and record keeping. UKCC, London

29 Mouth Care

Learning outcomes

By the end of this section, you should know how to:

- prepare the patient for this nursing practice
- collect and prepare the equipment
- carry out mouth care according to the individual needs of the patient in both a community and an institutional setting.

Background knowledge required

Revision of the anatomy and physiology of the mouth and pharynx, with special reference to the teeth, salivary glands and oral mucosa

Revision of pharmaceutical literature related to the mouthwashes and mouth-cleaning preparations in current use

Review of health authority policy related to mouth care in both community and institutional care.

Indications and rationale for mouth care

Mouth care is the use of a toothbrush and paste, a mouthwash or other mouth-cleaning preparation *to help the patient to maintain the cleanliness of his teeth or dentures* and *to encourage the flow of saliva to maintain a healthy oropharyngeal mucosa*. The condition of the teeth, gums and mouth is not only an indication of the general health of an individual, but may also influence overall health status (WHO 1988).

This nursing practice is also known as oral hygiene and may be required:

- for any patient who has not eaten for a period of time or whose diet is restricted, as the reduction in mastication decreases the flow of saliva; this may occur during the preoperative or postoperative period, especially in patients who have undergone oral or abdominal surgery
- for patients who are dehydrated for any reason as the normal flow of saliva will be reduced
- for patients suffering from nausea or vomiting as they will be reluctant to eat
- for patients being treated with oxygen therapy, particularly using unhumidified oxygen, which has a drying effect on the oral mucosa
- for patients who are having radiotherapy or cytotoxic medication for malignant disease as this may adversely affect the cells of the oral mucosa (Porter 1994)

- for patients with any form of facial paralysis or muscle weakness as the inability to masticate adequately reduces the flow of saliva and may cause food debris to be retained in the mouth. This may include an unconscious patient or one in the terminal stages of illness
- for patients who have poor manual dexterity or cognitive impairment (Field 1998a, b)
- for patients with an oral infection such as candidiasis.

There is a lack of research on the frequency of mouth care, which will vary for each individual. The use of an effective oral assessment tool is strongly advised to ensure the early detection of problems within vulnerable patient groups (Roberts 2000). Intensive mouth care may be carried out every 2 hours, whereas mouthwashes may only be required two or three times a day (Holmes 1996).

Equipment

Suitable tray or trolley
Plastic gloves (non-sterile)
Pencil torch
Spatula
Toothbrush
Toothpaste
Container for dentures (for institutional care this should be appropriately labelled)
Beaker
Bowl or receiver
Towel or other protective covering
Mouthwash solution
Soft tissues for wiping the mouth
Receptacle for disposable items.

Additional equipment for specialised mouth care as required

- mouth-care pack or equivalent equipment
- plastic gloves (non-sterile)
- foam sticks
- cotton buds
- prescribed medication, e.g. an antifungal agent if thrush is diagnosed
- solution for mouth cleaning
- lubrication for lips, e.g. petroleum jelly
- suction equipment.

Toothbrush and toothpaste

The patient's own equipment may be used if it is available; otherwise, a soft, small-headed nylon brush and toothpaste can be supplied. This is usually the most appropriate equipment for this nursing practice (Bowsher et al 1999, Clay 2000).

Foam sticks

These are ineffective in removing debris from the teeth and gums (Clay 2000), but they are useful for rinsing or refreshing the mouth (Nicol et al 2000). Care should be taken that the foam head does not become detached and obstruct the patient's airway (Field 1998a, b).

Solutions to be used as mouthwashes

Various solutions are available, professional knowledge or individual prescription and patient preference influencing the choice of preparation used (Hatton-Smith 1994). All the solutions used should be clearly labelled and diluted according to their instructions. The procedure for checking the preparation is as for 'Administration of medicines' (*see* p. 1).

There remains little general consensus over the efficacy of oral care agents (Holmes 1998).

Saline   This can be made up using common salt, one level teaspoon (approximately 4.5 g) in 500 ml of water, also being available in sterile sachets. This is an effective mouthwash for patients who have had oral surgery, especially dental extractions.

Thymol   This is prepared in solution and is the main component of most mouthwash tablets. It has a mild antiseptic effect and is well tolerated when diluted to suit the patient's taste.

Sodium bicarbonate   This may be made up immediately prior to use. One level teaspoon of powder in 500 ml of water is a useful mouthwash for dissolving mucus and debris. A stronger solution can be used for soaking dentures before cleaning them.

Chlorhexidene   This is the most effective chemical agent for maintaining oral hygiene and for dental plaque control (Bowsher et al 1999, Xavier 2000). Stronger solutions can, however, stain the teeth, and long-term use can cause mucosal damage (Field 1998a, b).

Water   This may be the most refreshing and appropriate mouthwash to use after brushing the teeth.

Other aids for mouth care (if permitted)

Soda water   This may be appreciated as an alternative mouthwash.

Ice cubes   These may be sucked, but the number should be limited if the patient has a restricted oral intake.

Fresh fruit   This can be sucked and then removed. Pineapple, if allowed, can be very refreshing and will stimulate the flow of saliva as it contains the enzyme ananase, which can help to clean a coated tongue (Gelbart 1998).

Saliva substitutes   These are useful for the treatment of a dry mouth (Holmes 1996).

Soft paraffin/lip salves   These prevent the lips becoming dry and cracked.

Glycerine, with or without lemon, should not be used as it can dehydrate the oral tissue and is an ineffective cleanser (Gelbart 1998). In addition, lemon is acidic and can lead to irritation and the decalcification of the teeth (Clay 2000).

Solutions for mouth cleaning

Any mouthwash solution can be used for mouth cleaning, as can solutions that actively stimulate the flow of saliva. The most efficient method of mouth cleaning remains, however, a mild toothpaste applied with a soft, small-headed toothbrush (Bowsher et al 1999, Clay 2000). The toothbrush may be dipped in any mouthwash or mouth-cleaning solution acceptable to the patient.

Mouth-care pack

This prepared sterile pack is used when intensive mouth care is needed for patients for whom a mouthwash alone, or tooth-brushing, is not appropriate. The pack may contain:

- a plastic tray divided into compartments to hold the mouth-cleaning solution
- cotton sticks
- foam sticks
- gauze swabs.

If a pack is not available, a sterile mouth-care tray can be assembled using:

- a foil tray
- a gallipot
- gauze swabs
- foam sticks
- cotton sticks.

The mouth-care pack should be covered, labelled with the patient's name and the date, cleaned and replenished after use, and replaced every 24 hours or as required. In the patient's own home, equipment can be adapted appropriately, maintaining a safe environment.

Guidelines and rationale for this nursing practice

- explain the nursing practice to the patient *to gain consent and co-operation, and to encourage participation in care, ensuring that there is some understanding of this practice*
- collect and prepare the equipment *to ensure an efficient use of time and resources*. Some solutions are more effective if prepared immediately before use
- ensure the patient's privacy *to respect his or her individuality and maintain self-esteem*
- help the patient into a comfortable sitting position, either in bed or on a chair *to help patient co-operation and promote as much independence as possible*. It is sometimes possible for patients to sit comfortably in front of a wash basin in either their own home or an institution
- place some protective material over the patient's chest and under the chin *to protect the clothes*. The patient's own towel can be used

- observe the patient throughout this activity *to monitor any adverse effects*
- don clean plastic gloves after efficient handwashing *to prevent contamination with body fluids and to maintain a safe environment*
- ask or help the patient to remove his or her dentures and place them in a bowl of clean water (labelled if necessary) *to gain access and a clear view of the oral cavity*
- examine the patient's mouth and tongue using the torch and spatula, *to observe the condition of the teeth, gums and mucosa. Note any food debris, any ulcers or sores and the condition of the lips* (Holmes & Mountain 1993)
- if possible, discuss with the patient the most suitable and acceptable mouth care for his or her particular needs *to promote individualised care and aid compliance*
- help patients to clean their teeth or dentures with their toothbrush and toothpaste
- offer a suitable mouthwash, explaining that it should not be swallowed, and help to hold the equipment as necessary *to rinse the mouth until all the debris and cleaning paste have been removed*
- offer tissues *for drying the mouth*
- help to apply lubrication to the lips as required *to maintain the integrity of the skin of the lips*. This can be done by placing the lubricant on a gloved finger and applying it directly, or patients may apply it themselves, *encouraging independence*
- return the patient's clean dentures in a bowl of clean water and encourage the patient to wear them *to maintain the shape of the oral cavity*
- ensure that the patient is left feeling as comfortable as possible. A period of rest should ideally be encouraged after this nursing practice
- dispose of equipment safely *to maintain a safe environment*
- document the nursing practice appropriately and immediately report any deterioration or improvement in the condition of the mouth, as well as abnormal findings. *This enables changes in practice to be implemented to maintain optimum mouth care for each patient*
- in undertaking this practice, nurses are accountable for their actions, the quality of care delivered and record-keeping according to the *Code of Professional Conduct* (UKCC 1992), *Guidelines for Professional Practice* (UKCC 1996) and *Guidelines for Records and Record Keeping* (UKCC 1998).

Intensive mouth care for dependent patients

- explain the nursing practice *to gain the patient's consent and co-operation if possible*
- ensure the patient's privacy *to respect individuality*
- help the patient into a comfortable position *so that he or she tolerates the practice*
- collect and prepare the equipment, including the mouth-cleaning pack or tray
- don clean plastic gloves *to prevent contamination with body fluids*
- remove dentures if present *to gain access and a clear view of the oral cavity*

Figure 29.1 *Cotton wool or foam stick for mouth cleaning*

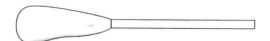

- examine the patient's mouth as before
- clean all round the mouth, gums and tongue with the mouth-cleaning solution, using a soft toothbrush if possible. *This will help to dislodge debris and remove plaque* (Buglass 1995). A cotton wool stick dipped into the solution may be used. Proprietary foam (Fig. 29.1) is a convenient and acceptable tool for mouth care if a toothbrush is not appropriate
- help the patient to use a mouthwash if possible, or rinse the mouth with a gauze swab soaked in mouthwash solution, allowing the patient to suck it. For patients with a wired mandible following oral surgery, a syringe of mouthwash in conjunction with suction may be used. This will require good co-operation from the patient and an adequate swallowing reflex *to prevent inhalation of the rinsing fluid*
- help the patient to clean the dentures, or clean them for him or her, using a toothbrush and toothpaste, under a running tap if possible, *to retain a healthy oral mucosa*
- proceed with the nursing practice as before.

Mouth care for an unconscious patient

Mouth-care guidelines are as for a dependent patient, with the following exceptions:

- position the patient on his or her side, with no pillow, and the head supported *so that no secretion or mouth-cleaning solution can flow into the trachea and be inhaled* (Kite & Pearson 1995)
- place waterproof material on the bed before placing tissues under the lower side of the face *to absorb solution and saliva draining from the mouth*
- check that suction equipment is at hand and in working order, and, if required, perform oral suction before commencing and during the nursing practice *to prevent any danger of fluid being inhaled.*

The dentures should have been removed, cleaned, appropriately labelled and stored with the patient's belongings on admission (*see* 'Unconscious patient', p. 367).

Relevance to the activities of living

Observations and further rationales for this nursing practice will be included within each activity of living as appropriate.

Maintaining a safe environment

The oral mucosa itself is part of the body's defence against infection. Mouth care, which helps to keep the teeth and oral mucosa in good condition, is important in maintaining a safe environment for the patient. Although mouth care does not require an aseptic technique, all the equipment should be clean or disposable, and all precautions should be taken to prevent cross-infection. The nurse should wash his or her hands before commencing and after completing mouth care for each patient.

The nurse should be protected from any blood-borne viral infection that might be present in the saliva, for example hepatitis B or HIV. It is advisable to wear gloves for all mouth care as it may involve direct contact with the oral mucosa and oral secretions (Thomas 1994).

Patients who are receiving cytotoxic medication for a malignant disease such as leukaemia may be at greater risk of infection than normal. The treatment itself may also affect the cells of the oral mucosa. A special mouth-care regime using mouthwashes, suspensions or creams may be prescribed for such patients. If possible, patients should, in order to minimise the risk of cross-infection, apply these themselves once the nurse has demonstrated the procedure. The importance of this care in the prevention of infection should be explained to the patient, and the nurse may use this time as an opportunity for patient education.

Mouthwashes should only be given to patients who are alert and well orientated, with a good cough reflex, otherwise there is a danger of accidental inhalation of the solution. For patients with a poor swallowing and cough reflex, oral suction equipment should be used to prevent any danger of aspiration of excess fluid in the oral cavity during this nursing practice.

Communicating

A patient who has a dry or infected mouth will find it uncomfortable to talk, and dry lips can also be painful when speaking, so appropriate mouth care can help with communication. Having a mouth that feels fresh can also help to raise the patient's morale and encourage him or her to take an interest in other people and the surroundings.

Breathing

Patients who have a cough and sputum may appreciate regular mouthwashes to clear mucus that may have lodged round the teeth and gums. A mouthwash should be given after chest physiotherapy to freshen the mouth and encourage a feeling of well-being, although an opportunity to clean the teeth may be even more welcome. Oxygen therapy dries the oral mucosa so patients receiving this treatment, either at home or in an institution, will appreciate regular mouth care.

Eating and drinking

The opportunity for mouth care should be available for all patients after meals. They should be encouraged to clean their teeth and/or dentures, as well as to rinse their mouth; the nurse may need to assemble the equipment and give appropriate help. This regular encouragement should form part of patient education in personal hygiene, and the importance of a healthy mouth, teeth and gums should be emphasised (WHO 1988).

A dry or 'dirty' mouth may discourage a patient from eating. Good mouth care can be a help in promoting the appetite and an encouragement to eat when this is important to aid recovery. Conversely, patients who are not allowed to eat via the oral route will need frequent mouth care as masticating food stimulates saliva, which helps to maintain a healthy mucosa. Some patients go home with nasogastric feeding or parenteral nutrition and may need assistance with mouth care from the community nurse for some time until they can manage their own mouth care. Adequate fluid intake is an additional help in maintaining a moist, healthy oral environment.

Some medicines, for example antihistamines, antidepressants, anticholinergics, antipsychotic and cytotoxic agents, and steroids, may have a negative effect on the mouth so regular assessment of the oral cavity is essential in these patients. Phenytoin can cause gum tenderness and gingival hypertrophy, whereas antibiotics can encourage oral Candida infections (Clay 2000, Gelbart 1998). Patients using oral steroid inhalers should be advised to rinse their mouth with water following each inhalation.

Personal cleansing and dressing

An important part of this activity of living is the patient's own oral hygiene. The nurse should be able to identify any associated problems during the assessment of the patient, and this may be an opportunity for patient education in relation to dental and oral hygiene. Giving a rationale for treatment and nursing care should enable the nurse to include the whole family in health promotion related to oral hygiene and dental care, for example using a toothbrush effectively (Trevelyan 1994).

Using a toothbrush effectively   Brushing the teeth loosens and removes debris trapped in the spaces and also prevents the growth of plaque, which harbours bacteria and may be a precursor of dental caries. Brushing also stimulates the blood circulation in the gums and helps to keep the soft tissue healthy. The teeth should be brushed with the toothbrush held at an angle of 45°. Vibrating strokes of the brush at gum level will help to dislodge plaque and debris. This is known as the 'Bass' method (Thurgood 1994). The inner aspects of the teeth should be brushed in the same way. Efficient tooth cleaning should not be hurried. The mouth should be well rinsed several times during and after tooth cleaning. Facilities for cleaning the teeth or dentures should be offered after meals to all patients who are not self-caring.

The correct use of dental floss can be included when discussing dental hygiene (Fig. 29.2). The importance of regular visits to the dentist should also be emphasised when the opportunity arises. This is an opportunity for the community nurse to extend health education to the whole family (Levine 1993).

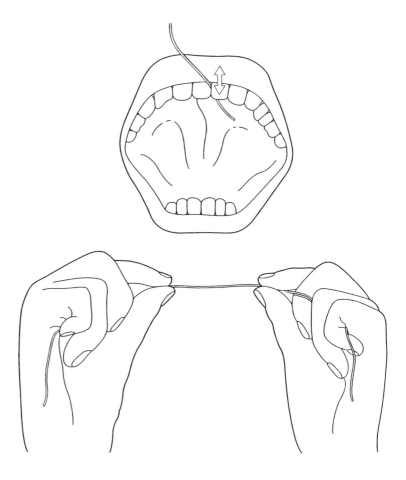

Figure 29.2 *Mouth care: use of dental floss*

Expressing sexuality

Sexuality can be expressed positively in the form of non-verbal communication. Smiling is, for example, an important way of projecting the self to other people: teeth and gums that are well cared for enhance the body image and the feeling of well-being. If a patient is feeling depressed, appropriate mouth care and a fresh mouthwash may encourage a male patient to agree to having a shave in preparation for meeting his sensitive visitors, whereas a female patient may feel encouraged to put on make-up, lipstick and perfume. At home, an increase in self-esteem will encourage the patient's interest in family events and aid rehabilitation.

Patient/carer education: key points

In partnership with the patient and/or carer, ensure that they are competent to carry out any practices required. Information should be given on an appropriate point of contact for any concerns that may arise.

Health education and health promotion with regard to mouth care should be multidisciplinary from childhood to old age: the health visitor, school nurse, practice nurse and district nurse, as well as the dentist and dental hygienist, may be involved. Advice should include:

- the importance of good care of the mouth, teeth and gums related to general health
- good tooth-cleaning technique and care of the dentures
- nutritional advice about the relationship of the incidence of dental caries to food and drink with a high sugar content
- the importance of removing debris from the teeth and fornices of the mouth after meals
- the influence of fluoride in the development of teeth
- the correct method of brushing and flossing the teeth.

Patients with a suppressed immune system should be taught oral hygiene procedures to prevent mucosal infection.

References

Bowsher J, Boyle S, Griffiths J 1999 Oral care. Nursing Standard 13(37): 31
Buglass E 1995 Oral hygiene. British Journal of Nursing 4(9): 516–519
Clay M 2000 Oral health in older people. Nursing Older People 12(7): 21–26
Field D 1998a Mouth care. 1. Nursing Times 94(7 suppl): 1–2
Field D 1998b Mouth care. 2. Nursing Times 94(8 suppl): 1–2
Gelbart M 1998 All mouth. Nursing Times 94(46): 26–28
Hatton-Smith C 1994 A last bastion of ritualised practice? A review of nurses' knowledge of oral health care. Professional Nurse 9(5): 304–308
Holmes S 1996 Nursing management of oral care in older patients. Nursing Times 92(9): 37–39
Holmes S 1998 Promoting oral health in institutionalised older adults: a nursing perspective. Journal of the Royal Society of Health 18(3): 167–172
Holmes S, Mountain E 1993 Assessment of oral status. Evaluation of three oral assessment guides. Journal of Clinical Nursing 2(1): 35–40
Kite K, Pearson L 1995 A rationale for mouth care: the integration of theory with practice. Intensive and Critical Care Nursing 11(2): 71–76
Levine R 1993 The scientific basis of dental health education. Health Authority, London
Nicol M, Bavin C, Bedford-Turner S, Cronin P, Rawlings-Anderson K 2000 Essential Nursing Skills. CV Mosby, London
Porter H 1994 Mouth care in cancer. Nursing Times 90(14): 27–29
Roberts J 2000 Developing an oral assessment and intervention tool for older people. 3. British Journal of Nursing 9(19): 2073–2078
Thomas L 1994 Glove story. Gloves, cost benefit analysis. Nursing Times 90(36): 31–35
Thurgood G 1994 Nurse maintenance of oral hygiene. British Journal of Nursing 3(7): 332–334, 351–353
Trevelyan J 1994 Oral traditions. Nursing Times 90(14): 24–27
United Kingdom Central Council for Nursing, Midwifery and Health Visiting 1992 Code of professional conduct. UKCC, London
United Kingdom Central Council for Nursing, Midwifery and Health Visiting 1996 Guidelines for professional practice. UKCC, London
United Kingdom Central Council for Nursing, Midwifery and Health Visiting 1998 Guidelines for records and record keeping. UKCC, London
World Health Organization 1988 Oral health: global indicators for health. WHO, Geneva
Xavier G 2000 The importance of mouth care in preventing infection. Nursing Standard 14(18): 47–51

30 Moving and Handling

Learning outcomes	By the end of this section, you should know how to:
	<ul><li>assess the requirements correctly</li><li>plan the safest method of moving the patient</li><li>adapt the principles of movement to suit each particular situation.</li></ul>

Background knowledge required	Revision of the anatomy and physiology of the spinal column and main joints and muscles of the body Revision of the current theories on safe and efficient moving and handling practices European Commission guidelines on moving and handling Royal College of Nursing guidelines on moving and handling Local policies on moving and handling patients.

Indications and rationale for moving and handling a patient	It may be necessary for one, two or more staff, with the help of mechanical aids, *to move patients when they are unable to move themselves* because of:
	<ul><li>severe injury</li><li>major surgery</li><li>paralysis</li><li>acute illness</li><li>weakness</li><li>unconsciousness</li><li>disability.</li></ul>

Outline of the procedure	It is important to understand the theories underlying safe and efficient moving and handling practices. In normal adults, the imaginary 'centre of gravity' point lies near the base of the spine. If suspended from this point, the body would, in theory, balance (Fig. 30.1). The feet form what is called the 'base'; if the centre of gravity moves beyond the area of the base, the body will become unbalanced and fall unless all the major muscles of the trunk and legs tense and hold the body upright. A prolonged period of imbalance can lead to stress and strain of these muscles and ultimately injury and pain (Fig. 30.2). Widening the base to keep the centre of gravity within the baseline will help to avoid this and lead to more safe and efficient movement.
	Most adults have developed unsafe movement habits, and their movements involve many unbalanced actions, so the re-education of the body to adopt safe

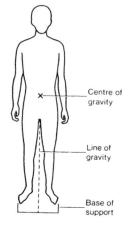

Centre of gravity

Line of gravity

Base of support

Figure 30.1   *Centre of gravity*

movement habits is to be encouraged. Such habits can be developed by increasing the awareness of how the body reacts to a variety of movements. The aim should be to achieve an acceptable balance between mobility and stability that will not place undue strain on the musculoskeletal system.

When preparing to move a patient or object, relax the knees, widen the base appropriately and point the leading foot in the direction of movement, then expand the spine by elevating the shoulders. Approach the load to be moved with open palms and hold it from underneath upwards to avoid a pinching grip on the load and unnecessary stress on the muscles of the fingers, hands and arms. Hold the load as near to your body as possible. Just before the 'effort' phase of the move, relax the spine so that the move begins with the spine in a non-fixed position; then lead with the top of the head in the direction of the move, and again expand the spine. The momentum caused by this action should allow the patient or object to come with you. If necessary, break the move into several stages, repositioning yourself after each move.

Equipment

Risk assessment forms
Mechanical aids, e.g. a lifting device (Fig. 30.3), patient sling or sliding sheets.

Guidelines and rationale for this nursing practice

- assess and plan the moving and handling requirements of patients with regard to their physical and psychological condition, weight and ability to help, the environment, the number of helpers and the most appropriate mechanical aids. This assessment and plan should be detailed in the patient's care plan and be frequently reviewed as the patient's condition changes
- if possible, clear the area of any obstacles, *for ease of movement*
- ensure an appropriate bed height *to reduce the risk of back injury*

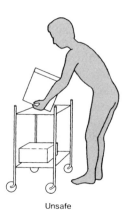

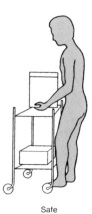

Figure 30.2   *Examples of safe and unsafe lifting*

Unsafe   Safe

- collect any help and/or mechanical aids required *to reduce any risk involved*
- explain fully to the patient and any helpers what is going to happen and what is expected of them *so that they can co-operate as much as possible*
- observe the patient throughout this activity *to detect any signs of distress.* When patients know exactly what is going to happen to them, they should be more relaxed and co-operative, and this should lessen the risk of injury for both them and staff

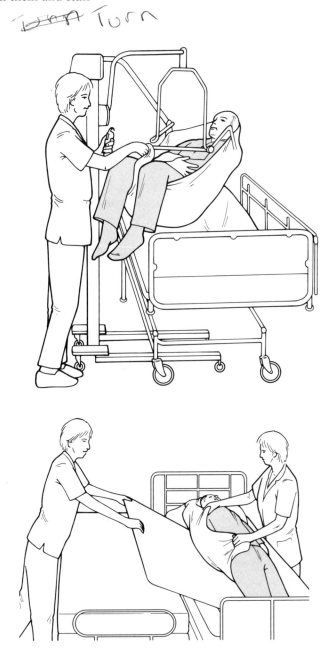

Figure 30.3 *Examples of mechanical aids*

(continued)

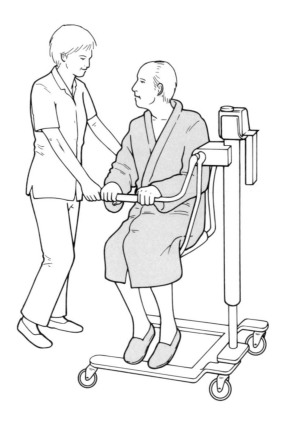

Figure 30.3
(continued)

- adopt a suitable position for the move, or manoeuvre the mechanical aid into position for the move
- apply the recommended theories of safe and efficient moving and handling practice when performing the move, *to protect nursing staff from back injury*
- carry out the move, one nurse acting as leader and giving instructions *so that everyone knows what is expected of them and can act together*
- ensure that the patient is left feeling as comfortable as possible
- clean any equipment used, *to reduce the risk of cross-infection*, and replace it in its *storage position so that it is accessible to other members of staff*
- in undertaking this practice, nurses are accountable for their actions, the quality of care delivered and record-keeping according to the *Code of Professional Conduct* (UKCC 1992), *Guidelines for Professional Practice* (UKCC 1996) and *Guidelines for Records and Record Keeping* (UKCC 1998).

There should always be a minimum of two nurses to move a patient when the person being moved cannot fully bear weight, and/or a mechanical aid such as a hoist should be used.

Relevance to the activities of living

Maintaining a safe environment

The safety of the patient and that of the carers is of equal importance. To avoid the danger of back injury to carers, mechanical aids should be used on all possible occasions. Patients who cannot bear weight must be moved using a hoist.

The latest edition of the guide to the moving and handling of patients produced by the Royal College of Nursing mentions some moves, for example the underarm drag lift, the Australian or shoulder lift, the top and tail or through-arm lift, the orthodox or cradle lift and team-lifting, which are potentially dangerous for patients and carers, and strongly advises against their use.

Know your own moving capacity, whether for patients or objects, and do not exceed it (RCN and Back Pain Association 1997). Ensure that you are up to date with the latest moving and handling guidelines; you should be required, by your employer, to attend regular training to update your moving and handling practices. Do not move patients unnecessarily.

A full assessment must be carried out prior to moving and handling patients. This should be detailed in the patient's care plan and should be frequently reviewed. In the community, liaison between the community nurse, occupational therapist and physiotherapist is essential in ensuring that equipment and appropriate moving and handling techniques are used. The physiotherapist will normally provide equipment such as walking sticks or frames, whereas the occupational therapist will offer such items as bathing equipment, seating and housing adaptations. The community nurse may provide nursing aids, for example hoists, commodes, monkey poles and special beds.

There are an increasing number of aids available, for example free-standing hoists, tracking hoists, tilting chairs, swivel cushions, bath aids, sliding sheets and boards, to help to move patients; the companies that develop them are always happy to demonstrate their latest models.

Communicating

Good communication between the carers, and between the carers and the patient, is very important for the successful and safe movement of the patient. Successful communication will enable the patient to feel safer and more confident in the carers' moving abilities.

Personal cleansing and dressing

Appropriate clothing and footwear for carers and patient can improve the success of a move.

Mobilising

Patients should be encouraged to move themselves as much as possible. Carers sometimes move patients unnecessarily because it is quicker than waiting for patients to move themselves.

Patient/carer education: key points

In partnership with the patient and/or carer, ensure that they are competent to carry out any practices required. Information should be given on an appropriate point of contact for any concerns that may arise.

Mechanical aids should be installed in the patient's home prior to transfer from the hospital to the community. This is usually arranged jointly by nursing staff, occupational therapists and physiotherapists.

Carers must be taught safe moving and handling techniques, and staff must also ensure that carers are proficient in the use of any mechanical aids provided. Patients should be encouraged to move themselves whenever possible.

To gain the patient's co-operation and to ensure that he or she will not react to move in an unexpected way, it is important to provide a full explanation of what is going to happen.

References

RCN and Back Pain Association 1997 Guidelines for the moving and handling of patients. RCN, London

Roper N, Logan W, Tierney A 1990 The elements of nursing. 4th edn. Churchill Livingstone, Edinburgh

United Kingdom Central Council for Nursing, Midwifery and Health Visiting 1992 Code of professional conduct. UKCC, London

United Kingdom Central Council for Nursing, Midwifery and Health Visiting 1996 Guidelines for professional practice. UKCC, London

United Kingdom Central Council for Nursing, Midwifery and Health Visiting 1998 Guidelines for records and record keeping. UKCC, London

31 Nebuliser Therapy

Learning outcomes

By the end of this section, you should know how to:

- prepare the patient for this nursing practice
- collect and prepare the equipment
- administer medication via a nebuliser, either in the community or in an institutional setting.

Background knowledge required

Revision of the respiratory system, with special reference to respiratory diseases associated with bronchospasm

Revision of 'Oxygen therapy' (*see* p. 271)

Revision of 'Administration of medicines' (*see* p. 1).

Indications and rationale for using nebuliser therapy

A nebuliser attached to a flow of air or oxygen converts a solution of a drug into an aerosol for therapeutic inhalation (*British National Formulary*). A nebuliser may be indicated for the following reasons:

- *to administer bronchodilators* for the relief of bronchospasm associated with respiratory disease, e.g.:
  — asthma
  — chronic obstructive airways disease (COAD) (Flynn 1993)
- *to administer mucolytic medication* to lower the viscosity of the secretions and aid expectoration, e.g.:
  — COAD
  — cystic fibrosis
  — bronchial carcinoma
- *to deliver an antibiotic* to a patient with chronic purulent infection, e.g. in cystic fibrosis.

The medication, as well as its administration by air or oxygen, is prescribed by a medical practitioner. It may need to be diluted with 2–3 ml of normal saline and is normally prescribed 3–4 times a day. The procedure may be co-ordinated with chest physiotherapy and may be administered by a nurse or physiotherapist. For the patient with asthma, an estimation of peak flow of tidal volume may be recorded before and after nebuliser therapy. If long-term treatment is needed, the patient may become efficient in his or her own self-care using nebuliser treatment at home, under the supervision of the community team (Tettersell 1993).

There are three main types of nebuliser (Porter-Jones 2000):

- jet
- ultrasonic
- high flow.

The symptoms and the effectiveness of the treatment regime are assessed by measuring the peak expiratory flow rate before and after the use of nebulisers or inhalers (Jevon et al 2000).

Equipment

Prescribed air supply: piped, in cylinders or via a portable air compressor
Prescribed oxygen supply, either piped or in cylinders
Peak flow meter
Adapter
Oxygen tubing
Nebuliser (Fig. 31.1)
Mouthpiece or appropriate oxygen mask, e.g. a Hudson mask (Fig. 31.1)
Prescribed medication (if dilution of drug is required, sodium chloride 0.9% normally being used)

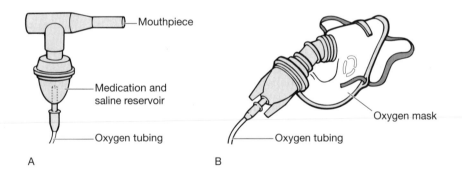

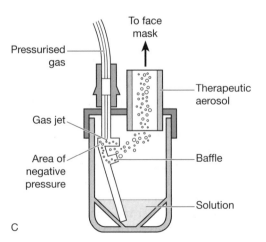

Figure 31.1 *Nebuliser*
A *Attached to a mouthpiece*
B *Attached to an oxygen mask*
C *Cross-section*

Sputum carton as required
'No Smoking' signs as appropriate (*see* 'Oxygen therapy', p. 271)
Receptacle for soiled disposable items.

For peak flow measurement

Peak flow meter (Fig. 31.2)
Disposable mouthpiece
Specific chart for documenting the results.

Guidelines and rationale for this nursing practice

- explain the nursing practice to the patient *to gain consent and co-operation, and to encourage participation in care*
- ensure the patient's privacy *to respect individuality and maintain self-esteem*
- prepare and assemble the equipment *so that everything is ready*
- explain the dangers of smoking to the patient and his or her visitors, positioning the 'No Smoking' signs as appropriate, thus *making sure that they understand that there is an increased risk of fire when oxygen is being administered*
- help the patient to estimate the peak flow of his or her tidal volume by recording the best of three results on the peak flow meter before commencing nebuliser therapy. This will *help to evaluate the efficiency of the treatment* (Kendrick & Smith 1992)
- help the patient into a comfortable position *so that he or she will tolerate the therapy without distress*
- observe the patient throughout the activity *to monitor the effects of the nebuliser therapy*

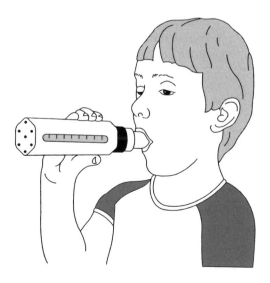

Figure 31.2 *Peak flow meter*

- identify and check the medication prescription (*see* 'Administration of medicines', p. 1). This is a *professional requirement for prescribed medication*
- prepare the prescribed dose in a suitable sterile syringe (diluting with sodium chloride 0.9% if required) *to ensure the correct administration procedure*
- separate nebulisers should be used for each drug prescribed, bronchdilators being given first (Edmond 2000)
- fill the nebuliser with the prepared medication (Fig. 31.3)
- adjust the flow meter to 5 L or turn on the air compressor *to ensure the efficient vaporisation of the medication*
- observe the fine spray from the nebuliser *to check that the equipment is working*
- encourage the patient to breathe the nebulised vapour through the mouthpiece *for maximum effect*; a mask may be used if a patient has difficulty with the mouthpiece
- remain with the patient until all the solution has been nebulised
- encourage the patient to expectorate *as the medication may help to loosen the bronchial secretions* (Hough 1992)
- ensure that the patient is left feeling as comfortable as possible. *Bronchospasm is further reduced if the patient is relaxed and reassured*
- help the patient to estimate the peak flow of his or her tidal volume by recording the best of three results on the peak flow meter. This should preferably be recorded half an hour after the completion of nebuliser therapy *as some bronchodilators have their maximum effect during this period* (Brewin & Hughes 1995)
- wash and dry the nebuliser, tubing and mask or mouthpiece *to maintain a safe environment*
- retain the equipment in a polythene bag *for the patient's next administration. To prevent infection, the equipment should be changed every 24 hours*
- document the nursing practice appropriately, monitor after-effects and report any abnormal findings immediately *to ensure safe practice and enable prompt, appropriate medical and nursing intervention to be initiated*
- in undertaking this practice, nurses are accountable for their actions, the quality of care delivered and record-keeping according to the *Code of Professional Conduct* (UKCC 1992), *Guidelines for Professional Practice* (UKCC 1996) and *Guidelines for Records and Record Keeping* (UKCC 1998).

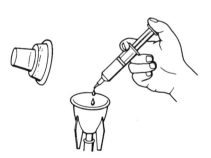

Figure 31.3 *Nebuliser taken apart to introduce a prepared medication*

Relevance to the activities of living

Observations and further rationale for this nursing practice will be included within each activity of living as appropriate.

Maintaining a safe environment

If oxygen is used, all precautions to prevent the risk of fire should be maintained, as with oxygen therapy (*see* p. 271).

This is not a sterile procedure, but adequate standards of cleanliness should be maintained. The nurse should wash his or her hands before commencing and on completing this nursing practice. The equipment for each patient should be kept clean and dry when not in use. It should be changed every 24 hours to prevent infection.

The prescription should be checked by a registered nurse or medical practitioner (*see* 'Administration of medicines', p. 1).

Regular maintenance checks of all equipment should be carried out as per local policy.

Communicating

During the nursing practice itself, the patient will not be encouraged to speak.

The solution is normally administered over a period of up to 10 minutes, which can be explained to the patient.

Breathing

Monitor the respiration rate and depth and type of respiration, taking readings as frequently as required. The patient should take deep regular breaths through the mouthpiece of the nebuliser to ensure that the medication reaches the mucosa of the bronchi and bronchioles rather than just the oropharynx (Everard et al 1993). Patients will often experience less dyspnoea after this procedure, and there may be a dramatic relief of bronchospasm for patients with asthma. This can be monitored by peak flow recording over a period of time.

Occasionally, two drugs are prescribed via the nebuliser; these should **NOT** be, unless it is specifically stated, mixed. They should be administered in separate nebulisers, one after the other, prescribed bronchodilators always being administered first. The nebulisers should be labelled appropriately and kept clean and dry for future use (Cattell & Jones 1995).

For efficient vaporisation, a flow of 4–5 L of oxygen on the flow meter is required. For patients with COAD, this will, however, provide a dangerously high percentage of oxygen (*see* 'Oxygen therapy', p. 271) so air should be prescribed for administration instead. This can take the form of a piped supply or one from an air compressor (Dodd et al 1995). For patients with asthma, an oxygen flow rate of 6–8 L is recommended unless otherwise advised by medical staff (Porter-Jones 2000).

For patients in intensive care areas, a nebuliser can be introduced into the ventilator circuit and medication administered as prescribed.

Observe and record the amount, colour and type of any sputum.

Eating and drinking

A healthy mouth and oropharyngeal mucosa is essential for maximum absorption of the medication. Frequent oral hygiene should therefore be performed as appropriate. A mouthwash after expectorating may be appreciated and should be available if desired.

Patient/carer education: key points

In partnership with the patient and/or carer, ensure that they are competent to carry out any practices required. Information should be given on an appropriate point of contact for any concerns that may arise. The reason for the nebuliser therapy should be carefully explained to the patient and his or her family so that compliance is continued (Coakley 2000).

If oxygen is used for nebulisation, information about fire risks and the precautions needed should be explained (*see* 'Oxygen therapy', p. 271).

If the patient is self-caring, instructions about preparing the medication and using the equipment should be given, and the nurse should ensure that these continue to be followed correctly. At home, the nurse should ensure that the patient and carers keep the equipment clean and separate from other household equipment, in order to maintain a safe environment.

The patient should understand the importance of immediately reporting any changes in respiratory function, such as increased dyspnoea, cough or sputum, or any general feeling of distress.

References

Brewin A, Hughes J 1995 Effect of patient education on asthma management. British Journal of Nursing 4(2): 81–82, 99–101

British National Formulary (current edition) Nebulisers. London

Cattell R, Jones S 1995 Nebuliser therapy and nursing knowledge. British Journal of Nursing 4(16): 954–957

Coakley A 2001 Helping patients to master correct inhaler techniques: the nursing role. British Journal of Nursing 10(7): 424–432

Dodd M, Hanley S, Johnson S, Webb A 1995 District nebuliser compressor service: reliability and costs. Thorax 50(1): 81–82

Edmond C 2000 The respiratory system. In: Alexander M, Fawcett J, Runciman P (eds) Nursing practice – hospital and home: the adult. 2nd edn. Churchill Livingstone, Edinburgh

Everard M, Hardy J, Milner A 1993 Comparison of nebulised aerosol deposition in the lungs of healthy adults following oral and nasal inhalation. Thorax 48(10): 1045–1046

Flynn M 1993 Management of chronic obstructive airways disease. British Journal of Nursing 2(14): 717–723

Hough A 1992 Making sense of – sputum retention, Nursing Times 88(36): 33–35

Jevon P, Ewens B, Manzie J 2000 Measuring peak expiratory flow. Nursing Times 96(38): 49–50

Kendrick A, Smith E 1992 Respiratory measurements. 2. Simple measurement of lung function. Professional Nurse 7(1): 748–754

Porter-Jones G 2000 Nebulisers. 1. Preparation. Nursing Times 96(36): 45–46

Tettersell MJ 1993 Asthma patients' knowledge in relation to compliance with drug therapy. Journal of Advanced Nursing 18(1): 103–113

United Kingdom Central Council for Nursing, Midwifery and Health Visiting 1992 Code of professional conduct. UKCC, London

United Kingdom Central Council for Nursing, Midwifery and Health Visiting 1996 Guidelines for professional practice. UKCC, London

United Kingdom Central Council for Nursing, Midwifery and Health Visiting 1998 Guidelines for records and record keeping. UKCC, London

32 Neurological Examination

Learning outcomes	By the end of this section, you should know how to: - prepare and support the patient for a neurological examination - collect and prepare the equipment - if required, assist the medical practitioner during the neurological examination.
Background knowledge required	Revision of the anatomy and physiology of the nervous system Revision of 'Care of the unconscious patient' (*see* p. 367).
Indications and rationale for neurological examination	Neurological examination is a method of obtaining some objective data on the functioning of a patient's nervous system (Brunner & Suddarth 1992). This may be required: - *to aid in the diagnosis of a neurological disease* - *to monitor the effect of a neurological disease* - *to aid in the assessment of treatment during the course of a neurological disease.*
Outline of the procedure	This procedure is carried out by a medical or skilled nurse practitioner, usually in conjunction with an examination of the motor and sensory function of the patient's trunk and limbs. The ophthalmoscope and pencil torch are used to assess the function of the optic, oculomotor, trochlear and ophthalmic branch of the trigeminal cranial nerves. The auriscope and tuning fork are used to examine the ears and assess the function of the vestibulocochlear cranial nerve respectively. An assessment of the patient's sensation to pain, touch and temperature is made using a sterile needle, a cotton wool ball and test tubes of hot and cold water. The olfactory cranial nerve is assessed when the patient is asked to identify the odours of various strong-smelling substances. The tendon hammer is used by the medical practitioner when testing a spinal reflex such as the knee jerk. Assessment for an upper motor neurone lesion will also require the use of a tendon hammer for stroking the lateral aspect of the sole of the patient's foot. The function of the facial cranial nerve is assessed by asking the patient to identify various substances, that is, salt, sugar, vinegar and lemon juice. To prevent inaccurate results, the patient will be asked to use a mouth rinse after each substance has been tasted.

Equipment

Ophthalmoscope
Pencil torch
Auriscope
Tuning fork
Sterile injection needle
Non-sterile cotton wool balls
Test tubes filled with hot and cold water
Small containers of various strong-smelling substances, e.g. peppermint
    and oil of cloves
Tendon hammer
Small samples of salt, sugar, lemon juice and vinegar
Glass of water for rinsing the patient's mouth
Trolley or tray for equipment
Receptacle for used mouth rinse
Receptacle for soiled disposable items.

Guidelines and rationale for this nursing practice

- help to explain the procedure to the patient *to gain consent and co-operation*
- wash the hands *to reduce cross-infection* (Horton 1995)
- prepare the equipment *to ensure that all the equipment is available and ready for use*
- ensure the patient's privacy *to reduce anxiety*
- observe the patient throughout this activity *to note any signs of distress*
- help the patient into a comfortable position *to allow the patient to maintain the position and to provide easy access for the practitioner*
- assist the medical practitioner during the examination *to enhance the overall quality of the procedure* (Pemberton 1988)
- ensure that the patient is left feeling as comfortable as possible, thus *maintaining the quality of this nursing practice*
- dispose of the equipment safely *to reduce any health hazard*
- document the nursing practice appropriately, monitor the after-effects and report any abnormal findings immediately, *providing a written record and assisting in the implementation of any action should an abnormality or adverse reaction to the practice be noted*
- in undertaking this practice, nurses are accountable for their actions, the quality of care delivered and record-keeping according to the *Code of Professional Conduct* (UKCC 1992), *Guidelines for Professional Practice* (UKCC 1996) and *Guidelines for Records and Record Keeping* (UKCC 1998).

Relevance to the activities of living

Maintaining a safe environment

All equipment should be clean or disposable, and all precautions should be taken to prevent cross-infection. The nurse should wash his or her hands before commencing and on completing the nursing practice (Horton 1995).

A second practitioner is not always present during a neurological examination, but assistance may be required by the examiner, for example with a paralysed patient.

Communicating

The practitioner who carries out the examination gives the patient an explanation of the procedure, but the nurse may be required to repeat the explanation (Brunner & Suddarth 1992).

Depending on the nature of the disease condition that has demanded the neurological examination (as these are many and diverse), any of the patient's activities of living may be affected, but the examination itself does not have any adverse effects on these.

Patient/carer education: key points

In partnership with the patient and/or carer, ensure that they are competent to carry out any practices required. Information should be given on an appropriate point of contact for any concerns that may arise.

The patient should be given an initial explanation of the procedure by the medical practitioner, but the nurse may need to repeat this. The patient should have the initial results of the examination explained and discussed (Pemberton 1988).

References

Brunner L, Suddarth D (eds) 1992 The textbook of adult nursing. Chapman & Hall, London
Horton R 1995 Handwashing: the fundamental infection control principle. British Journal of Nursing 4(16): 926–933
Pemberton L 1988 Assessment of the nervous system. In: Allan D (ed.) Nursing and the neurosciences. Churchill Livingstone, Edinburgh
United Kingdom Central Council for Nursing, Midwifery and Health Visiting 1992 Code of professional conduct. UKCC, London
United Kingdom Central Council for Nursing, Midwifery and Health Visiting 1996 Guidelines for professional practice. UKCC, London
United Kingdom Central Council for Nursing, Midwifery and Health Visiting 1998 Guidelines for records and record keeping. UKCC, London

33 Nutrition

There are three parts to this section:

1 Feeding a dependent patient
2 Enteral feeding
3 Parenteral nutrition.

1 Feeding a dependent patient

Learning outcomes

By the end of this section, you should know how to:

- prepare the patient for this nursing practice
- collect and prepare the equipment
- carry out the feeding of a dependent patient.

Background knowledge required

Revision of the anatomy and physiology of the mouth and oesophagus, with special reference to the physical acts of mastication and swallowing.

Indications and rationale for the feeding of a dependent patient

The nurse may be required to feed a dependent patient *to maintain adequate nutrition in*:

- a patient who is unable to use his or her upper limbs because of paralysis or serious illness
- a patient who has lost upper limb co-ordination because of a physical or mental disease
- a patient who has recently lost his or her eyesight
- a patient who has an injury around the mouth.

Equipment

Feeding utensils such as a fork, knife, spoon, drinking cup with a spout or cup with an angled straw
A cloth, disposable napkin or paper towel
Diet, as ordered by the patient
Trolley or tray for equipment
Receptacle for soiled disposable items.

Guidelines and rationale for this nursing practice

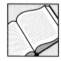

In hospital or at home, this practice may be undertaken by the patient's relatives or carers.

- explain the nursing practice to the patient *to gain consent and co-operation*
- collect and prepare the equipment *to ensure that all the equipment is available and ready for use*
- help the patient into a comfortable position *to allow easy access to the patient by the nurse and also allow the patient to maintain his or her position during the practice*
- observe the patient throughout this activity *to note any signs of distress*
- wash the hands and put on an apron *for general hygiene purposes and to reduce the risk of cross-infection*
- *for patient satisfaction and enjoyment*, keep the food not being eaten at a suitable temperature
- remind the patient of his or her ordered menu *to permit psychological preparation for the food*
- when possible, the nurse should sit down while feeding the patient *so that this is made an enjoyable social occasion*
- ask the patient which food he or she wishes to eat first, thereby *giving the patient some control over the activity*
- offer the food to patients at a rate set by them *as hurrying them while they are eating may induce nausea or vomiting*
- *to prevent gagging or choking*, place the spoon or fork accurately into the patient's mouth
- offer sips of fluid during the meal *to aid in the mastication and swallowing of the food*
- discontinue feeding when asked by the patient in order *to prevent a feeling of distension and excessive fullness*
- assist the patient with mouth care following the meal *as this will promote dental health and may reduce the incidence of dental caries*
- ensure that the patient is left feeling as comfortable as possible, thus *maintaining the quality of this nursing practice*
- dispose of equipment safely *to reduce any health hazard*
- document the nursing practice appropriately, monitor the after-effects and report any abnormal findings immediately, thus *providing a written record and assisting in the implementation of any action should an abnormality or adverse reaction to the practice be noted*
- in undertaking this practice, nurses are accountable for their actions, the quality of care delivered and record-keeping according to the *Code of Professional Conduct* (UKCC 1992), *Guidelines for Professional Practice* (UKCC 1996) and *Guidelines for Records and Record Keeping* (UKCC 1998).

reference

Relevance to the activities of living

Maintaining a safe environment

All equipment should be clean and all precautions be taken to prevent cross-infection. Nurses should wash their hands before commencing and on completion of the nursing practice. A coloured apron or tabard may be worn by staff for meal service to reduce the risk of cross-infection (Nicol et al 2000).

The nurse will need to check the temperature of the food with the patient to prevent burning of the mouth, lips or tongue.

Communicating

Patients should be assisted to choose and order their own food from the menu. Eating is a pleasant social occasion for most people so the nurse must help to maintain this atmosphere. Patients should whenever possible have the choice to eat their meals in a dining area (ACHC 1997). The addition of background music and the use of tablecloths, cloth napkins, place mats, condiments and table decorations, particularly in long-stay care, can make mealtimes a more pleasant experience (Caroline Walker Trust 1995).

Patient preferences and special dietary needs should be identified and observed (Sampson 2000). This includes cultural, ethnic and religious requirements (ACHC 1997, Caroline Walker Trust 1995).

Continuous verbal prompting may be required while feeding a patient who has a degree of dementia, and consistency of care-giver can improve eating behaviour in patients with severe dementia (McGillivary & Marland 1999). A blind patient should be told what food to expect in order to prevent surprise at an unexpected flavour. Other patients should be shown the food to be eaten as this will assist in its digestion.

Breathing

The nurse should observe the patient for difficulty in swallowing, which may precede choking. Placing the spoon or fork too far back in the patient's mouth may lead to gagging or choking. A patient who has temporarily lost the ability to swallow, such as a stroke victim, may be assisted by a skilled speech therapist to regain the swallowing reflex.

Eating and drinking

Completing a nutritional assessment on admission will highlight any potential problems with nutrition. A variety of risk assessment tools are available, and staff should follow their particular local policy.

Sips of fluid will assist a patient to swallow food and also rid the mouth of the taste of one food prior to a different taste.

The patient should, when appropriate, be given the choice of feeding utensil to be used. Some patients do not like to use a feeding cup with a spout but prefer a straw and a cup or glass. A plate guard, a non-slip mat or adapted cutlery may help to promote independence (Nicol et al 2000).

A patient who has a motor or sensory loss on one side of the face will need to be fed on the unaffected side of the mouth. The nurse should check that food does not accumulate in the cheek of the affected side.

Staff should identify any other fuctional problems with eating, such as poorly fitting dentures (ACHC 1997) and mouth infections. Ensure that any lack of appetite is noted and acted upon. Unpleasant smells, frequent interruptions and poorly presented food can have a detrimental effect on food intake (Wood 1999), as can the effect of some medicines (Holmes 1998).

When possible, patients should be assisted to put the food into their own mouth as this may help them to feel less dependent on the nurse.

Drinks and other foods, such as pieces of fruit, should be frequently offered between meals.

Relatives of the patient may wish to assist the patient in eating his or her food. This should be encouraged as it is of great psychological benefit both to the patient and the relatives. Information and education on the constituents of a healthy diet should be discussed with the patient, relatives and carers.

Personal cleansing and dressing

On ending the meal, the nurse should ask patients whether they wish their face to be washed and whether mouth hygiene is desired. The nurse and carer have a role in the prevention of dental caries by the provision and maintenance of good oral care.

Ensure that all visible traces of food debris, spillages and soiled napkins are removed from the patient, thereby maintaining a positive body image, which may enhance the patient's self-esteem.

Patient/carer education: key points

Advice on a healthy dietary intake and the benefits of such a diet should be given by the nurse to both the patient and the carers. The nurse should provide information and education on the constituents of any special diet that is required by the patient.

Information regarding the maintenance of oral health should also be given by the nurse.

2 Enteral feeding

There are two parts to this section:

A Enteral feeding via a nasogastric tube and intermittent bolus or a continuous drip system
B Enteral feeding via a gastrostomy/jejunostomy tube.

The concluding subsection 'Relevance to the activities of living' refers to the two practices together.

Learning outcomes	By the end of this section, you should know how to:

- prepare the patient for this nursing practice
- collect and prepare the equipment
- describe the principles of enteral feeding
- outline some of the problems of enteral feeding.

Background knowledge required	Revision of the anatomy and physiology of the gastrointestinal tract Revision of the nutritional requirements of the human body.

Indications and rationale for enteral feeding	Enteral feeding is the introduction of the daily nutritional requirements, in liquid form, directly into a patient's stomach or small intestine by means of a tube. The tube may be inserted through the nostril and passed down into the stomach, or introduced directly into the stomach or small intestine via a surgical incision made in the abdominal wall.

Enteral feeding may be performed ***to maintain adequate nutrition*** in the following circumstances:

- obstruction of the oesophagus, e.g. by a neoplasm
- loss of the swallowing reflex
- oesophageal fistula
- preoperative preparation of malnourished patients
- during radiotherapy treatment
- postoperatively for patients who have had some types of oral surgery, or oesophageal surgery
- some unconscious patients
- patients who have severe burns.

Enteral feeding can be administered in several ways. It may be given through a fine tube, for example Clinifeed, with its own administration set and container for the feed, or it can be channelled through a pump. Enteral feeds may also be introduced via a self-retaining tube such as a Foley's catheter or percutaneous endoscopic gastrostomy tube via a surgical opening in the abdominal wall into the stomach, duodenum or jejunum.

2A *Enteral feeding via a nasogastric tube and intermittent bolus or continuous enteral feeding*

Equipment	Enteral feeding tube and introducer

Lubricant, e.g. iced water or jelly
Hypoallergenic tape
Container with prepared feed
Enteral feed administration set
Intravenous infusion stand

Gravity or volumetric pump if required
Water
Syringe (50 ml)
Gallipot, syringe and pH indicator strips
Stethoscope
Receptacle for soiled disposable items.

The second syringe should be a 10 ml size if a fine-bore tube is being used
or a 50 ml catheter-tip syringe for a Ryles-type tube.

Guidelines and rationale for this nursing practice

- explain the nursing practice to the patient *to gain consent and co-operation*
- collect and prepare the equipment *for efficiency of practice*
- help the patient into a comfortable position, ideally sitting upright (Smith et al 1999) but otherwise at an angle of 30–45° (Murray 2000)
- observe the patient throughout this activity *to detect any signs of discomfort or distress*
- insert the enteral feeding tube as described in 'Gastric aspiration' (*see* p. 161) and then remove the introducer or assist the qualified practitioner as requested
- before commencing the feed, an X-ray is necessary *to confirm the position of the tube* as the lumen is too narrow to allow the usual tests to be carried out and it is necessary to ascertain that the tube has been correctly positioned. If a Ryles-type tube has been used the correct positioning of the tube can be checked by flushing the tube with 20 ml of air to ensure that it is clear (Mallett & Dougherty 2000). A small amount of stomach contents is then aspirated and placed in the gallipot. The pH-sensitive paper can then be dipped into it. A pH of 3 or less indicates stomach contents. The introduction of 5–10 ml of air via the syringe while listening over the epigastrium for a gurgling sound will indicate that the air is reaching the stomach and also confirm the correct positioning of the tube
- attach the prepared feed in the container to the infusion stand
- join the administration set to the container using a non-touch technique (Smith et al 1999) and allow the feed to run through to the end of the set before it is connected to the feeding tube *so that as little air as possible is introduced to the patient's stomach*
- adjust the flow rate as required or connect to the appropriate pump and ensure the rate of flow is as prescribed *so that the patient's stomach does not become overdistended and produce feelings of nausea*
- when intermittent bolus feeding is the method of choice, run some water through at the end of the feed *to clear the tube*
- ensure that the patient is left feeling as comfortable as possible, thus *maintaining the quality of this practice*
- record appropriately the time of commencement of feeding and the amount and type of feed given, monitor the after-effects and report any abnormal findings immediately, *providing a written record and assisting in the*

*implementation of any action should an abnormality or adverse reaction
to the practice be noted*

- in undertaking this practice, nurses are accountable for their actions, the
  quality of care delivered and record-keeping according to the *Code of
  Professional Conduct* (UKCC 1992), *Guidelines for Professional
  Practice* (UKCC 1996) and *Guidelines for Records and Record Keeping*
  (UKCC 1998).

Narrow-bore tubes for continuous enteral feeding are made of silicone or
polyurethane, with a diameter ranging from 1 to 3 mm. They are more
comfortable for the patient than the wide-bore tube and less likely to cause
ulceration, inflammation, stricture, haemorrhage and erosion of the mucosa
(Woods 1998). They do, however, become blocked more easily, and it is almost
impossible to clear them by aspiration.

2B Enteral feeding via a gastrostomy/jejunostomy tube (Fig. 33.1)

Equipment

Water
Syringe
Prepared feed in its container
Enteral feed administration set
Enteral feed pump if required
Intravenous infusion stand if required
Receptacle for soiled disposable items.

**Guidelines and
rationale for this
nursing practice**

- explain the nursing practice to the patient *to gain consent and co-operation.*
  Patients should be encouraged to be active partners in care
- assist the patient into a suitable position, for example semi-recumbent,
  *to allow easy access to the gastrostomy site and to lessen the risk of a kink
  in the tube.* The patient should ideally not lie flat as this increases the risk
  of reflux and aspiration
- observe the patient throughout this activity *to detect any signs of discomfort
  or distress*
- collect and prepare the equipment *for efficiency of practice*
- insert the administration set into the feed bottle in an aseptic manner *to
  prevent infection*
- allow the feed to run through the set in order to expel all the air *as
  unnecessary air introduced into the stomach can cause pain and distension*
- the plastic cap at the end of the administration set should remain in place at
  this time *to prevent infection*
- flush the tube with about 10–50 ml of water via a syringe *to ensure that the
  tube is patent*
- insert the administration set into the tube (via the pump if used)

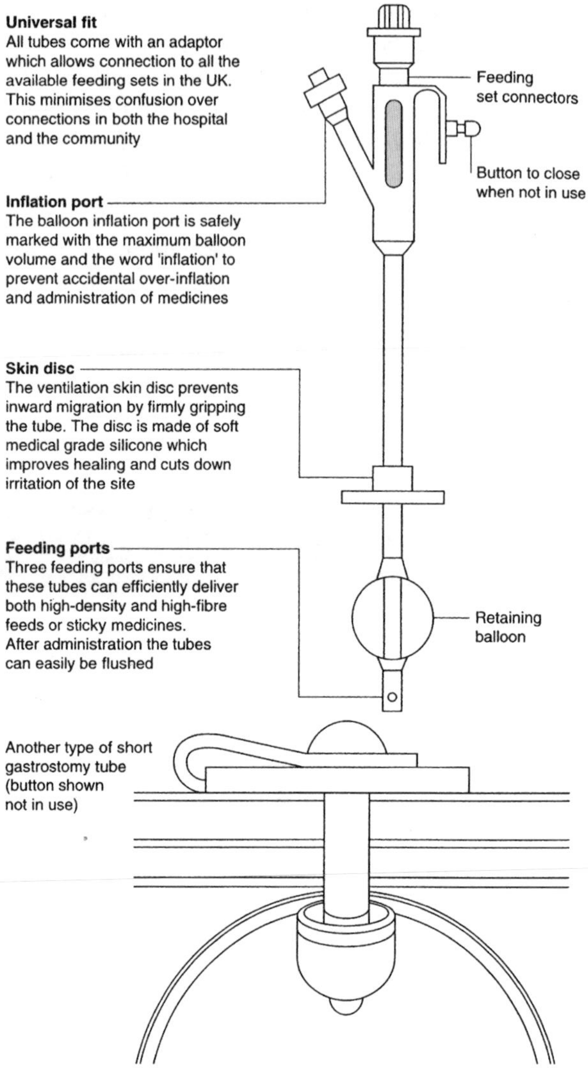

Universal fit
All tubes come with an adaptor which allows connection to all the available feeding sets in the UK. This minimises confusion over connections in both the hospital and the community

Feeding set connectors

Button to close when not in use

Inflation port
The balloon inflation port is safely marked with the maximum balloon volume and the word 'inflation' to prevent accidental over-inflation and administration of medicines

Skin disc
The ventilation skin disc prevents inward migration by firmly gripping the tube. The disc is made of soft medical grade silicone which improves healing and cuts down irritation of the site

Feeding ports
Three feeding ports ensure that these tubes can efficiently deliver both high-density and high-fibre feeds or sticky medicines. After administration the tubes can easily be flushed

Retaining balloon

Another type of short gastrostomy tube (button shown not in use)

Figure 33.1 *Enteral feeding: examples of gastrostomy tubes*

- start the flow by switching on the pump or adjusting the administration set
- disconnect the administration set when all the feed has been delivered
- flush the tube through with water *to clear the tube*
- ensure that the patient is left feeling as comfortable as possible, thus *maintaining the quality of this practice*
- dispose of the equipment safely *to reduce any health hazard*
- record appropriately the time and amount and type of feed administered, monitor the after-effects and report any abnormal findings immediately, *providing a written record and assisting in the implementation of any action should an abnormality or adverse reaction to the practice be noted*

- in undertaking this practice, nurses are accountable for their actions, the quality of care delivered and record-keeping according to the *Code of Professional Conduct* (UKCC 1992), *Guidelines for Professional Practice* (UKCC 1996) and *Guidelines for Records and Record Keeping* (UKCC 1998).

Relevance to the activities of living

Maintaining a safe environment

Although an aseptic technique is not necessary when administering enteral feeding, a good standard of hygiene must be maintained to prevent the patient developing a gastrointestinal infection. A strict aseptic technique is necessary when re-dressing the gastrostomy site in order to prevent the wound becoming infected. When the gastrostomy site has healed (usually about 10 days after insertion of the tube), a dressing is no longer required (Nicol et al 2000). The tube should be rotated through a complete circle on a daily basis to encourage the formation of a smooth stoma and prevent overgranulation (Reeves & Cubbs 2000). The guard should be lifted and the site washed with mild soap and water, the guard then being replaced. Creams, dressings and talcum powder should be avoided (Reeves & Cubbs 2000). The administration set for enteral feeding should be changed daily to reduce the risk of infection (Smith et al 1999, Woolfrey et al 1997).

No feed should be administered via a nasogastric tube until the nurse has checked that the tube is in the correct position. It can become displaced by severe retching, coughing or vomiting, and following endotracheal suctioning (Colagiovanni 2000). There is no single completely reliable method of checking whether a nasogastric tube is in position apart from an X-ray. Aspiration of the stomach contents and checking for acidity, indicating gastric contents (pH < 3) as opposed to bronchial secretions (pH > 6), combined with listening via a stethoscope to a small amount of air being introduced into the stomach through a syringe and down the tube, are considered by many practitioners to be currently the most reliable methods when an X-ray is not available. The pH method cannot be used successfully on patients who are receiving acid-inhibiting medication (Mallett & Dougherty 2000).

Eating and drinking

The patient may be allowed a small amount of liquid orally; this can help to stimulate secretion of some of the digestive juices. It is necessary to ensure that the patient receives an adequate amount of fluid over each 24 hour period, as well as all the essential nutrients (BAPEN 1996, 1999). The identification of any food allergies should be documented (Sampson 2000). A formal nutritional assessment should be carried out (Murray 2000) and the patient's nutritional requirements discussed with a nutritionist. A poor nutritional intake may result from the effects of trauma, surgery and/or disease (Dennis 2000).

Nausea, distension and diarrhoea can be a problem, these often being caused by the feed being administered too rapidly; the continuous drip system helps to overcome this (Colagiovanni 1999). Intermittent bolus feeding is waning in popularity for this reason, although it is highly convenient for community patients as it allows them to carry on their normal routine between feeds and also means that they can conform to family mealtimes. Medication should never be added to the feed (Naysmith & Nicholson 1998, Woolfrey et al 1997). It should be given in liquid form whenever possible, or via dispersible tablets, and the tube flushed through with water before, after and between each medicine. The advice of a pharmacist should be sought.

Flushing nasogastric tubes is currently as effective using water as using any other solution (Colagiovanni 2000).

Eliminating

Diarrhoea can be a problem and is usually caused by feeding that is too rapid or administering a feed that is too concentrated. A feed contaminated by pathogens will also lead to diarrhoea (Murray 2000).

Personal cleansing and dressing

Frequent oral hygiene should be offered to the patient receiving enteral feeding because his or her lips, tongue and oral mucosa will rapidly become dry and cracked if no fluid is passing over them.

The patient with a gastrostomy can bathe or shower safely provided the tube is closed (Nicol et al 2000).

Sleeping

Patients may prefer to receive their food by the continuous drip system while they are asleep at night. This allows them more freedom of movement during the day.

Expressing sexuality

A gastrostomy tube can have a negative effect on body image (Woods 1998). A gastrostomy button that lies flush with the skin can be inserted once the gastrostomy site has been established. This prevents snagging on clothing and reduces interference with sexual activity (Holmes 1996).

Patient/carer education: key points

A clear explanation of the necessity of this form of feeding will help to gain the patient's co-operation. If the patient is self-administering feeds, the importance of hygiene needs to be stressed. The feeding pattern also need to be agreed with the patient.

3   Parenteral nutrition

Learning outcomes

By the end of this section, you should know how to:

- prepare and support the patient for this nursing practice
- collect and prepare the equipment
- assist the medical practitioner with the insertion of a central venous catheter
- maintain an infusion of parenteral nutrition for a period of time in an institutional or community setting.

Background knowledge required

Revision of the anatomy and physiology of the cardiopulmonary system, with special reference to the circulation of the blood, and the veins of the neck and upper thorax

Revision of the nutritional needs required to maintain health

Revision of 'Intravenous therapy' (*see* p. 181) and 'Care of a Hickman catheter' (*see* p. 191).

Revision of 'Aseptic technique' (*see* p. 407)

Review of health authority policy regarding parenteral nutrition in both community and institutional care.

Indications and rationale for parenteral nutrition

Parenteral nutrition is the intravenous infusion of essential nutrients into patients who are unable to maintain an adequate nutritional intake by the oral or nasogastric route (Burnham 1999). *It may be indicated for anyone who is unable to ingest, digest or absorb sufficient oral or enteral feeding,* for example:

- patients who have had surgery involving major resection of the intestine as they will have a reduced ability to digest food
- patients who have extensive inflammatory disease of the alimentary system as inflammation of the gut reduces the efficiency of the digestive process
- patients who have malabsorption problems because, despite a reasonable intake, an inadequate amount of nutrients will be absorbed and be available for the cells
- patients who have severe nausea and vomiting, e.g. following chemotherapy for malignant disease. The appetite is reduced, and food will not remain in the stomach long enough for digestion to occur.

'Total parenteral nutrition' (TPN) is the term used when all the patient's nutritional requirements are given by intravenous infusion. Parenteral nutrition may also be given as a supplement to nasogastric or oral feeding (Zainal 1994).

Outline of the procedure

This procedure should be performed ideally in the operating theatre. If it is performed in the ward, it should take place in the treatment room.

The insertion of the intravenous catheter for the infusion of parenteral nutrition is performed by a medical practitioner using an aseptic technique. A cap and theatre mask are worn. Having washed his or her hands, the medical practitioner dons a theatre gown and gloves, and prepares the sterile equipment on the trolley, maintaining asepsis. When the patient is in the correct position, sterile drapes are placed round the area of the access site. A local anaesthetic may be administered. The skin area of the access site is cleansed prior to the insertion of an intravenous catheter through the subclavian or internal jugular vein to allow the tip of the catheter to lie in the superior vena cava. A flow of prescribed infusion fluid is established, and the distal end of the catheter is stitched in position. The access site is covered with a sterile dressing.

A catheter will occasionally be tunnelled subcutaneously so that the entry site to the vein is separated from the skin entry site; this will reduce the risk of infection. It is performed when long-term parenteral nutrition is envisaged (RCN 1992).

The concentration of the nutrients is irritant to peripheral vessels and could cause damage to peripheral veins, so parenteral nutrition should always be infused through a central venous catheter. The infusion fluid enters the circulation at the superior vena cava, is rapidly diluted by the volume of blood entering the heart and is quickly distributed by the circulation, thus reducing any problems of irritation of the vessels involved (Springett & Murray 1994).

The position of the patient is important during this procedure and depends on the choice of entry site for catheterisation. There are three main entry sites.

The subclavian vein   The patient lies supine with no pillow, the neck being extended. The head of the bed is lowered by 10°.

The internal jugular vein   The patient lies supine with no pillow, and the neck is extended. The head is rotated away from the site of entry and is well supported in position. The head of the bed is lowered by 10°. This position is important to prevent the development of an air embolus.

The median cephalic vein   The patient lies supine. The chosen arm is extended with the palm upwards and the elbow supported. Peripherally inserted central catheters, introduced via the cephalic or basilic vein, are increasingly being used as technology advances (Gabriel 1994).

Equipment

As for intravenous infusion (*see* p. 181).

Additional equipment

Theatre cap and mask
Sterile gown
Sterile gloves
Sterile minor operation pack or sterile drape and towels
Waterproof protection for the bed
Alcohol-based lotion for cleansing the skin
Prescribed infusion fluid for parenteral nutrition
An appropriate sterile catheter depending on the site of entry used,
    e.g. a Hickman catheter or double- or triple-lumen catheter

Sterile needles and black silk sutures
ECG monitoring equipment if required
Volumetric infusion pump
Cassette for priming the infusion pump or a specialised infusion set
Dark bag for excluding light from the prepared infusion fluid.

Infusion fluid for parenteral nutrition

This will be prescribed by the medical practitioner for each 24 hour period as to the patient's nutritional needs and related blood chemistry. A combination of nutrients will be used to give a balanced intake, and vitamins and trace elements will be included in the prescription (Gobbi & Torrance 2000).

In areas where pharmacy services are available, the intravenous feeding regime is prepared as prescribed for each patient in 2 or 3 L bags under laminar flow conditions every 24 hours. Everything for parenteral nutrition, including vitamins and trace elements, is added individually. This reduces the risk of infection that might occur when an infusion of several different fluids in separate containers were prescribed; a series of taps, or Y-connectors, are thus needed for the infusion.

A combination of the following intravenous fluids may be prescribed. All are usually available in 500 ml containers (see the current pharmaceutical literature) (*British National Formulary*):

- carbohydrates, e.g. dextrose 20%
- fats, e.g. Intralipid 10% or 20%
- proteins, e.g. Vamin 14 EF, Vamin 18 EF.

Many other products are available, the choice depending on the patient's needs and the medical practitioner's preference.

The following may also be added:

- vitamins, e.g. Multibionta. Some vitamins are destroyed by sunlight so if these are added to a 24 hour parenteral infusion, the container must be covered by a dark bag to exclude light
- electrolytes, e.g. potassium and phosphates
- trace elements, e.g. zinc and magnesium.

Hickman catheter

A Hickman intravenous catheter may be chosen by the medical practitioner for a parenteral infusion that is needed over a period of weeks. This radio-opaque silastic catheter has a small sponge-like Dacron cuff at its distal end. The line is tunnelled subcutaneously, the cuff helping to retain the line in position as fibrous tissue forms round it. Patients may go home with this catheter in situ and become proficient in self-care under the supervision of the primary health-care team (Corbett et al 1993). Patients will require extensive training in the care and maintenance of parenteral nutrition, the British Association for Enteral and Parenteral Nutrition (1994a) suggesting that this should be provided only in specialised centres where a co-ordinated multidisciplinary service is available (BAPEN 1994b).

The Hickman catheter is also used for infusions of intravenous cytotoxic medication that are prescribed over a long period and are not suitable for a peripheral infusion because of their irritant properties.

Volumetric infusion pumps

Parenteral nutrition should be infused using a continuous volumetric infusion pump. This ensures that a steady flow of prescribed nutrients is infused at a rate suitable for the patient's metabolism. If a pump is unavailable, a burette administration set should be used. Infusion pumps are primed with a special cassette and introduced into the infusion circuit between the administration set from the infusion fluid and the infusion catheter. There are clear manufacturer's instructions for all infusion pumps, which should be followed when setting up infusions.

Infusion pumps can be set to give an hourly flow rate of between 1 and 999 ml per hour. All pumps are fitted with alarm systems that monitor for any occlusion of the lines, air bubbles and completion of the available fluid. Recent equipment has a digital readout of details of the infusion and the alarm system. New equipment for the controlled administration of intravenous infusion is continually being developed. There are different types of infusion pump and gravity-feed infusion set on the market, and the choice of use may depend on health authority policy.

Guidelines and rationale for this nursing practice

- help to explain the procedure to the patient *to gain consent and co-operation, and to encourage participation in care* (Hamilton 1993)
- ensure the patient's privacy, respecting *individuality and maintaining self-esteem*
- collect and prepare the equipment *for efficiency of practice*
- check the prescribed intravenous fluid for parenteral nutrition (*see* 'Administration of medicines', p. 1)
- wash hands *to reduce cross-infection* (Horton 1995)
- prime the equipment (*see* 'Intravenous infusion', p. 187)
- help the patient into the appropriate position, depending on the site of entry used for the insertion of the central venous catheter, *so that optimum safety is maintained for the patient*
- observe the patient throughout this activity *to monitor any adverse effects*. The central line enters the large veins adjacent to the heart and may occasionally cause arrhythmias so monitoring the patient's ECG may be helpful
- adjust the tilt of the bed to lower the patient's head if necessary in order *to minimise the risk of an air embolus*
- remain with the patient and help to maintain his or her position. Reassurance will be needed *as the patient may find this part frightening*
- assist the medical practitioner as required *to ensure a safe outcome for this practice*
- commence the infusion of parenteral nutrition at the prescribed rate once the catheter is in position and the sterile dressing has been applied to the access site

- cover the infusion with a dark bag *to protect any vitamins from light, which may cause their deterioration*
- ensure that the patient is left feeling as comfortable as possible. The patient should ideally have a period of rest after this nursing practice *to reduce anxiety and stress*
- dial the required number of millilitres per hour on the infusion pump (see the manufacturer's instructions), or fill the burette chamber hourly with the prescribed volume of fluid, *to maintain the infusion as prescribed*
- dispose of the equipment safely *to maintain a safe environment*
- document the nursing practice appropriately, monitor the after-effects and report any abnormal findings immediately. *This ensures safe practice and enables prompt and appropriate medical and nursing intervention to be initiated*
- in undertaking this practice, nurses are accountable for their actions, the quality of care delivered and record-keeping according to the *Code of Professional Conduct* (UKCC 1992), *Guidelines for Professional Practice* (UKCC 1996) and *Guidelines for Records and Record Keeping* (UKCC 1998).

Relevance to the activities of living

Observations and further rationale for this nursing practice will be included within each activity of living as appropriate.

Maintaining a safe environment

All precautions and observations for the prevention of infection should be maintained. The whole infusion and the administration set should be changed every 24 hours, maintaining asepsis.

The lines should be observed for air bubbles, the connections being regularly checked and the lines supported to prevent any disconnection, thus helping to avoid the development of an air embolus. The alarm systems of the infusion pumps should be familiar to the staff using the equipment, and appropriate action should be taken when they are activated.

The nurse should ensure that the catheter site is dressed using an aseptic technique (*see* p. 407) and that interventions are conducted in the knowledge of recent research on this invasive procedure (Roberts 1994).

The nurse may help with patient education in maintaining a safe environment. Learning an aseptic technique of wound cleaning and dressing will allow some independence for patients discharged home with long-term TPN (Stillwell 1992) (*see* 'Hickman catheter', p. 191).

Breathing

Respiration should be observed, and all the vital signs recorded 4 hourly or as frequently as is necessary. Breathlessness accompanied by a moist cough and frothy sputum may indicate pulmonary oedema caused by circulatory overload. Any abnormality should be reported so that the rate of the prescribed infusion can be adjusted (*see* 'Intravenous therapy', p. 181).

A rare complication is the development of a pneumothorax; this is more likely to occur at the time of insertion of the catheter. Any sudden change in the patient's general condition or respiratory function should be reported immediately.

Eating and drinking

Accurate fluid balance recordings should be maintained. Fluid intake should be recorded as frequently as necessary – hourly, 2 hourly or 4 hourly – depending on the patient's condition. Details of the intravenous nutrients infused should be recorded accurately and any adverse effects reported.

The patient's blood sugar level may initially be monitored regularly while parenteral nutrition is in progress, the result indicating the patient's ability to metabolise the nutrients infused. Blood glucose estimation (*see* p. 39) should be performed 4 hourly or as ordered. A continuous infusion of insulin is occasionally prescribed for patients who need a large calorie intake but whose metabolism is temporarily deficient. This may occur when a patient has suffered severe trauma, burns or scalds.

A patient receiving parenteral nutrition has little or nothing to eat or drink by mouth so frequent oral hygiene should be performed to maintain a healthy oral mucosa until a normal diet is resumed. With appropriate health education, patients receiving long-term TPN may be helped to become independent in keeping their oral mucosa healthy.

Eliminating

Fluid output should be recorded to maintain accurate fluid balance charts and help to monitor renal function.

The patient may need help when using a commode in order to support the infusion lines and prevent any disconnection.

Personal cleansing and dressing

Light, comfortable clothing will allow access to the infusion site; the reason for this should be explained to the patient. Help may be needed with washing and showering. Some patients may be discharged home with TPN, support being given by carers and the district nurse.

Expressing sexuality

A continuous infusion and a long-term central line will result in an altered body image, but perceptive and supportive nursing care and good communication skills will help to alleviate the effects of this.

At home, the adaptation of normal clothes, as well as counselling and help from the primary health-care team, will enable normal activities to resume as far as possible, restoring the patient's self-esteem.

Mobilising

In some instances, parenteral nutrition may continue when patients are up and about in the ward, and staff can help them to take their infusion with them. A light mobile pole and supportive explanations in relation to maintaining a safe environment will give the patient confidence to be more independent and visit other patients or the television room as his or her condition allows. Patients are occasionally discharged home while still receiving parenteral nutrition; with supervision and counselling from the primary health-care team, they can resume many normal activities.

Sleeping

The normal sleeping posture may have to be adapted to accommodate the infusion lines, and the patient should be helped into a comfortable position.

Patients receiving long-term home TPN may choose the times of their nutritional infusion period. TPN may be given overnight so that a more normal lifestyle can be resumed during the day.

Patient/carer education: key points

In partnership with the patient and/or carer, ensure that they are competent to carry out any practices required. Information should be given on an appropriate point of contact for any concerns that may arise.

Explanations given before, during and after the line has been inserted, as well as the rationale for continuing parenteral nutrition, will help the patient to understand and interpret the condition and its treatment. The nurse should be sensitive to the timing and relevance of the information for each stage of this practice.

The community team will help to encourage the independence of the person receiving TPN at home. This will include teaching the relevant aspects of:

- aseptic technique
- care of the central venous catheter
- observation of the site
- preparation of the intravenous feed
- use of the volumetric infusion pump
- mouth care.

Patients requiring long-term care should understand the importance of reporting redness, swelling or pain at the catheter site or any feeling of being generally unwell. Their independence may be increased if they are taught the principles of blood glucose monitoring.

Patient education should be part of the discharge planning and should commence well before the patient goes home. It is helpful to have a liaison nurse working between the community and the institution, written information in the form of an education leaflet reinforcing the patient's and carer's knowledge and confidence.

A contact telephone number to use as a 'help-line' will improve the patient's confidence and independence.

References

Association of Community Health Councils for England and Wales 1997 Hungry in hospital. ACHC, London

British Association for Parenteral and Enteral Nutrition 1994a Enteral and parenteral nutrition in the community. BAPEN, Maidenhead

British Association for Parenteral and Enteral Nutrition 1994b Organisation of nutritional support in hospitals. BAPEN, Maidenhead

British Association for Parenteral and Enteral Nutrition 1996 Standards and guidelines for nutritional support of patients in hospital. BAPEN, Maidenhead

British Association for Parenteral and Enteral Nutrition 1999 Current perspectives on enteral nutrition in adults. BAPEN, Maidenhead

British National Formulary (current edition) British Medical Association and Royal Pharmaceutical Society of Great Britain, London

Burnham W 1999 Parenteral nutrition. In: Dougherty L, Lamb J (eds) Intravenous therapy in nursing practice. Churchill Livingstone, Edinburgh

Caroline Walker Trust 1995 Eating well for older people. CWT, London

Colagiovanni L 1999 Nutrition: taking the tube. Nursing Times 95(21): 63–64, 67, 71

Colagiovanni L 2000 Preventing and clearing blocked feeding tubes. Nursing Times 96 (17 suppl): 3–4

Corbett K, Meehan L, Sackey V 1993 A strategy to enhance skills. Developing intravenous skills for community nursing. Professional Nurse 9(1): 60–63

Dennis M 2000 Nutrition after stroke. British Medical Bulletin 56(2): 466–475

Gabriel J 1994 An intravenous alternative. Nursing Times 90(31): 39–41

Gobbi M, Torrance G 2000 Nutrition. In: Alexander M, Fawcett J, Runciman P (eds) Nursing practice – hospital and home: the adult. Churchill Livingstone, Edinburgh

Hamilton H 1993 Care improves, while costs reduce. The clinical nurse specialist in total parenteral nutrition. Professional Nurse 8(9): 592–596

Holmes S 1996 Percutaneous endoscopic gastrostomy: a review. Nursing Times 92(17): 34–35

Holmes S 1998 Food for thought. Nursing Standard 12(46): 23–27

Horton R 1995 Handwashing: the fundamental infection control principle. British Journal of Nursing 4(16): 926–933

McGillvary T, Marland GR 1999 Assisting demented patients with feeding problems in a ward environment. A review of the literature. Journal of Advanced Nursing 29(3): 608–614

Mallett J, Dougherty L (eds) 2000 Royal Marsden manual of clinical nursing procedures. 5th edn. Blackwell Science, Oxford

Murray A 2000 Enteral tube feeding: helping to provide nutritional support. Community Nurse (May): 13–17

Naysmith NR, Nicholson J 1998 Nasogastric drug administration. Professional Nurse 13(7): 424

Nicol M, Bavin C, Bedford-Turner S, Cronin P, Rawlings-Anderson K 2000 Essential nursing skills. CV Mosby, London

Reeves J, Cubbs H 2000 Caring for people with PEG in the community. Community Nurse (March): 21–22

Roberts P 1994 Simply a case of good practice. Professional Nurse 8(12): 775–779

Royal College of Nursing 1992 Skin tunnelled catheters. Guidelines for care. RCN, London

Sampson H 2000 Food anaphylaxis. British Medical Bulletin 56(4): 925–935

Smith L, Baker F, Stead L, Soulsby C 1999 Feeding via a nasogastric tube. Nursing Times 95(8 suppl): 1–2

Springett J, Murray C 1994 Direct input. Nursing Times 90(17): 48–52

Stillwell B 1992 Skills update: central venous lines (using Hickman lines). Community Outlook 2(5): 22–23

United Kingdom Central Council for Nursing, Midwifery and Health Visiting 1992 Code of professional conduct. UKCC, London

United Kingdom Central Council for Nursing, Midwifery and Health Visiting 1996 Guidelines for professional practice. UKCC, London

United Kingdom Central Council for Nursing, Midwifery and Health Visiting 1998 Guidelines for records and record keeping. UKCC, London

Wood S 1999 Nutrition in the ward. Nursing Times 95(11): 54–55

Woods S 1998 Use of enteral and parenteral feeding. Professional Nurse 14(1): 44–46

Woolfrey S, Geddes A, Hussain A, Cox J 1997 Percutaneous endoscopic gastrostomy. Pharmaceutical Journal 257: 181–184

Zainal G 1994 Nutrition of critically ill people. Intensive and Critical Care Nursing 10(3): 165–169

34 Oxygen Therapy

Learning outcomes	By the end of this section, you should know how to: ■ prepare the patient for this nursing practice ■ collect and prepare the equipment ■ administer oxygen therapy at home or in an institutional setting.

Background knowledge required	Revision of the anatomy and physiology of the cardiopulmonary system, with special reference to the exchange of gases and the mechanism of respiration Revision of the dangers of the use of oxygen Review of health authority policies regarding fire precautions and oxygen therapy, in both institutional and community care.

Indications and rationale for oxygen therapy	Oxygen therapy is the introduction of increased oxygen to the air available for respiration *to prevent hypoxia,* a condition in which insufficient oxygen is available for the cells of the body, especially those in the brain and vital organs (Armstrong 2000). Hypoxia may occur in the following circumstances:

- respiratory disease in which the area available for respiration is reduced by, for example:
  — infection
  — chronic conditions such as chronic obstructive airways disease (COAD) and carcinoma
  — pulmonary infarction or embolus
  — asthma
- chest injuries following trauma, when the mechanism of respiration may be impaired
- heart disease, when the cardiac output is reduced by, for example:
  — myocardial infarction
  — congestive cardiac failure
- haemorrhage, reducing the oxygen-carrying capacity of the blood
- preoperatively and postoperatively when analgesic drugs, e.g. narcotics, may have an effect on respiratory function
- in emergency situations, e.g. cardiac or respiratory arrest and cardiogenic, bacteraemic or haemorrhagic shock, as the cardiac output will fall, reducing the amount of oxygenated blood available to the vital organs
- head or spinal injuries.

Except in emergency situations, oxygen therapy will be prescribed by a medical practitioner, who will specify both the percentage of oxygen and the method of administration. The administration of oxygen is one of the specific medical treatments: patients will have individually assessed requirements related to their particular medical problem (*British National Formulary*).

Oxygen therapy can be administered in the patient's own home under the care of the community nurse or in an institutional setting, but the principles underlying this nursing practice remain the same wherever it takes place. At home, the oxygen cylinder and its associated equipment will be delivered regularly to the patient's home from a central supply, depending on policy of the individual health board, as prescribed and ordered by the general practitioner. Alternatively, oxygen may be administered via an oxygen concentrator, which is an effective and economical way to deliver therapy to a patient who requires long-term intervention (*British National Formulary*). Guidelines on the monitoring of patients outside institutional settings is provided by the Royal College of Physicians (1999).

Equipment

Oxygen supply, e.g. piped oxygen or oxygen cylinder
Oxygen concentrator (for use in the community)
Reduction gauge as required
Flow meter
Oxygen mask or nasal cannulae as appropriate
Oxygen tubing
Humidifier as appropriate
'No Smoking' signs
Receptacle for soiled disposable items.

Oxygen masks

Oxygen masks are designed to provide an accurate percentage of oxygen by entraining an appropriate amount of air for a specific flow rate of oxygen (Place 1997). Instructions are available for each type of mask and these should be used accordingly (Bambridge 1993).

Edinburgh mask   The percentage of oxygen is adjusted solely by the flow rate of the flow meter.

Hudson mask and Venturi mask   With these masks, there are various attachments that can be used to give a more specific percentage of oxygen if one has been prescribed (Fig. 34.1). The required flow of oxygen for the prescribed percentage is given for each attachment, which may be colour coded.

Nasal cannulae

These are light plastic tubes inserted into each nostril and shaped to fit over the ears to maintain their position (Fig. 34.2). Patients find them less claustrophobic than a conventional mask, but they are not suitable for all patients as lower oxygen percentages are not accurately obtained and, at higher percentages, humidification is inadequate.

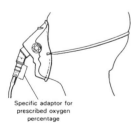

Specific adaptor for
prescribed oxygen
percentage

Figure 34.1 *Oxygen therapy: mask in position*

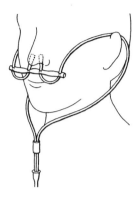

Figure 34.2 *Oxygen therapy: nasal cannulae in position*

T-piece

Oxygen may be delivered directly into an endotracheal tube or tracheostomy tube via wide corrugated tubing and a T-piece. Adequate humidification is essential here.

Oxygen tents

These are used mainly in paediatrics, when babies and young children would not tolerate masks. The danger of fire is increased further using this method, because of the larger area of concentration of oxygen within the oxygen tent, and the difficulty of confining the gas to a small area when nursing the patient.

Emergency situations

For emergency resuscitation procedures, oxygen may be administered via an Ambubag and resuscitation mask for a higher percentage of oxygen to be given with assisted ventilation (*see* 'Cardiopulmonary resuscitation', p. 79).

Humidifiers

It is important that the oxygen administered is adequately humidified to prevent drying of the mucosa of the respiratory tract. Various humidifiers are available. When percentages of oxygen above 35% are prescribed, humidifiers that nebulise and warm the water vapour should be used to help to maintain a healthy bronchial mucosa.

Humidifier bottles should be changed according to local policy or manufacturer's instructions (Sheppard & Davis 2000).

Guidelines and rationale for this nursing practice

- identify and check the prescription for oxygen therapy *to ensure that the correct percentage is administered* (Baxter et al 1993)
- explain the nursing practice to the patient *to gain consent and co-operation, and encourage participation in care*
- explain the dangers of smoking to the patient, family and friends, and display appropriate 'No Smoking' signs, *making sure that all understand the increased risk of fire when oxygen is administered*
- at home, hang the notice on the oxygen cylinder, *as a reminder for all the family and visitors*
- collect and assemble the equipment as required *so that everything is at hand*
- help the patient into a comfortable position *so that he or she will tolerate the oxygen therapy without distress*
- observe the patient throughout this activity *to monitor any adverse effects as well as any improvement in respiratory function*
- fill the humidifier with sterile water to the correct level *so that there is efficient humidification of the inspired oxygen*
- adjust the flow rate of oxygen as prescribed *so that the correct percentage is administered* (Bell 1995)

- observe the flow of oxygen and water vapour through the mask or cannulae before administration *to check that the equipment is working efficiently*
- place the mask in the correct position, and adjust it to fit firmly and comfortably over the patient's nose and mouth (*see* Fig. 34.1 above) *so that all the oxygen prescribed is administered and as little as possible escapes from the mask*
- remain with the patient as necessary *and help him or her to keep the equipment in position*
- top up the level of water in the humidifier as required *to maintain humidification*
- check the oxygen tubing regularly for any build up of condensation, *which may reduce the flow* (Sheppard & Davis 2000)
- assist the medical practitioner with the estimation of arterial blood gases as required *to evaluate the efficiency of the treatment*
- monitor the saturation levels using pulse oximetry if required *to evaluate the effect of the oxygen administered* (Jones 1995)
- observe all fire precautions *to minimise the risk of fire throughout the practice while oxygen is being used*
- ensure that the patient is left feeling as comfortable as possible *so that he or she will continue to tolerate the oxygen therapy* (Ashurst 1995)
- dispose of the equipment safely *to prevent any transmission of infection*
- document the nursing practice appropriately, monitor the after-effects and report any abnormal findings immediately, *ensuring safe practice and enabling prompt appropriate medical and nursing intervention to be initiated as soon as possible*
- in undertaking this practice, nurses are accountable for their actions, the quality of care delivered and record-keeping according to the *Code of Professional Conduct* (UKCC 1992), *Guidelines for Professional Practice* (UKCC 1996) and *Guidelines for Records and Record Keeping* (UKCC 1998).

Pulse oximetry

It is possible to measure the oxygen saturation level (SaO_2) by a non-invasive technique. An electronic device called a pulse oximeter measures the absorption of red and infrared light passing through living tissue. The equipment is normally a specialised, sensitive electronic clip that fits comfortably on a finger, a toe or an earlobe (Fig. 34.3), the result being recorded on the patient's electronic monitor. The oximeter reading responds closely to the arterial blood gas level, so fewer blood samples are needed for monitoring the arterial blood oxygen level. The fact that a continuous readout of the level can be observed helps to evaluate the effect of oxygen therapy and, being non-invasive, aids maintaining a safe environment for both patient and staff (Coull 1992).

Arterial blood gas estimation

In intensive care areas and accident and emergency units, and during perioperative care, the effectiveness of oxygen therapy may be monitored by the medical practitioner assessing the arterial blood gases. The results are recorded

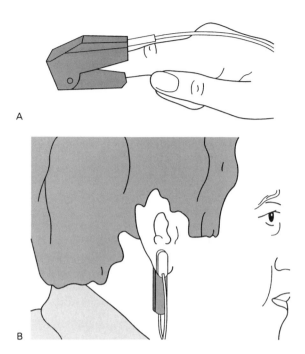

Figure 34.3 *Oxygen therapy: pulse oximeter*
A *Hand sensor*
B *Earlobe sensor*

in relation to the percentage of oxygen administered, changes in the percentage of oxygen or method of administration being made accordingly. Samples of arterial blood are usually obtained from the radial artery, either from an indwelling arterial cannula or by individual sampling, performed by the medical practitioner. The nurse should maintain observations of the arterial puncture site. There is less need for this type of assessment now that pulse oximetry is available (Stoneham et al 1994).

Relevance to the activities of living

Observations on and further rationale for this nursing practice will be included within each activity of living as appropriate.

Maintaining a safe environment

The patient's general condition should be observed to identify any deterioration or improvement in the hypoxic state, for example degree of drowsiness, level of orientation or level of consciousness. The colour and condition of the patient's skin should be observed for cyanosis, clamminess or sweating.

Oxygen is a gas that readily supports combustion, so in areas where it is used, the risk of fire is greatly increased. Every precaution to prevent fire should be taken. The patient should, if possible, be aware of the problem and help in maintaining a safe environment. The dangers of smoking should be explained to the patient, family and visitors. 'No Smoking' signs can help to reinforce this precaution. Health authority policy on fire precautions should be familiar to all staff and carers.

Alcohol-based solutions, oils and grease should not be used in areas where oxygen is being administered as these volatile substances are readily flammable and the presence of oxygen increases the risk of fire. All such precautions should also be part of patient education when therapy is being administered in a community setting, involving all the family and the associated carers as well.

The administration of oxygen does not require an aseptic technique, but an adequate level of cleanliness should be maintained to prevent cross-infection, and equipment should be replaced as necessary. The nurse should wash his or her hands before commencing and on completing this nursing practice, and when handling body fluids such as sputum.

Communicating

Oxygen masks can be a barrier to communication by making it more difficult for the patient to speak and be heard, so there is a risk of misunderstanding (Place 1997). This may cause the patient to remove the mask so the nurse needs good communication skills to help the patient tolerate the procedure while it is necessary. The use of closed (direct) questions, to which only a 'yes' or 'no' answer is needed, may be of help.

Breathing

A need for oxygen therapy usually indicates that the patient has some difficulty with breathing. This dyspnoea may be relieved by helping the patient into an appropriate and comfortable position as the condition allows, for example sitting upright, leaning over a bed table supported on a pillow, or sitting in a chair.

The respiration rate should be recorded as frequently as necessary, noting the type and depth of the respirations (Kendrick & Smith 1992).

Patients who have bronchospasm can be helped by medications that induce bronchodilation, either systemically or via a nebuliser as prescribed (see 'Nebuliser therapy', p. 241).

Patients who have COAD have permanently altered respiratory physiology. The respiratory drive or stimulus for respiration responds only to a low arterial blood level of oxygen so only low percentages of oxygen, for example 24–28%, should be prescribed and administered; raising the arterial blood oxygen level too high in these patients could cause respiratory arrest. It is important that the patient and family understand the importance of not altering the prescribed flow rate and the danger of increasing the amount of oxygen administered.

Eating and drinking

The removal of the mask for drinking should be supervised by the nurse and will depend on the patient's condition. It may be possible to change to nasal cannulae at mealtimes, using a mask at other times to maintain the accuracy of the oxygen percentage being administered.

Oxygen, even when adequately humidified, causes the mouth and nasal passages to become dry. Frequent oral and nasal hygiene will therefore be required for the patient's comfort and to maintain a healthy oropharyngeal mucosa. Oral fluids should be encouraged as to counteract the drying effect on the mucosa (Sheppard & Davies 2000).

Personal cleansing and dressing

The patient may need help with both washing and dressing, depending on his or her condition.

The inside of the oxygen mask may become wet with condensation so the patient's face can be washed and the inside of the mask dried as appropriate. This will greatly increase the patient's comfort and tolerance of this nursing practice.

Expressing sexuality

The use of a face mask has an adverse effect on the patient's self-image so the nurse should use good communication skills to counteract this.

Male patients should be helped to shave daily as this enables the mask to fit comfortably, as well as preserving self-esteem; aftershave should not, however, be used as it is often alcohol based.

An explanation about the dangers of using perfume or make-up during this procedure should be given to female patients. Extra opportunities for washing and drying the face may help to alleviate the feeling of neglect of body image.

Patient/carer education: key points

In partnership with the patient and/or carer, ensure that they are competent to carry out any practices required. Information should be given on an appropriate point of contact for any concerns that may arise.

The reason for the administration of oxygen therapy should be explained to the patient and the family and carers involved. They should understand that it is a specific part of the treatment.

At home, the patient and carers should be shown how to adjust the flow rate to the prescribed rate only, how to fill the humidifier, maintaining a safe environment, and how to connect the mask and tubing. The procedure for changing oxygen cylinders or using an oxygen concentrator, and the personnel involved, will depend on health authority policy; carers may in some instances be instructed in this.

The increased risk of fire should be explained and simple instructions about fire precautions given. The danger of smoking when oxygen is used should be continually reinforced: patient and family co-operation is needed for this. They can choose where 'No Smoking' signs should be displayed.

For patients with COAD, everyone should understand the importance of never increasing the prescribed flow of oxygen delivered to the patient. This may need reinforcing if there is a change of carer in the community setting. The reason for this should be part of patient education.

The patient should understand the importance of immediately reporting any changes in respiratory function such as increased dyspnoea, cough, sputum or a general feeling of distress.

References

Armstrong DJ 2000 Shock. In: Alexander M, Fawcett J, Runciman P (eds) Nursing practice – hospital and home: the adult. Churchill Livingstone, Edinburgh

Ashurst S 1995 Oxygen therapy. British Journal of Nursing 4(9): 508–515

Bambridge A 1993 An audit of comfort and convenience of oxygen masks and nasal catheters in the provision of post operative oxygen therapy. Professional Nurse 8(8): 513–518

Baxter K, Nolan K, Winyard J, Goldhill D 1993 Are they getting enough? Meeting the oxygen therapy needs of post-operative patients. Professional Nurse 8(5): 310–312

Bell C 1995 Is this what the doctor ordered? Accuracy of oxygen therapy prescribed and delivered in hospital. Professional Nurse 10(5): 295–300

British National Formulary (current edition) Oxygen. London, British Medical Association and the Royal Pharmaceutical Society of Great Britain

Coull A 1992 Making sense of pulse oximetry. Nursing Times 88(32): 42–43

Jones S 1995 Getting the balance right. Pulse oximetry and inspired oxygen concentration. Professional Nurse 10(6): 368–372

Kendrick A, Smith E 1992 Respiratory measurements. 2. Simple measurements of lung function. Professional Nurse 7(1): 748–754

Place B 1997 The skill behind the mask. Nursing Times 93(26): 31–32

Royal College of Physicians 1999 Domiciliary oxygen therapy services: clinical guidelines and advice for prescribers. Royal College of Physicians, London

Sheppard M, Davis S 2000 Oxygen therapy. 2. Nursing Times 96(30): 43–44

Stoneham M, Saville G, Wilson I 1994 Knowledge about pulse oximetry among medical and nursing staff. Lancet 344: 1339–1342

United Kingdom Central Council for Nursing, Midwifery and Health Visiting 1992 Code of professional conduct. UKCC, London

United Kingdom Central Council for Nursing, Midwifery and Health Visiting 1996 Guidelines for professional practice. UKCC, London

United Kingdom Central Council for Nursing, Midwifery and Health Visiting 1998 Guidelines for records and record keeping. UKCC, London

35 Paracentesis: Abdominal

Learning outcomes	By the end of this section, you should know how to:
	• prepare the patient for this procedure • collect and prepare the equipment • assist the medical practitioner with abdominal paracentesis as required.

Background knowledge required	Revision of the anatomy and physiology of the abdominal organs, with special reference to the peritoneum Revision of 'Aseptic technique' (*see* p. 407).

Indications and rationale for abdominal paracentesis	Abdominal paracentesis is the removal of fluid from the peritoneal cavity through a sterile cannula or needle. Medication is sometimes introduced into the peritoneal cavity by the same route. The procedure may be performed for the following reasons:

- *to obtain a specimen of abdominal fluid for diagnostic purposes*
- *to relieve intra-abdominal pressure* caused by increased fluid within the abdominal cavity. This is called ascites and may occur in association with several conditions:
  — congestive cardiac failure involving dysfunction of the right side of the heart
  — chronic hepatic disease
  — malignant disease with metastases in the liver
- *to introduce medication into the peritoneal cavity*, e.g. cytotoxic therapy for malignant disease.

Outline of the procedure	Abdominal paracentesis is carried out by the medical practitioner using an aseptic technique. A mask and sterile gown, as well as sterile gloves, should be worn.

The site of insertion is midway between the umbilicus and the symphysis pubis along the midline. The skin is cleansed with antiseptic lotion and a local anaesthetic is administered, the area round the site being covered with sterile towels. A small skin incision is made with a sterile blade, and a trocar and cannula are inserted into the peritoneal cavity. The trocar is removed, allowing fluid to flow through the cannula. The specimens of abdominal fluid required for investigation are collected at this stage by holding the appropriately labelled sterile containers under the flow of fluid, maintaining asepsis. The cannula may be removed and a sterile dressing applied, or it may be stitched in position and attached to sterile tubing and a closed drainage bag if drainage is to be maintained. A suitable sterile dressing should be applied around the cannula.

The flow of drainage fluid is regulated with a gate clamp or roller clamp to prevent too rapid a reduction of intra-abdominal pressure. Initially, only 1 L of fluid should be allowed to drain, before regulating the flow to 100 ml per hour or as prescribed by the medical practitioner. This should prevent the patient developing symptoms of shock because of the sudden lessening of pressure in the abdominal cavity.

Equipment	Trolley Theatre mask Sterile gown Sterile gloves Sterile dressings pack Sterile towels Sterile bowl Sterile specimen containers, appropriately labelled, completed laboratory forms and a plastic specimen bag for transportation Antiseptic lotion Sterile abdominal paracentesis set containing: — a specialised trocar and cannula — forceps — a blade and holder — tubing Local anaesthetic and equipment for its administration Sterile sutures and a needle for stitching the cannula in position Sterile drainage bag Gate clip or roller clamp Disposable tape measure Measuring jug Receptacle for soiled disposable items.
Guidelines and rationale for this nursing practice	<ul><li>help to explain the procedure to the patient *to gain consent and co-operation, and encourage participation in care*</li><li>ask the patient to empty his or her bladder immediately prior to the procedure. This will ensure that the bladder remains within the pelvis, thus *preventing any risk of perforation when the trocar is inserted*</li><li>ensure the patient's privacy, *respecting individuality and maintaining self-esteem*</li><li>measure and record the patient's abdominal girth before commencing the procedure *to compare with measurements taken after abdominal paracentesis*</li><li>help to collect and prepare the equipment, *making good use of time and resources*</li></ul>

- help the patient into a suitable, comfortable position. He or she may sit upright with the back well supported. The legs should if possible be lowered *to allow easier access to the insertion site and to increase the patient's comfort.* A bed that can be adjusted to allow only the lower limbs to be lowered is the most suitable. In some instances, the medical practitioner may prefer the patient to lie flat. The position chosen depends on the reason for the abdominal paracentesis
- help to adjust the patient's clothing *to expose the site of insertion*
- observe the patient throughout this activity *to monitor any adverse effects*
- help to prepare the sterile field as required *to maintain asepsis*
- assist the medical practitioner as required during the procedure
- measure the amount of drainage and adjust the flow of drainage fluid as required *to ensure that the volume drawn does not cause a sudden reduction in intra-abdominal pressure.* Initially only 1 L of fluid should be removed, then regulating the flow to 50–150 ml per hour as prescribed
- ensure that the patient is left feeling as comfortable as possible in a sitting position *so that drainage is encouraged*
- dispose of equipment safely *to prevent the transmission of infection*
- dispatch labelled specimens of abdominal fluid to the appropriate laboratory with their completed forms immediately *so that investigations can be commenced as soon as possible*
- document the procedure appropriately, monitor the after-effects and report any abnormal findings immediately *to ensure safe practice and enable prompt, appropriate medical and nursing intervention to be initiated*
- in undertaking this practice, nurses are accountable for their actions, the quality of care delivered and record-keeping according to the *Code of Professional Conduct* (UKCC 1992), *Guidelines for Professional Practice* (UKCC 1996) and *Guidelines for Records and Record Keeping* (UKCC 1998).

Relevance to the activities of living

Observations on and further rationale for this nursing practice will be included within each activity of living as appropriate.

Maintaining a safe environment

This is an invasive procedure giving direct access to the peritoneal cavity so all precautions to minimise the risk of infection should be taken. Asepsis should be maintained, and an adequate handwashing technique should be practised.

After the procedure, the site should be observed for any redness or swelling, which may indicate infection; this should be reported immediately. Dressings should be changed as required, using an aseptic technique (*see* 'Wound care', p. 405).

Any leakage of fluid round the cannula should be noted and reported as this may indicate that the cannula is blocked or has become dislodged.

The safety of staff transporting specimens should be maintained by enclosing the containers in plastic specimen bags (*see* 'Specimen collection', p. 317).

Communicating

Patients do not normally find this procedure too uncomfortable, even during a period of continuous drainage. When the abdominal paracentesis is performed to relieve pressure caused by excess fluid in the peritoneal cavity, the patient is usually much more comfortable after the procedure has been performed. A prescribed analgesic medication should be administered if required.

Breathing

Following this procedure, the patient's blood pressure, pulse and respiration rate should be recorded 4 hourly for 24–48 hours. The frequency of recording will depend on the patient's condition and the reason for the abdominal paracentesis.

When a patient has had severe ascites, with a raised intra-abdominal pressure, the blood pressure and pulse should be recorded every half hour for 2 hours immediately after this procedure as a sudden drop in intra-abdominal pressure can cause cardiogenic shock as a result of rapid vasodilatation. A low blood pressure recording should be reported immediately, and the rate of flow of the drainage fluid should be reduced to a minimum.

Initially only 1 L of fluid should be removed before regulating the flow as prescribed by the medical practitioner. This may be 50–150 ml per hour, depending on the patient's condition.

Eating and drinking

The fluid intake should be recorded and accurate fluid balance charts maintained. This will enable any reduction or increase in the volume of peritoneal fluid to be monitored in relation to fluid intake and urinary output.

The patient's appetite may have been poor because of the feeling of fullness and discomfort caused by the ascites; patients often experience indigestion as a result of pressure on the stomach. Depending on the situation, they may have to be encouraged to eat following this procedure in order to make up the protein that has been lost with the peritoneal fluid. Advice from the dietitian may help with the choice of nourishing foods, and the family may be encouraged to help provide favourite treats if appropriate.

Eliminating

The colour and viscosity of the peritoneal fluid should be noted. The presence of blood should be noted and reported as it may indicate trauma to the abdominal organs during the insertion of the trocar.

The amount of fluid drained should be accurately measured and recorded, and fluid balance charts should be maintained throughout this procedure. Appropriate arrangements for measuring urinary output should be made, with the patient's co-operation. The patient may be helped to the toilet, or to use a commode, depending on his or her condition.

Fluids and electrolytes pass across the peritoneal membrane so electrolytes may also be lost in the drained ascitic fluid. This may cause hypokalaemia (a low potassium level) or hyponatraemia (a low sodium level). The medical practitioner will monitor the patient's blood chemistry and prescribe replacement potassium and sodium as required. A loss of protein, often present in ascitic fluid, may also be a concern.

The drainage of a large amount of excess peritoneal fluid is not routinely performed as the fluid will reform from the circulation unless the cause itself can be treated. Volumes sufficient to relieve distressing pressure and associated symptoms can be removed without causing problems. When ascites is caused by abdominal metastases, the patient may gain some relief from a continuous drainage of the excess peritoneal fluid; this will be prescribed as appropriate.

Measurement of the abdominal girth may help to monitor developing or improving ascites. The bladder should be emptied before the daily measurement, which should be taken at the same position each time. To facilitate accurate measurement, and with the patient's permission, lines may be drawn on each side of the abdomen outlining the path of the tape measure for 1 or 2 cm.

Personal cleansing and dressing

Depending on the patient's condition, he or she may be able to have a shower while this procedure is in progress; a waterproof dressing can be used to protect the cannula site.

The patient's clothes may have to be adapted to accommodate the cannula and drainage bag.

Controlling body temperature

Body temperature should be recorded 4 hourly during and after this procedure to monitor any change that might indicate a developing infection. Any abnormality should be reported immediately.

Mobilising

Immediately after this procedure, the patient should remain in bed to enable observations of his or her condition to be made. Mobilising may then be encouraged as the condition allows. Patients with a continuous drainage system may need help to maintain a safe environment when mobilising in order to prevent infection or disconnection of the tubing.

Expressing sexuality

The presence of an abdominal catheter will give the patient the feeling of an altered body image (Roper et al 2000). The nurse's attitude and communication skills, both verbal and non-verbal, can help the patient to accept this. The relief of abdominal pressure from excess ascites should, however, help the patient's acceptance.

Patient/carer education: key points

In partnership with the patient and/or carer, ensure that they are competent to carry out any practices required. Information should be given on an appropriate point of contact for any concerns that may arise.

Explain the reason for the procedure and the importance of the patient's position during the insertion of the catheter. Reassure the patient that he or she should feel more comfortable once some of the abdominal fluid has drained away.

If the catheter is to remain in situ for some time, explain how the patient can cope with toileting, personal cleansing and dressing, and outline the help he or she will be given with this.

The patient should understand the importance of reporting redness, swelling, pain or discomfort at the access site, even after the catheter has been removed.

References

Roper N, Logan W, Tierney A 2000 The Roper–Logan–Tierney model of nursing. Churchill Livingstone, Edinburgh

United Kingdom Central Council for Nursing, Midwifery and Health Visiting 1992 Code of professional conduct. UKCC, London

United Kingdom Central Council for Nursing, Midwifery and Health Visiting 1996 Guidelines for professional practice. UKCC, London

United Kingdom Central Council for Nursing, Midwifery and Health Visiting 1998 Guidelines for records and record keeping. UKCC, London

36 Preoperative Nursing Care

The guidelines in this nursing practice apply to both patients experiencing day surgery and those undergoing surgery that requires a longer stay in hospital.

Learning outcomes

By the end of this section, you should know how to:

- explain the standard preoperative preparation of a patient who is scheduled for surgery
- describe the nurse's role in looking after a patient prior to surgery.

Background knowledge required

Revision of the cardiopulmonary system
Review of health authority policy on the preoperative preparation of patients.

Indications and rationale for preoperative care

Preoperative nursing care is required *to promote the optimum physical and psychological condition of patients undergoing surgical procedures* (Scott et al 1999).

Guidelines and rationale for this nursing practice

- explain the pre- and postoperative routines to the patient and answer any questions appropriately; the discussion of any fears or anxieties that the patient may have should be encouraged. Studies have demonstrated that patients' *anxiety levels are reduced by receiving information and explanations*
- record the temperature, pulse, respiration rate, blood pressure and urinalysis results *to give baseline findings with which to compare postoperative observations*
- carry out an evacuation of the patient's bowel using suppositories or the specific bowel preparation requested by the surgeon. This is usually requested if the surgical procedure involves the bowel *as evacuation helps to reduce the risk of contamination of the wound by intestinal organisms*
- offer the sedative that was ordered by medical staff the night before surgery *in order to help the patient sleep well*
- fast the patient for 4–6 hours prior to surgery so that the stomach is empty *in order to avoid the risk of regurgitation and the inhalation of gastric contents while under the anaesthetic*
- prepare the skin according to health authority policy. This may involve the removal of an area of body hair by shaving or depilatory cream, showering or

bathing using an antiseptic soap, and putting on a theatre gown and perhaps socks and paper pants. These preparations are used *to reduce the risk of a postoperative infection*. Research into the removal of body hair and the use of antiseptic preparations in baths and showers has, however, produced contradictory findings

- ensure that all underwear has been removed, although paper pants may be worn on some occasions. Nail varnish should be removed from fingernails and toenails *so that they can be examined by the anaesthetist for signs of hypoxia*, and make-up should be removed for the same reason. Dentures must be removed *because of the danger of inhaling them, causing asphyxiation*. Health authority policies on the removal of spectacles, hair grips, contact lenses, hearing aids and other prostheses, e.g. wigs and artificial eyes or limbs, vary

- tape the wedding ring to the patient's finger. All other jewellery and valuables that the patient has brought into hospital should be recorded, put into an envelope, labelled appropriately and placed in a valuables box or safe. Pay special attention to any body piercing that patient may have. It may not be possible to remove some piercings, so these should be taped. Document on the preoperative assessment chart any body piercing, whether taped or untaped. Metal jewellery may be accidentally lost or may be a cause of harm to the patient, e.g. a diathermy burn

- check the patient's identification verbally and from the identification band, and confirm that the form of consent for the operation has been signed. This is done *to comply with legal requirements and hospital policy*

- after the patient has had the opportunity to micturate, administer the premedication ordered by the anaesthetist. Premedication can *help to relax the patient and may dry up any secretions*

- help the patient to put on anti-embolic stockings if these have been recommended. This is *to reduce the risk of deep vein thrombosis*

- leave the patient to rest quietly when the premedication has been given, but observe him or her for any reaction to the drugs. Request that the patient does not get out of bed unsupervised after the administration of premedication *to reduce the risk of falls when a sedative drug has been given*. Rest may also *encourage relaxation and maximise the effect of the premedication*. In day surgery units, premedication is often only offered to patients who appear to have a high anxiety level

- when the porter from the theatre reception area arrives to collect the patient, accompany them to the theatre reception area and hand the patient over to the care of a theatre nurse. There is usually a checklist that the ward nurse and theatre nurse complete. The patient may travel to theatre on a hospital bed or a theatre trolley, according to health authority policy. Ensure that all the relevant documentation, e.g. case notes, medicine prescription chart, X-rays, ECG tracings and reports, accompanies the patient to theatre. Research studies have demonstrated that a known person accompanying the patient *helps to reduce anxiety*. Appropriate relevant information should have been given to the relatives beforehand so that they can, with the patient's permission, telephone to check progress

- in undertaking this practice, nurses are accountable for their actions, the quality of care delivered and record-keeping according to the *Code of Professional Conduct* (UKCC 1992), *Guidelines for Professional Practice* (UKCC 1996) and *Guidelines for Records and Record Keeping* (UKCC 1998).

Relevance to the activities of living

Maintaining a safe environment

Preoperative skin care may vary, as individual surgeons have their own theories on any skin preparation necessary to minimise infection of the wound. Putting clean linen on the bed for the patient's return from theatre is another measure that helps to prevent infection.

It is essential that the patient is carefully identified to ensure that the correct patient has the correct operation. All patient identification must be clearly printed, legible and accurate, and contain all the details specified in the Trust's policies and protocols.

Patient safety while under the influence of premedication is the nurse's responsibility. It is also the nurse's responsibility to ensure that the patient's valuables are listed and safely stored.

Communicating

Information and explanations are an important part of the nurse's responsibility for patients in surgical wards. Research has shown that explanations prior to surgery can help to reduce the incidence of postoperative pain and complications. Information booklets are essential for all patients undergoing surgery. Patients should also be given time to formulate any questions. For patients experiencing day surgery, preadmission booklets are essential as much of the information given at the outpatient clinic may be forgotten or misunderstood by the patient.

A brief description of what to expect in the immediate postoperative period can often be reassuring to the patient, especially if equipment such as a urethral catheter, wound drain or intravenous infusion will be in use.

When the patient is being anaesthetised, hearing is the last sense to disappear so staff should ensure that the content of conversation in the vicinity of the patient will not increase his or her anxiety.

Breathing

The patient should be encouraged to stop smoking some time before surgery to enable the lung fields to be as clear as possible and lessen the susceptibility to pulmonary infection. Stopping smoking immediately before surgery may increase pulmonary secretions and increase the risk of a chest infection developing in the immediate postoperative period.

Breathing exercises should be explained to the patient. These consist of encouraging the patient to sit as upright as possible and to breathe in deeply through the nose, expanding the chest and abdominal wall as much as possible.

This allows a good inflation of the lungs. On exhaling, the chest and abdominal walls should be allowed to relax and then extra air pushed out of the lungs. The wound can be supported if necessary.

Eating and drinking

As mentioned above, the patient should be fasted for 4–6 hours prior to surgery to avoid the danger of inhaling the gastric contents while the cough reflex is suppressed during general anaesthesia. If this has not been possible, for example in an emergency admission, it may be necessary to pass a nasogastric tube and aspirate the stomach contents (*see* 'Gastric aspiration', p. 161).

It is especially important for day surgery patients to know the length of time they have to fast and the reasons for this.

Research has shown that prolonged periods of fasting reduce the blood glucose level to below normal range and also cause the patient to become dehydrated. This can impair the healing process and reduce the body's ability to cope with the trauma of surgery.

Eliminating

It is necessary for the patient to have an empty bladder and rectum, especially if muscle relaxing drugs are going to be used during surgery, because of the risk of contaminating the theatre table with excrement and the attendant risk of infecting the surgical wound. In addition, a full bladder is more liable to be damaged during abdominal surgery; in emergency surgery, the bladder may be catheterised to obviate this potential complication.

Patients undergoing day surgery may have to carry out the required bowel preparation at home if this is prescribed by the surgeon; nurses need to ensure that the patient knows how to use any suppositories or enema supplied for this purpose.

Personal cleansing and dressing

As mentioned above, special skin preparation may be required, although some research has shown that the bacterial skin count is lower when skin cleansing is carried out in theatre rather than some hours prior to surgery.

The discussion surrounding the removal of, and method of removal of, body hair from around the site of surgery is ongoing and unresolved.

Mobilising

The patient should receive some preoperative teaching about postoperative exercises to prevent such complications as pressure sores, deep venous thrombosis and chest infections. Nursing staff should ensure that the physiotherapist has visited the patient to give this teaching or, in the case of day surgery patients, that they have a knowledge of these exercises.

Patients considered to be at risk of developing a deep vein thrombosis may be fitted with anti-embolic stockings as a prophylactic measure. Preventive heparin therapy may be administered to patients who are considered to have a high risk of developing a deep vein thrombosis.

Expressing sexuality

Having to remove all their personal clothing, jewellery, make-up, nail varnish and dentures can make patients feel that their personality and personal dignity are under threat (Matiti & Sharman 1999). An explanation for these procedures should be given, together with an assurance that the patient's wishes regarding cleansing and dressing will be met as soon as possible after surgery. Cultural considerations related to removing underwear, headscarves and jewellery should be made (Roper et al 2000). With prior arrangement and consent, these may be taken off after the patient has been anaesthetised and replaced before he or she regains consciousness. This practice highlights true individualised care.

Sleeping

The patient's normal sleeping pattern may be disturbed by the unaccustomed noise of the ward, the change of environment or anxiety, and every possible means should be used to reduce or remove the cause of anxiety and promote comfort. Medication may be ordered to promote sleep on the night prior to surgery.

Dying

It is not uncommon for a patient to worry about dying while anaesthetised. The patient should be helped to verbalise and discuss this fear, and to realise that, with modern technology, such an occurrence is rare.

Many patients facing surgery benefit from attention to their spiritual needs from the hospital chaplain, who is a member of the caring team.

Patient/carer education: key points

In partnership with the patient and/or carer, ensure that they are competent to carry out any practices required. Information should be given on an appropriate point of contact for any concerns that may arise.

It is important that patients undergoing day surgery should have obtained beforehand all the information and knowledge necessary for them to undergo their surgery successfully. This will probably involve nurses at the outpatient clinic, in the community and in the day surgery unit. Written material should be provided to reinforce the verbal information given. Patients will need to carry out at home many of the preoperative preparations, such as bowel preparation, skin preparation and fasting.

References

Matiti M, Sharman J 1999 Dignity: a study of preoperative patients. Nursing Standard 14(13–15): 32–35
Roper N, Logan W, Tierney A 2000 The Roper–Logan–Tierney model of nursing. Churchill Livingstone, Edinburgh

Scott E et al 1999 Understanding perioperative nursing. Nursing Standard 13(49): 49

United Kingdom Central Council for Nursing, Midwifery and Health Visiting 1992 Code of professional conduct. UKCC, London

United Kingdom Central Council for Nursing, Midwifery and Health Visiting 1996 Guidelines for professional practice. UKCC, London

United Kingdom Central Council for Nursing, Midwifery and Health Visiting 1998 Guidelines for records and record keeping. UKCC, London

37   Postoperative Nursing Care

In the case of day surgery, many of the guidelines described here will be carried out by the community nurse, the patient or the carers at home.

Learning outcomes

By the end of this section, you should know how to:

- explain the general postoperative care of a patient
- describe the nurse's role in carrying out general postoperative care.

Background knowledge required

Revision of the clinical features of shock
Revision of the physiology of wound healing
Review of health authority policy on postoperative care.

Indications and rationale for postoperative care

Postoperative nursing care is required to monitor the patient's condition *in order to prevent and identify any problems that may occur after a surgical procedure.*

Guidelines and rationale for this nursing practice

When receiving the patient back into the ward

- check that the airway is patent and that the patient is breathing adequately. The patient is usually conscious before leaving the recovery room, but if he or she is heavily sedated, *the tongue may slip back and obstruct the airway, so this should be checked for*
- monitor oxygen saturation *to ensure adequate perfusion*
- record the temperature, pulse and blood pressure, and compare the results with the patient's preoperative recordings. *This will give some indication of the stability of the patient's condition*
- observe the wound and any drains, e.g. a Redivac or corrugated drain, that may be present *to ensure there are no problems such as haemorrhage*
- if an intravenous infusion is present, check that it is functioning according to medical staff instructions
- read the patient's theatre notes to confirm the surgical procedure that has been carried out and ascertain any instructions from the surgeon or anaesthetist, e.g. the positioning of the patient or any oxygen therapy required
- ensure that the patient is lying in as comfortable a position as possible and that the limbs are positioned in a manner that will not endanger muscle and nerve tissue. These measures can *help to control the level of pain*

- administer analgesics as required by the patient and as prescribed by the medical staff *to relieve pain and anxiety*: several research studies have demonstrated that patients rate being in pain as the most anxiety-provoking issue when undergoing surgery.

Continuing postoperative nursing

- record blood pressure, pulse and respiration rate until these are within the normal range and stable. *This usually indicates the reduction of physiological stress induced by the surgery*
- assist the patient to wash and change into his or her own nightwear and offer a mouthwash, *to aid comfort and the recovery of a sense of individuality*. If the patient has been wearing anti-embolic stockings, the continued benefit of these is to be emphasised
- encourage the patient to sit up in bed well supported by pillows (unless contraindicated) and move around as much as possible, helping him or her out of bed when the blood pressure recordings are satisfactory. These measures *help to minimise the risk of complications such as skin breakdown and deep venous thrombosis*
- unless contraindicated (e.g. by the presence of a nasogastric tube), allow a graduated amount of fluid; then gradually introduce solid food if there is no vomiting and if bowel sounds are present, *in order to rehydrate the patient and to help restore the blood glucose level to within the normal range*
- observe the wound regularly for leakage, bleeding or haematoma
- record the amount and time when the patient passes urine and has a first bowel movement *as constipation is a common postoperative problem because of immobility, dehydration and the use of narcotic analgesics*
- arrange an ongoing pain control assessment *to reduce unnecessary distress to the patient*
- ensure that the patient has adequate periods of rest *as this will aid recovery*
- give encouragement and support to the patient and any explanation or information that may be requested
- the breathing exercises described on page 287 should be encouraged *to help avoid the problems mentioned above*
- in undertaking this practice, nurses are accountable for their actions, the quality of care delivered and record-keeping according to the *Code of Professional Conduct* (UKCC 1992), *Guidelines for Professional Practice* (UKCC 1996) and *Guidelines for Records and Record Keeping* (UKCC 1998).

Relevance to the activities of living

Maintaining a safe environment

All precautions must be taken to prevent infection; for example, a strict aseptic technique should be used when carrying out wound care. An appropriate wound dressing that will promote an ideal healing environment should be prescribed.

While the patient is under the influence of anaesthesia and analgesics, safety is of prime importance and is a nursing responsibility.

Communicating

Hearing is one of the first senses to return after anaesthesia.

Adequate explanations, support and encouragement must be available to the patient at all times. Patient education on surgery and its after-effects must be well planned and carried out by an appropriately qualified memberof staff, preferably prior to surgery, being reinforced in the postoperative period (Coll et al 1999).

Pain control should be well planned and frequently evaluated (Nendick 2000).

Breathing

Chest infections and pulmonary embolism are potential problems for patients undergoing surgery; patient education prior to surgery about suitable exercises and deep breathing can help to prevent these.

The complication of haemorrhage should be detected by monitoring the wound, the pulse rate, the blood pressure and the patient's colour.

Eating and drinking

Fluid should be limited to 3 L for the first 24 hours after surgery because of the excess production of antidiuretic hormone as a result of surgery; thereafter, unless contraindicated, fluid intake should be encouraged. A gradual return to a normal diet, high in protein and vitamins, should be encouraged to promote wound healing.

Anti-emetics may be prescribed if the patient is suffering from nausea and vomiting (Jolley 2000).

Eliminating

Anaesthesia can alter bladder muscle tone and may cause difficulty with micturition. It has been demonstrated that anaesthesia can lead to an excess secretion of antidiuretic hormone, and it may take 24–48 hours for renal function to return to normal. If the patient's bladder becomes very distended, catheterisation may be necessary, although all other activities to encourage micturition will be attempted first.

If the surgery has involved handling the intestine, abdominal distension caused by large amounts of flatus can result, causing extreme discomfort. A paralytic ileus may develop, the clinical features of this being abdominal distension, vomiting and an absence of bowel sounds; this must be reported immediately.

As with the bladder muscle, some forms of anaesthesia can have an effect on the muscle layer of the bowel, and bowel function may take 24–48 hours to return to normal. If the patient has not had a bowel movement by the third postoperative day, a bulk-forming laxative or evacuant suppositories may be administered.

Personal cleansing and dressing

Adequate assistance should be given in the immediate postoperative period, but the patient should be encouraged to be independent as soon as possible.

The appearance of the skin over the pressure areas and around the wound site should be observed.

Mobilising

The patient should have been taught preoperatively about the importance of movement in bed to prevent pressure sores and the development of a deep vein thrombosis. Anti-embolic stockings may be appropriate. The rate of mobilisation will vary depending on the type of surgery carried out, the general condition of the patient and the personal response to the stress of surgery. A nursing assessment should enable the nurse and patient to plan the most suitable programme of mobilisation for that individual.

Working and playing

Surgery may affect the patient's ability to return to his or her former employment, hobbies or sport. Encouragement and support should be maintained while alternatives are found.

Expressing sexuality

If surgery results in an altered body image, the patient may require ongoing support and encouragement to adjust to and accept the change.

Sleeping

The patient's normal sleeping patterns may be altered after surgery because of observations being carried out or because of pain, anxiety, discomfort, noise or a connection to unusual equipment. Medication to induce sleep may be prescribed but only after other measures, for example helping the patient to find a more comfortable position, relieving pain, giving a hot soothing drink or listening to the patient's concerns, have been tried.

Patient/carer education: key points

In partnership with the patient and/or carer, ensure that they are competent to carry out any practices required. Information should be given on an appropriate point of contact for any concerns that may arise.

Depending on the surgical procedure performed, the hospital patient may require a planned education programme delivered by an appropriately experienced nurse. All patients should be informed of ways of reducing the risk of occurrence of the common postoperative complications.

Day surgery patients and their carers assume a large degree of responsibility for postoperative care, and staff must ensure that they are able to cope with this before allowing the patient to be discharged. Close liaison should be maintained with the community nursing service (*see* 'Transfer of patients between care settings', p. 359).

Discharge medications should be clearly explained, especially if they are new to the patient. Involvement of the family and carers can help to ensure compliance.

References

Coll AM, Moseley L, Torrance C 1999 Fine tuning the day surgery process. Nursing Standard 14(4): 38–41

Jolley S 2000 Postoperative nausea and vomiting: a survey of nurses' knowledge. Nursing Standard 14(23): 32–34

Nendick M 2000 Patient satisfaction with postoperative analgesia. Nursing Standard 14(22): 32–37

United Kingdom Central Council for Nursing, Midwifery and Health Visiting 1992 Code of professional conduct. UKCC, London

United Kingdom Central Council for Nursing, Midwifery and Health Visiting 1996 Guidelines for professional practice. UKCC, London

United Kingdom Central Council for Nursing, Midwifery and Health Visiting 1998 Guidelines for records and record keeping. UKCC, London

38 Pulse

Learning outcomes	By the end of this section, you should know how to:

- prepare the patient for this nursing practice
- locate, assess, measure and record the radial pulse
- locate the major pulse points of the body.

Background knowledge required	To help you to palpate the pulse and interpret the results, it is necessary to have some knowledge of the structure, function and pathology of the cardiovascular system, particularly the heart, the conduction system and the arteries.

Indications and rationale for assessing the radial pulse	A pulse is the rhythmic expansion and recoil of the elastic arteries caused by the ejection of blood from the left ventricle. It can be palpated where an artery near the body surface can be pressed against a firm structure such as bone. Three aspects are usually noted when a pulse is being palpated – its rate, rhythm and quality.

The pulse may be assessed for the following reasons:

- on admission *to ascertain the patient's pulse and assess whether or not it falls within the normal range for the person's age*
- preoperatively *to ascertain the patient's baseline pulse rate, rhythm and quality so that comparisons can be made with postoperative assessments*
- postoperatively *to monitor the rate, rhythm and quality as indicators of the patient's cardiovascular stability and to compare the findings with the preoperative baseline data*
- *to help to estimate, in general terms, the degree of fluid loss when the level of body fluids is lowered*, e.g. after excessive vomiting, excessive diarrhoea or haemorrhage. In the event of a large fluid loss from the body, the pulse is thready and rapid. Severe electrolyte imbalance causes impaired cell function and cardiac arrhythmias
- *to compare with baseline admission assessments to help to evaluate the effect of treatment on patients who have cardiovascular or pulmonary disease.* The majority of patients with these problems will have pulse irregularities that should stabilise with treatment
- *to monitor the patient who is receiving a blood or blood product intravenous infusion.* Elevated pulse and temperature are among the first signs of reaction to the infusion.

Equipment

Watch with a second hand.

Guidelines and rationale for this nursing practice

- explain the nursing practice to the patient *to obtain consent and co-operation.* Patients should be encouraged to be active partners in their care
- ensure that the patient is in a position that is as comfortable and relaxed as possible. *This will help the nurse to obtain a true baseline measurement*
- observe the patient throughout this activity for any signs of discomfort or distress. *This should allow the nurse to intervene immediately in the event of an adverse reaction*
- locate the radial artery, place the first and second fingers along it and press gently. Sufficient pressure should be applied to allow the artery to be against an underlying bone *so that the pulse of blood passing through the artery can be felt*, but care must be taken not to press too hard or the artery may be occluded. See 'Relevance to activities of living', below
- count the pulse for 60 seconds *to allow sufficient time to detect any irregularities or other defects.* See 'Relevance to activities of living', below
- document the findings appropriately, comparing past recordings, and report any abnormal findings immediately *to enable early intervention to improve the problem*
- in undertaking this practice, nurses are accountable for their actions, the quality of care delivered and record-keeping according to the *Code of Professional Conduct* (UKCC 1992), *Guidelines for Professional Practice* (UKCC 1996) and *Guidelines for Records and Record Keeping* (UKCC 1998).

Sites of major pulse points of the body

Although the pulse assessment is usually made using the radial artery, there are other sites where an artery near the body surface can be pressed against an underlying bone or other firm body structure. The major pulses (Fig. 38.1) are the:

- temporal
- carotid
- brachial
- radial
- femoral
- popliteal
- posterior tibial
- dorsalis pedis.

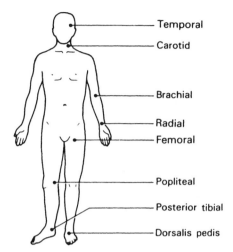

Figure 38.1 *Major pulse points*

Temporal
Carotid
Brachial
Radial
Femoral
Popliteal
Posterior tibial
Dorsalis pedis

Relevance to the activities of living

Breathing

Rate   The resting adult usually has a pulse rate of 60–100 beats per minute. Tachycardia (a rapid pulse rate) can be the result of pain, anger, fear or anxiety, all of which stimulate the sympathetic nervous system and cause the release of adrenaline (epinephrine). It can also occur in some heart diseases, anaemia and fever, and during exercise, all of which require a greater amount of oxygen and thus increase the cardiac output (Alexander et al 2000).

Bradycardia (a slow pulse rate) occurs in any condition, for example raised intracranial pressure, that stimulates the parasympathetic nervous system. Specific heart conditions such as damage to the conducting mechanism after a myocardial infarction can also cause bradycardia. It also occurs in fit athletes, who develop a very efficient heart muscle action.

Rhythm   The rhythm should be regular; any irregularities should be noted. It should be observed whether the irregularities occur at regular or irregular intervals. A normal regular irregularity may occur, particularly in younger people, in conjunction with inspiration and expiration.

Quality   The pulse pressure is the difference between the systolic and the diastolic pressure. The force is a reflection of the pulse strength. The pulse is usually recorded as being normal, bounding, weak and thready, or absent (Goodall 2000).

Elasticity   The elastic recoil of the artery wall should be noted. The artery of a healthy young adult feels flexible and non-tortuous, quite different from that of an elderly patient suffering from a condition such as arteriosclerosis, whose artery will feel hard and cord-like.

The pulse rate is much higher in babies and young children than adults because they have a higher metabolic rate. A pacemaker occasionally 'fires' before the sinoatrial node; the resulting decrease in filling time of the heart chambers causes a pause in the rhythm, which can be detected when assessing the pulse.

Eating and drinking

The level of the body fluids can affect the pulse rate, as can an electrolyte imbalance. A drop in the level of body fluids, for example as a result of haemorrhage, will lead to a rapid, thready and weak pulse.

Controlling body temperature

Fever causes the pulse rate to be raised because of the need for a greater supply of oxygen. Hypothermia can cause a slowing of the rate because of the need to keep the body's core temperature as high as possible (Roper et al 2000).

Mobilising

Exercise increases the rate of the pulse because of the increased demand from muscles for oxygen and nutrients, and the increased production of waste products.

Working and playing

Occupations that demand physical exertion result in an increased pulse rate, as do hobbies such as an active participation in sport.

Dying

The peripheral pulses are often difficult to palpate in the dying patient because of the gradual non-functioning of the various cardiopulmonary mechanisms; they may be absent in the period immediately prior to death.

Patient/carer education: key points

In partnership with the patient and/or carer, ensure that they are competent to carry out any practices required. Information should be given on an appropriate point of contact for any concerns that may arise.

It is helpful to explain to patients that their pulse rate will increase with exercise. If they wish to palpate their own pulse, they should be shown the correct way to do this, staff monitoring the results until the patient has been shown to be competent.

References

Alexander M, Fawcett J, Runciman P (eds) 2000 Nursing care – hospital and home: the adult. 2nd edn. Churchill Livingstone, Edinburgh

Goodall S 2000 Peripheral vascular disease. Nursing Standard 14(25): 48–52

Marieb E 1989 Human anatomy and physiology. Benjamin Cummings, Redwood City, California

Roper N, Logan W, Tierney A 2000 The Roper–Logan–Tierney model of nursing. Churchill Livingstone, Edinburgh

United Kingdom Central Council for Nursing, Midwifery and Health Visiting 1992 Code of professional conduct. UKCC, London

United Kingdom Central Council for Nursing, Midwifery and Health Visiting 1996 Guidelines for professional practice. UKCC, London

United Kingdom Central Council for Nursing, Midwifery and Health Visiting 1998 Guidelines for records and record keeping. UKCC, London

39 Rectal Examination

Learning outcomes	By the end of this section, you should know how to: • prepare the patient for this procedure • collect and prepare the equipment • assist the medical practitioner as requested.
Background information required	Revision of the anatomy and physiology of the sigmoid colon, rectum and anus.
Indications and rationale for rectal examination	Rectal examination is used as a diagnostic aid when there is: • *rectal bleeding* • *severe constipation* • *severe diarrhoea* • *pain in the anal or rectal area* • *a suspected enlarged prostate gland* • *a suspected rectocele.*
Outline of the procedure	The medical practitioner will put a disposable glove on the dominant hand and apply some lubricant to the fingertips. He or she will then insert one or two fingers into the patient's rectum and perform the examination. On completing the examination, the doctor will remove the glove by turning it inside out as he or she takes it off. A lubricated rectal speculum may be inserted and, using the light source, a visual examination carried out. An anal or rectal swab may also be taken for laboratory examination.
Equipment 	Tray Disposable gloves Sterile rectal speculum (Fig. 39.1) Water-soluble lubricant Protective covering for the bed Receptacle for soiled disposable items Swabs Sterile laboratory swab in a container Light source.

Guidelines and rationale for this nursing practice

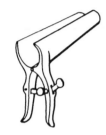

Figure 39.1   *Rectal speculum*

- help to explain the procedure to the patient *to gain consent and co-operation*
- collect and prepare the equipment *for efficiency of practice*
- assist the patient into the position requested by the medical practitioner, ensuring privacy. This is usually the left lateral position
- observe the patient throughout this activity *to detect any signs of discomfort or distress*
- assist the medical practitioner as requested
- ensure that the patient is left feeling as comfortable as possible. If any bleeding is likely as a result of the examination, ensure that the patient's underwear is protected
- dispose of the equipment safely *for the protection of others*
- document the examination in the patient's records, monitor the after-effects and report any abnormal findings immediately *to provide a written record and assist in the implementation of any action should an abnormality or adverse reaction to the practice be noted*
- in undertaking this practice, nurses are accountable for their actions, the quality of care delivered and record-keeping according to the *Code of Professional Conduct* (UKCC 1992), *Guidelines for Professional Practice* (UKCC 1996) and *Guidelines for Records and Record Keeping* (UKCC 1998).

Relevance to the activities of living

Maintaining a safe environment

The nurse and medical practitioner should wash their hands before commencing and on completing the procedure.

Communicating

This can be a painful and embarrassing procedure for the patient so a careful explanation of the need for this examination should be given (Roper et al 2000).

Breathing

It should be explained to patients that they can help themselves to relax while the examination is taking place by breathing in and out slowly and deeply.

Eliminating

An empty rectum facilitates the examination, but when there is rectal bleeding it is not advisable to administer suppositories or an enema (Alexander et al 2000).

Personal cleansing and dressing

Always ensure that the patient's anal area is clean and dry after this examination.

Expressing sexuality

This procedure can be embarrassing for the patient so the nurse must ensure that there is maximum privacy while the examination is being conducted.

Patient/carer education: key points

In partnership with the patient and/or carer, ensure that they are competent to carry out any practices required. Information should be given on an appropriate point of contact for any concerns that may arise.

A careful explanation should help to gain patients' co-operation and aid relaxation, which will in turn reduce the discomfort of the examination.

The patient should be informed of whom to contact if severe pain, discharge or bleeding is experienced after the examination.

References

Alexander M, Fawcett J, Runciman P (eds) 2000 Nursing practice – hospital and home: the adult. 2nd edn. Churchill Livingstone, Edinburgh

Roper N, Logan W, Tierney A 2000 The Roper–Logan–Tierney model of nursing. Churchill Livingstone, Edinburgh

United Kingdom Central Council for Nursing, Midwifery and Health Visiting 1992 Code of professional conduct. UKCC, London

United Kingdom Central Council for Nursing, Midwifery and Health Visiting 1996 Guidelines for professional practice. UKCC, London

United Kingdom Central Council for Nursing, Midwifery and Health Visiting 1998 Guidelines for records and record keeping. UKCC, London

40   Respiration

Learning outcomes	By the end of this section, you should know how to: • prepare the patient for this nursing practice • assess, measure and record the respirations • recognise any abnormalities.
Background knowledge required	To help you to assess, record and interpret respiration, it is necessary to have some knowledge of the respiratory system, particularly the physiology of the bronchi, bronchioles and alveoli.
Indications and rationale for assessing respiration	The basic activity of the respiratory system is to supply sufficient oxygen for the body's metabolic needs and remove carbon dioxide. This is achieved through inspiration and expiration. One respiration consists of an inspiration and an expiration. Respiration may be assessed for the following reasons: • to obtain a baseline measurement *so that any alteration in the patient's breathing pattern can be promptly noticed* • to monitor a patient who has breathing problems *to help in diagnosis* • to compare against baseline measurements *to help evaluate the effect of treatment on patients who have pulmonary disease.*
Equipment 	Watch with a second hand.
Guidelines and rationale for this nursing practice 	• this is the one assessment that is best carried out without the patient's knowledge *because if the patient becomes aware that the respiration rate is being assessed, this can cause the rate to change* • ensure that the patient is in a comfortable position and is as relaxed as possible *as this will help to ensure an accurate assessment* • observe the patient throughout for any signs of discomfort or distress *in order to monitor any adverse effects* • this practice is usually carried out immediately after the assessment of the patient's pulse while the nurse still has his or her finger in position to palpate

the radial pulse. *This helps to reduce the risk of the patient becoming aware that the respiration rate is being assessed*

- count the respirations for 60 seconds by observing the rise and fall of the patient's chest. One respiration consists of an inspiration and an expiration. Assessment for 60 seconds *enables the nurse to become aware of any irregularities or abnormalities in the patient's breathing pattern*
- document the findings appropriately, comparing them against past recordings. Report any abnormal findings immediately and be aware of any possible complications *so that remedial action can immediately be taken*
- in undertaking this practice, nurses are accountable for their actions, the quality of care delivered and record-keeping according to the *Code of Professional Conduct* (UKCC 1992), *Guidelines for Professional Practice* (UKCC 1996) and *Guidelines for Records and Record Keeping* (UKCC 1998).

Relevance to the activities of living

Breathing

Rate   The normal rate of respiration for a resting adult is accepted as being between 12 and 20 respirations per minute. This rate increases with exercise.

Rhythm   Certain disease processes can affect the rhythm of respiration. The rhythm should be regular, and any irregularities should be noted. Many nursing textbooks that specialise in diseases of the respiratory system will provide the reader with a detailed explanation of several irregular breathing patterns and their causes (Alexander et al 2000).

Quality   The quality of respiration can be affected by, for example, a fractured rib, the patient attempting to reduce the discomfort of breathing by taking very shallow inspirations.

Personal cleansing and dressing

The clothing may have to be adjusted to allow the nurse to observe the rise and fall of the patient's chest. Patients who are having breathing problems may need to have their clothing moved to facilitate their respiration (Roper et al 2000).

Controlling body temperature

An elevated body temperature usually results in an increased rate of respiration as the body loses heat through expiration.

Mobilising

Patients who have breathing problems may have restricted mobility and may need to sit in an upright or slightly forward position to facilitate their breathing. Postoperative patients should be encouraged to breathe deeply and move around as much as possible to help to avoid the potential problem of a chest infection.

Patient/carer education: key points

In partnership with the patient and/or carer, ensure that they are competent to carry out any practices required. Information should be given on an appropriate point of contact for any concerns that may arise.

Explain techniques that may help to ease breathing difficulties to patients who have respiratory problems. Such advice may include the avoidance of restricive clothing, resting positions and breathing techniques. The effects of exercise on breathing rates and patterns should also be explained.

References

Alexander M, Fawcett J, Runciman P (eds) 2000 Nursing practice – home and hospital: the adult. 2nd edn. Churchill Livingstone, Edinburgh

Roper N, Logan W, Tierney A 2000 The Roper–Logan–Tierney model of nursing. Churchill Livingstone, Edinburgh

United Kingdom Central Council for Nursing, Midwifery and Health Visiting 1992 Code of professional conduct. UKCC, London

United Kingdom Central Council for Nursing, Midwifery and Health Visiting 1996 Guidelines for professional practice. UKCC, London

United Kingdom Central Council for Nursing, Midwifery and Health Visiting 1998 Guidelines for records and record keeping. UKCC, London

41 Skin Care

Learning outcomes

By the end of this section, you should know how to:

- prepare the patient for this nursing practice
- collect the equipment
- carry out skin care.

Background knowledge required

Revision of the anatomy and physiology of the skin
Revision of the predisposing factors for the development of a pressure sore
The health authority policy regarding risk assessment, pressure sore
  classification, care implementation and criteria for the use of aids to prevent
  pressure sores should be reviewed
Revision of moving and handling a patient (*see* p. 235) and active and passive
  exercises (*see* p. 145).

Indications and rationale for skin care

This care involves the maintenance of a patient's skin viability by ensuring skin
cleanliness, relieving skin capillary pressure, ensuring adequate nutritional status
and monitoring potential problems. Skin care is indicated for every patient,
but specific circumstances increase the need for care when:

- *the patient is incontinent*
- *the patient's mobility is temporarily or permanently impaired*, e.g. a bedfast,
  paralysed or unconscious patient
- *the patient has a poor nutritional status*
- *the patient has impaired peripheral circulation.*

Equipment

Appropriate risk assessment scale, e.g. the Norton (Fig. 41.1), Waterlow
  (Fig. 41.2) or Braden (Bergstrom et al 1987) Scale
Pressure-relieving devices (Bale 2000).

Guidelines and rationale for this nursing practice

- explain the nursing practice to the patient *to gain consent and co-operation*
- ensure the patient's privacy *to reduce anxiety*
- wash the hands *to reduce the risk of cross-infection* (Horton 1995)
- observe the patient throughout this activity *to note any signs of distress
  or discomfort*
- assess the risk factor of the patient developing a pressure sore, utilising
  one of the assessment scales, such as the Norton (Fig. 41.1) or Waterlow

		A		B		C		D		E		Total Score
		Physical Condition		Mental Condition		Activity		Mobility		Incontinent		
		Good	4	Alert	4	Ambulant	4	Full	4	Not	4	
		Fair	3	Apathetic	3	Walk/help	3	Sl. limited	3	Occasionally	3	
		Poor	2	Confused	2	Chairbound	2	V. limited	2	Usually/ur.	2	
Name	Date	V. bad	1	Stuporous	1	Bedfast	1	Immobile	1	Doubly	1	

Instructions for use

1. Identify the most appropriate description of the patient (4, 3, 2, 1) under each of the five headings (A to E) and total the result.

2. Record the 'score' with its date in the patient's notes or on a chart.

3. Assess weekly and whenever any change in the patient's condition and/or circumstances.

With a 'score' of 14 and below the patient is 'At Risk' denoting need for intensive care, i.e. 1–2 hourly changes of posture and the use of pressure-relieving aids.

Note: When oedema of the sacral area has been present a rise of score above 14 does not indicate less risk of a lesion.

Figure 41.1 *Norton Scale. From Roper et al (1985), with permission*

Build/weight for height		Visual skin type		Continence		Mobility		Sex Age		Appetite	
Average	0	Healthy	0	Complete	0	Fully mobile	0	Male	1	Average	0
Above average	2	Tissue paper	1	Occasionally	1	Restricted/	1	Female	2	Poor	1
Below average	3	Dry	1	incontinent		difficult		14–49	1	Anorectic	2
		Oedematous	1	Catheter/	2	Restless/	2	50–64	2		
		Clammy	1	incontinent		fidgety		65–75	3		
		Discolour	2	of faeces		Apathetic	3	75–80	4		
		Broken/spot	3	Doubly incontinent	3	Inert/traction	4	81+	5		

Special risk factors:
(1) Poor nutrition eg terminal cachexia	8		
(2) Sensory deprivation eg diabetes, paraplegia, cerebrovascular accident	5	**Assessment value**	
(3) High dose anti-inflammatory or steroids in use	3	At risk =	10
(4) Smoking 10+ per day	1	High risk =	15
(5) Orthopaedic surgery/fracture below waist	3	Very high risk =	20

Directions for use:

1 Assess the patient, circling the number in each category in which the patient fits

2 Add up all the numbers, including 'special risk factors'

3 If the total places the patient within the 'at risk', 'high risk' or 'very high risk' areas, turn the card over and read the suggested preventive aids listed on the back

4 Record the circled numbers in the patient's documentation, giving the total and the date

5 Assess each patient every third day, unless the need to reassess the patient earlier becomes evident

Figure 41.2 *Waterlow Scale*

(Fig. 41.2) Scale *to permit preventive care to be implemented*. This should be performed as part of the initial assessment process and at regular intervals throughout care when the patient's condition alters (Bale 2000, Waterlow 1992)

- assess the patient using a nutritional risk assessment tool
  Score (Russell 2000) *to assess the patient's nutritional status*
  increases the risk of skin breakdown
- identify individual patient problem areas, such as a patient with peripheral
  vascular disease whose affected limb may be at greater risk than the rest of his
  or her body *as there will be increased risk of the development of a pressure
  sore* (Davies 1994)
- when a risk factor is noted, institute preventive skin care (Davies 1994),
  which will reduce the risk of development of a pressure sore
- relieve the pressure exerted on the skin surface by regularly changing the
  patient's body position (Lowthian 1987) and using pressure-relieving devices
  (Bale 2000) *to prevent or reduce devitalisation of the healthy tissue*
- support the patient's body and limbs in natural positions *to promote comfort
  and prevent damage*, and *maintain joint and muscle movement* with
  passive and active exercises (*see* p. 145)
- a patient who is assessed as having a high risk factor will require frequent, for
  example 2 hourly, changes of position *to relieve the pressure of the soft tissues
  against bone* (Bale 2000). A turning chart may be used to record the time,
  position of the patient and signature of the nurse or carer
- reduce the pressure, friction and shearing forces on the skin by the use of
  any of the recommended aids available, such as static load distribution,
  posture changing or dynamic load distribution beds or mattresses
  (Lowthian 1995), which *reduce the factors contributing to pressure sore
  development*
- cleanse the skin of an incontinent patient or a patient who is perspiring
  profusely *as the number of micro-organisms will be greatly increased*. Use
  soap with caution *as the alkaline content tends to dry the skin and deplete
  it of its natural oils*
- thoroughly dry the skin by patting gently. These measures will *decrease the
  number of skin micro-organisms and lessen the development of infected
  skin tissue*
- examine and classify (Box 41.1) the patient's skin during the nursing practice
  for signs of hyperaemia or loss of integrity, *which signifies the development
  of a pressure sore* (Reid & Morison 1994)
- *reduce the shearing and friction forces exerted on a patient's skin* by using a
  skilled moving and handling technique when repositioning him or her, and
  proper positioning of the patient to prevent sliding down in the bed or chair
  (Culley 1998)
- maintain, or improve when appropriate, the patient's nutritional status, using
  the services of a dietitian if necessary, *as poor nutritional and hydration
  status greatly increases the risk of pressure sore development* (Bale 2000,
  Russell 2000)
- educate the patient about preventive care for pressure sore development when
  his or her condition permits (Thomas et al 1990); a patient nursed in traction
  can, for example, assist in pressure relief measures. Co-operation on the part
  of and care by the patient are vital in the overall prevention of pressure sores
  (Morison 1992)

Box 41.1 The UK consensus classification of pressure sore severity (From Reid & Morison (1994), with permission)

Stage 0
No clinical evidence of a pressure sore
0.0 Normal appearance intact skin
0.1 Healed with scarring
0.2 Tissue damage, but not assessed as a pressure sore

Stage 1
Discoloration of intact skin (light finger pressure applied to the site does not alter the discoloration)
1.1 Non-blanchable erythema with increased local heat
1.2 Blue/purple/black discoloration. The sore is at least stage 1

Stage 2
Partial-thickness skin loss or damage involving epidermis and/or dermis
2.1 Blister
2.2 Abrasion
2.3 Shallow ulcer, without undermining of adjacent tissue
2.4 Any of these with underlying blue/purple/black discoloration or induration. The sore is at least stage 2

Stage 3
Full-thickness skin loss involving damage or necrosis of subcutaneous tissue but not extending to underlying bone, tendon or joint capsule
3.1 Crater, without undermining of adjacent tissue
3.2 Crater, with undermining of adjacent tissue
3.3 Sinus, the full extent of which is not certain
3.4 Full-thickness skin loss but wound bed covered with necrotic tissue (hard or leathery black/brown tissue or softer yellow/cream/grey slough) which masks the true extent of tissue damage. The sore is at least stage 3. Until debrided it is not possible to observe whether damage extends into muscle or involves damage to bone or supporting structures

Stage 4
Full-thickness skin loss with extensive destruction and tissue necrosis extending to underlying bone, tendon or joint capsule
4.1 Visible exposure of bone, tendon or capsule
4.2 Sinus assessed as extending to bone, tendon or capsule

Third digit classification
For the nature of the wound bed
x.x0 Not applicable: intact skin
x.x1 Clean, with partial epithelialisation
x.x2 Clean, with or without granulation, but no obvious epithelialisation
x.x3 Soft slough, cream/yellow/green in colour
x.x4 Hard or leathery black/brown necrotic (dead/avascular) tissue

Fourth digit classification
For infective complications
x.xx0 No inflammation surrounding the wound bed
x.xx1 Inflammation surrounding the wound bed
x.xx2 Cellulitis bacteriologically confirmed

- after giving any of the forms of care above, ensure that the patient is left feeling as comfortable as possible *to ensure quality of patient care*
- dispose of used equipment safely *to reduce any health hazard*
- document the nursing practice appropriately, monitor the after-effects and report any abnormal findings immediately, *providing a written record and assisting in the implementation of any action should an abnormality or adverse reaction to the practice be noted*
- in undertaking this practice, nurses are accountable for their actions, the quality of care delivered and record-keeping according to the *Code of Professional Conduct* (UKCC 1992), *Guidelines for Professional Practice* (UKCC 1996) and *Guidelines for Records and Record Keeping* (UKCC 1998).

Relevance to the activities of living

Maintaining a safe environment

The prevention of pressure sores requires a multidisciplinary approach to the care of the patient (Culley 1998).

Risk assessment tools and pressure sore classification scales are numerous, and their use will vary throughout the health-care system. Nurses must ensure that they are knowledgeable regarding the tools specified within their working area and are able to begin critically to analyse their use.

All equipment should be clean or disposable and all precautions taken to prevent cross-infection. Nurses should wash their hands before commencing and on completing the nursing practice (Horton 1995).

Equipment that is used to relieve pressure must be checked at regular intervals to maintain its working condition. The equipment should be kept clean and dry, both when in use and when in storage, to reduce microbial growth that could act as a source of infection for the patient.

If a pressure sore develops, the cleansing and dressing of this wound must involve an aseptic technique (*see* p. 407). A sore is a break in skin continuity and is therefore at risk of infection. Numerous dressing materials and agents are available. The dressing of choice should be one that will provide maximum patient comfort and promote wound healing.

Sensory impairment to the skin, such as occurs in an unconscious or paralysed patient, may predispose to the development of a pressure sore.

In some local authorities, the responsibility for the regular pressure area care of a chronically ill individual at home has been deemed social care and is delivered by home carers (Nazarko 1995).

To ensure that quality care is delivered, a regular audit of risk assessment processes may be of benefit (Douglas & Watret 1995).

Communicating

It is important that the patient and, when appropriate, the relatives are educated on pressure sores and their prevention. The preventive and educational process should be a team approach involving the nurse, physiotherapist, occupational therapist, dietitian, social worker and doctor (Culley 1998). An educational leaflet such as that suggested by Morison (1992) or the Department of Health (1994) will assist in the information and education process of both patients and carers.

Breathing

A patient who has an impairment of the cardiovascular system, even for a short time, is at increased risk of developing a pressure sore as a result of the reduced perfusion of the skin tissue.

Eating and drinking

The patient's nutritional status must be assessed by the dietitian and appropriate intervention implemented as a poor nutritional status will increase the risk of pressure sore development (Bale 2000, Russell 2000). Unless otherwise instructed, the nurse may offer the patient high-calorie, high-protein drinks to supplement the diet that he or she is already eating. At home, the nurse will require the assistance of the carer in monitoring and encouraging the patient to maintain or improve his or her nutritional status. If the patient is unable to maintain a satisfactory nutritional status via the oral route, nasogastric or parenteral nutrition may be required.

Eliminating

A patient who is incontinent must have the skin kept as free of contamination as possible. Problems of eliminating may be overcome by bladder or bowel training programmes or by treating the underlying cause; urinary retention with overflow can, for example, manifest as urinary incontinence. Following incontinence, the skin should be washed and dried thoroughly without vigorous rubbing as this can cause maceration of the skin tissue. Soap should be used with caution because it has drying and oil-reducing effects, and skin that is dry and lacking in natural oils will break down more readily. A barrier cream may be used, but with caution as it may interfere with the oxygen and moisture exchange of the skin. The patient who is identified as incontinent must be assessed by a knowledgeable professional in continence care who can plan and implement individualised care (Swaffield 2000).

Personal cleansing and dressing

Nurses should use the form of assessment with which they are familiar to calculate the patient's risk factor for the development of a pressure sore.

When a patient is confined to bed, the use of a bed cage can greatly reduce the pressure created by the bed linen on the body. Sheets and blankets should be left loose at the edges of the bed, and using of a duvet can greatly reduce the weight of bed linen on the patient's body. Bed linen should be maintained in a clean, dry and wrinkle-free state.

Capillary pressure, shearing and friction forces are known to be some of the predisposing factors in the development of a pressure sore, and care must be instituted to reduce them. The capillary pressure can be relieved by altering the patient's body position at regular intervals, such as 2 hourly, or more frequently depending on the individual patient's 'at risk' assessment (Lowthian 1987). The shearing and friction forces exerted on the patient's skin tissue can be reduced by a skilled moving and handling technique, and by the positioning of the patient to prevent sliding in any direction while in bed or in a chair (Waterlow 1992). Adjusting the mattress to maintain the patient's knees in a slightly flexed position while the thighs remain supported, or using a padded footboard, can help to reduce slipping.

Attention must be paid to the patient's clothing: buttons, zips, belts and even hard objects such as loose change in the pocket have been known to produce a pressure sore.

Controlling body temperature

A patient suffering from hypothermia has an increased risk of developing a pressure sore because of the effect of the temperature change on the cardiovascular system and the perfusion of the skin.

Mobilising

Early ambulation is of great benefit in the prevention of a pressure sore.

A patient who is using a mobility aid is susceptible to the development of a pressure sore at the point of contact between the aid and the body. A patient who uses a pair of crutches may, for example, develop redness of the hands because of the alteration in distribution of the body weight. Involuntary muscle movements and joint contracture interfere with body positioning and can create an increase in the shearing and friction forces on the patient's skin, resulting in increased risk of a pressure sore developing.

Working and playing

A pressure sore may increase the patient's rehabilitation period and may have a resulting effect on his or her social status. The nurse must implement care to prevent patient boredom, depression and anxiety about the family's social needs. The social worker may need to be involved in this intervention.

Expressing sexuality

The nurse must provide adequate privacy during the nursing practice. The patient's individual wishes should be observed to help maintain self-esteem. Some patients may wish to personalise the pressure-relieving aid to boost their self-esteem and body image.

Sleeping

Skin care for the prevention and treatment of a pressure sore must be maintained throughout the 24 hour period. At home, this may require the assistance of the carer when the community nurse is not present.

Patient/carer education: key points

In partnership with the patient and/or carer, ensure that they are competent to carry out any practices required. Information should be given on an appropriate point of contact for any concerns that may arise. The patient and carers should also be given information on the care implemented to reduce the risk of pressure sore development.

A patient who is permanently at risk of pressure sore development must take an active role in the preventive care. This may involve the nurse in teaching the patient how to inspect the skin tissue regularly, for example using a mirror to assess skin areas that are difficult to access.

When a prolonged or permanent use of pressure-relieving aids by a patient is implemented, the patient and carers should be given information on the safe, continued care of the equipment and on appropriate action should a fault occur.

References

Bale S 2000 Wound healing. In: Alexander M, Fawcett J, Runciman P (eds) Nursing practice – hospital and home: the adult. 2nd edn. Churchill Livingstone, Edinburgh

Bergstrom N, Braden B, Laguzza A 1987 The Braden scale for predicting pressure sore risk. Nursing Research 36(4): 205–210

Culley F 1998 Nursing aspects of pressure sore prevention and therapy. British Journal of Nursing 7(15): 879–886

Davies K 1994 Pressure sores: aetiology, risk factors and assessment scales. British Journal of Nursing 3(6): 256–262

Department of Health 1994 Relieving the pressure: your guide to pressure sores. HMSO, London

Douglas D, Watret L 1995 Auditing pressure sore risk assessment. Journal of Wound Care 4(4): 189–191

Horton R 1995 Handwashing: the fundamental infection control principle. British Journal of Nursing 4(16): 926–933

Lowthian P 1987 The practical assessment of pressure sore risk. Care, Science and Practice 5(4): 3–7

Lowthian P 1995 Pegasus Airwave and Bi-Wave Plus. British Journal of Nursing 4(17): 1020–1024

Morison M 1992 A colour guide to the nursing management of wounds. Wolfe, London

Nazarko L 1995 Community care de-skilling. Nursing Management 2(4): 9–10

Reid J, Morison M 1994 Towards a consensus: classification of pressure sores. Journal of Wound Care 3(3): 157–160

Roper N, Logan W, Tierney A 1985 The elements of nursing. 2nd edn. Churchill Livingstone, Edinburgh

Russell L 2000 Malnutrition and pressure ulcers: nutritional assessment tools. British Journal of Nursing 9(4): 194–204

Swaffield J 2000 Continence. In: Alexander M, Fawcett J, Runciman P (eds) 1994 Nursing practice – hospital and home: the adult. 2nd edn. Churchill Livingstone, Edinburgh

Thomas A, Krowskop S, Noble G, Noble P 1990 Pressure sore management and the recumbent person. In: Bader D (ed.) Pressure sores: clinical practice and scientific approach. Macmillan, London

United Kingdom Central Council for Nursing, Midwifery and Health Visiting 1992 Code of professional conduct. UKCC, London

United Kingdom Central Council for Nursing, Midwifery and Health Visiting 1996 Guidelines for professional practice. UKCC, London

United Kingdom Central Council for Nursing, Midwifery and Health Visiting 1998 Guidelines for records and record keeping. UKCC, London

Waterlow J 1992 A policy that protects: the Waterlow pressure sore prevention/treatment policy. In: Horne E, Cowan T (eds) Staff nurse's survival guide. 2nd edn. Wolfe, London

42 Specimen Collection

General information is given on the collecting of specimens, followed by specific additional information. The section 'Relevance to the activities of living' refers to all types of specimen collection.

Learning outcomes

By the end of this section, you should know how to:

- identify the need for laboratory investigations
- facilitate the obtaining of the necessary specimens
- know the appropriate containers for each type of specimen
- arrange the correct storage and delivery of the specimens to the laboratory.

Background knowledge required

Revision of appropriate microbiology and pathology
Review of local policies referring to the collection and transportation of specimens.

Indications and rationale for collecting specimens

A specimen may be required:

- *as an aid to the diagnosis of disease*
- *for the purposes of screening in health to facilitate cancer diagnosis, staging and typing*
- *to monitor the effect of treatment*
- to permit laboratory culture *to identify pathogenic micro-organisms and determine drug sensitivity.*

Equipment

Appropriate container clearly labelled with the patient's details
Equipment to enable the collection of the specimen
Laboratory form
Plastic specimen bag for transportation.

General guidelines and rationale for · this nursing practice

- explain the nursing practice to the patient *to gain consent and co-operation. Patients should be encouraged to be active partners in care*
- ensure the patient's privacy *to help to maintain dignity and a sense of self*
- the nurse and the patient (if he or she is involved in the collection of the specimen) should wash their hands *to reduce the risk of cross-infection* (Horton 1995)

- ensure that the appropriate precautions are observed *to reduce the risk of contact with body fluids during the collection and transportation of the specimen* (Roberts 2000)
- collect the specimen at the most appropriate time *to facilitate obtaining accurate results*. This time will vary depending on the specimen; the optimum time for the collection of a specimen of urine for culture is, for example, from the first voiding of the bladder in the morning
- *to avoid interference with accurate results*, ensure that no substance that might cause an inaccurate result has been used prior to collection. A specimen of sputum could, for example, be adversely affected by the patient using an antiseptic mouthwash before giving the specimen
- ensure that sufficient quantities of the specimen have been collected *to allow accurate results*
- avoid contamination of the specimen by the hands of the nurse or patient *as this could invalidate the results of the culture and be a hazard to the individuals' health*
- avoid contamination of the outside of the container with the specimen substance *as this could pose a health risk to anyone handling the specimen*
- ensure that the patient is left feeling as comfortable as possible after collecting the specimen
- immediately dispatch the labelled specimen container to the laboratory with the completed form; *any delay may alter the reliability of any results obtained*. If a delay is unavoidable, the specimen can usually be stored in a specimen refrigerator until it can be sent for analysis
- document this nursing practice appropriately, monitor the after-effects and report any abnormal findings immediately *so that appropriate measures can be instigated to relieve the problem*
- in undertaking this practice, nurses are accountable for their actions, the quality of care delivered and record-keeping according to the *Code of Professional Conduct* (UKCC 1992), *Guidelines for Professional Practice* (UKCC 1996) and *Guidelines for Records and Record Keeping* (UKCC 1998).

Swab collection

Specific equipment

Sterile swab
Disposable gloves
Sterile water for a nose swab
Sterile vaginal speculum for a vaginal swab
Sterile lubricating jelly for a vaginal swab
Spatula for a throat swab.

Specific guidelines and rationale for these nursing practices

Wound swabs
- obtain a specimen before the wound is washed *so that the specimen material is not contaminated by the washing agent*

- rotate the swab in the wound *to obtain a sufficient quantity for examination.*

Throat swabs
- help the patient to sit in an appropriate position *to facilitate a good view of the faucial tonsils*
- depress the patient's tongue with a spatula *to facilitate access to the site*
- speedily and gently rub the swab over the faucial area
- avoid touching any other area of the mouth as the swab is being removed *so that the specimen will not be contaminated.*

Ear swabs
- help the patient to sit in a comfortable position with the head slightly tilted to the unaffected side
- gently pull the adult's pinna upwards and backwards to straighten the external canal. *This facilitates the insertion of the swab to obtain a specimen of the discharge*
- insert the swab into the external canal and rotate gently *to ensure that the swab is well coated with the discharge.*

Nasal swabs
- help the patient to sit in a comfortable position *to allow access to the nasal cavity*
- moisten the swab in sterile water before insertion into the nose *to make the procedure more comfortable for the patient* as the nasal cavity can be dry
- insert the swab into the nose, rotating it as it moves upwards towards the tip of the nose.

Vaginal swabs
- help the patient into an appropriate position *to allow access to the vagina*
- gently insert a lubricated speculum into the vagina to separate the vaginal walls. *This allows the area to be swabbed to be visualised*
- introduce the swab into the high vaginal area and gently rotate it. Charcoal-impregnated swabs should be used if a Trichomonas infection is suspected *as the organism survives for longer in this medium.*

Penile swabs
- help the patient into a comfortable position *to allow access to the penis*
- retract the prepuce *to allow the area to be swabbed to be visualised*
- rotate the swab gently in the urethral meatus *to collect a sample of the secretions.*

Faeces

Specific equipment

Disposable gloves
Bedpan
Sterile spatula
Sterile container
Receptacle for soiled disposable items.

Specific guidelines and rationale for this nursing practice

- ask the patient to defaecate into a clean bedpan, ensuring that the faecal matter does not become contaminated with urine *as this could affect the analysis results*
- use a spatula or implement provided to fill about one-third of the specimen container with faecal material
- if the faeces are being tested for occult blood, follow the instructions on the packaging in which the occult blood testing equipment is supplied.

Urine

Specific equipment

Sterile container
Disposable gloves
Bedpan or urinal may be necessary
Sterile receiver may be necessary to receive the specimen
Washing equipment to wash the surrounding tissue
Midstream specimens of urine: a sterile tinfoil bowl
Catheter specimens of urine: a sterile needle, syringe and alcohol-impregnated
    swab (Fig. 42.1)
24 hour urine collection: a large glass sterile container with a lid.

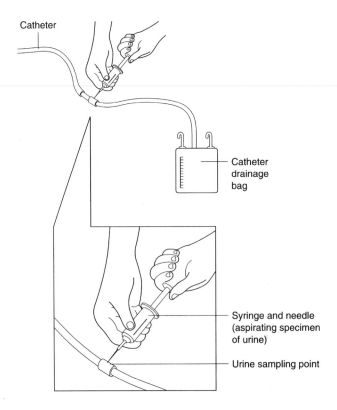

Figure 42.1 *Collecting a specimen of urine when a catheter is in position*

Specific guidelines and rationale for this nursing practice

- to facilitate the collection of a midstream specimen of urine, ask the patient to start passing urine to flush out the urethra *so that urethral organisms will not interfere with the analysis*
- collect the middle section of the stream directly into the container or, for a female, into a sterile bowl, then pouring this into the container
- to facilitate the collection of a catheter specimen of urine, wipe the catheter with an alcohol-impregnated swab
- connect the needle to the syringe and insert it into the specially marked section of the collecting bag tube. This section is made of a self-sealing material *so that the needle will not damage it.* Some collecting tubes now have a special port to which the syringe connects directly
- withdraw the required amount of urine into the syringe and then transfer it to the sterile container
- to commence a 24 hour collection, ask the patient to void his or her bladder and discard the urine *so that the patient and staff know the exact time the collection commences*
- collect all the urine passed in the next 24 hours.

Cervical smear

Specific equipment

Disposable gloves
Lubricating gel
Vaginal speculum
Container with appropriate fixative
Glass slide
Cervical spatula or brush
Medical wipes/tissues.

Specific guidelines and rationale for this nursing practice

- help the patient into the most appropriate position *to facilitate the collection of the specimen*
- put on the disposable gloves
- lubricate the spatula
- gently insert it into the vagina and open it slowly until the cervix can be visualised
- insert the brush or spatula and rotate it twice round the cervix, ensuring that it is at the entrance (Fig. 42.2)
- immediately transfer the cells to the glass slide and insert this into the container holding the fixative
- close the speculum and withdraw it gently
- offer tissues to the patient for her to clean the outside of her vagina and then provide privacy for dressing
- allow the patient time to recover from this procedure before sitting her upright, *as handling the cervix can cause a feeling of faintness as the result of a vasovagal response.*

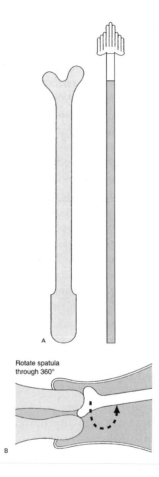

Figure 42.2 *Cervical smear*
A *Cervical spatula and brush*
B *Correct use of cervical spatula*

Relevance to the activities of living

Maintaining a safe environment

All staff who are involved in the collection, delivery and analysis of a human tissue or body fluid specimen must apply universal precautions (DoH 1998). Handwashing is an extremely easy way of reducing cross-infection when health-care staff are involved in specimen collection (Horton 1995).

A thorough cleansing of the patient's genitalia must be carried out prior to the collection of the specimen in order to reduce the number of contaminants from outside the urinary and intestinal systems. Antiseptics should not be used for cleansing as they will alter the number of pathogenic micro-organisms, leading to inaccurate laboratory results.

Human tissue, and body fluids such as urine and faeces, acts as a health hazard to the staff handling the specimens so gloves should be worn during collection to prevent staff contamination (Roberts 2000). The specimen container should only be a half to a third full, and must be checked for lid security to reduce the problem of leakage. The use of a plastic specimen container bag for transportation will help to prevent any risk to the staff should an accidental breakage of the specimen container occur. When a patient requires source isolation, all precautions prior to, during and following specimen collection must be maintained.

Once it has been collected, the specimen should immediately be dispatched to the laboratory. Should there be a delay, the specimen must be stored at 4°C in a special refrigerator to reduce further growth of the pathogenic micro-organisms. Urine specimen containers that contain boric acid crystals can be used when a delay in the dispatch of the specimen is anticipated, as boric acid acts as a urinary preservative.

A catheter specimen of urine should not be collected by disconnecting the drainage bag from the catheter or by taking the specimen from the outlet tap of the urine drainage bag. The former method has the potential to allow pathogenic micro-organisms access to the urinary system; the latter will not provide a specimen of urine that contains the 'true' pathogenic micro-organisms present in the urinary system. Care has to be taken during the collection of a catheter specimen of urine to prevent the accidental stabbing of the nurse's finger by advancing the needle too far and pushing it through the drainage tubing.

Communicating

The patient should be given an easily understood explanation of how and why the specimen collection is required. The laboratory results should be conveyed to the patient as soon as possible. Both of these tactics will reduce patient anxiety.

A patient who has a urinary tract infection, or has just had surgery to the urinary system, may suffer urinary muscle spasm and/or pain. The medical practitioner may prescribe appropriate analgesics and antispasmodics, which can be of great benefit.

Eating and drinking

A patient who is suspected of having a bacterial or viral infection of the urinary or intestinal system may suffer from thirst, nausea, vomiting and/or loss of appetite. The nurse will need to initiate the appropriate nursing interventions to help the patient.

Eliminating

Frequent micturition should be encouraged when a urinary infection is suspected. This will reduce the time the pathogenic micro-organisms have for multiplication within the patient's urinary system.

When collecting a specimen, the urine and/or faeces should be observed for colour, amount, consistency and any obvious abnormality.

A faecal specimen may be requested for bacterial or viral studies but can be taken for biochemical analysis such as testing for the presence of faecal occult blood. This test is now carried out at ward level by a nurse using a commercial biochemical testing kit such as Haemoccult. Nurses should acquaint themselves with the manufacturer's recommendations for use.

A stool chart may be initiated when the patient has a suspected intestinal infection. This records the frequency, colour, consistency and amount of faecal matter passed by the patient. The stool chart can be used as an aid to diagnosis and assists in the assessment of the effect of treatment.

Sleeping

A patient with a suspected infection of the urinary or intestinal system may suffer from an increase in or urgency of micturition and defaecation, which may interrupt sleep. The nurse should assist the patient with this problem by initiating the appropriate nursing interventions.

Expressing sexuality

A clear explanation of the reason for taking the specimen should be given to the patient, and he or she should be allowed as much privacy as possible.

Many patients will not have had any sexual experience so sufficient time must be provided for explanations and counselling to be given to these patients.

A skilled nurse may be involved in taking cervical smears as a screening process (McQueen 2000). This practitioner must be knowledgeable and must be able to understand and interpret the results, communicate the results to women, arrange the appropriate follow-up and implement fail-safe recommendations (RCN 1994).

Permitting other people to be involved in body functions such as eliminating is alien to many people's culture, and this needs to be handled with great sensitivity.

Patient/carer education: key points	In partnership with the patient and/or carer, ensure that they are competent to carry out any practices required. Information should be given on an appropriate point of contact for any concerns that may arise.
	An explanation of the method and reasons for collecting the specimen will help the patient to understand how and why the practice is necessary. This is particularly important if the patient is in the community and the specimen is being collected in his or her home. If the specimen is collected at home, the patient will need clear instructions on the storing of the specimen and where and when to deliver it so that it arrives at the laboratory in optimum condition.

References

Department of Health 1998 Guidance for clinical healthcare workers: protection against infection with blood-borne viruses. HMSO, London

Horton R 1995 Handwashing: the fundamental infection control principle. British Journal of Nursing 4(16): 926–933

McQueen A 2000 The reproductive systems. In: Alexander M, Fawcett J, Runciman P (eds) Nursing practice – hospital and home: the adult. Churchill Livingstone, Edinburgh

Roberts C 2000 Universal precautions: improving the knowledge of trained nurses. British Journal of Nursing 9(1): 43–47

Royal College of Nursing 1994 Cervical screening guidelines for good practice. Issues in nursing and health, factsheet No. 28. RCN, London

United Kingdom Central Council for Nursing, Midwifery and Health Visiting 1992 Code of professional conduct. UKCC, London

United Kingdom Central Council for Nursing, Midwifery and Health Visiting 1996 Guidelines for professional practice. UKCC, London

United Kingdom Central Council for Nursing, Midwifery and Health Visiting 1998 Guidelines for records and record keeping. UKCC, London

43   Stoma Care

Learning outcomes

By the end of this section, you should know how to:

- prepare the patient for this nursing practice
- collect and prepare the equipment
- carry out stoma care for the patient
- help patients to accept and care for their stoma themselves, both at home and in an institutional setting.

Background knowledge required

Revision of the anatomy and physiology of the digestive system, with special reference to the small and large intestines

Review of health authority policy regarding the role of the stoma care nurse and the literature available for patient education in an institutional and a community setting

Knowledge of the information and level of counselling given to the patient before the operation to create a stoma.

Indications and rationale for stoma care

A stoma is an opening from the small or large intestine onto the surface of the abdomen through which the bowel contents are diverted for excretion (Fig. 43.1). The stoma is formed after surgical intervention *for the treatment of intestinal disease*. Different names are used according to the site of the stoma (Crooks 1994).

Stoma care involves cleansing the stoma and surrounding skin, and providing a suitable appliance for the safe collection and disposal of excreta, *in order to enable the person to resume the normal activities of living as soon as possible.*

A **colostomy** is an opening from the colon, usually the transverse or descending colon, and may be required:

- *for patients who have malignant disease of the rectum or colon*
- *for patients who have diverticular disease of the colon*
- *for patients who have inflammatory disease of the intestine*, e.g. Crohn's disease or ulcerative colitis (Kelly 1994).

An **ileostomy** is an opening from the ileum and may be formed for the same reasons as a colostomy, although it is more often seen in *patients who have inflammatory disease of the intestine,* for example Crohn's disease or ulcerative colitis. In some cases, a temporary stoma may be formed so that once the disease has resolved, the stoma may be closed and the intestine anastomosed to function as before.

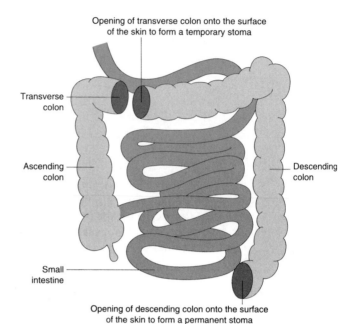

Opening of transverse colon onto the surface
of the skin to form a temporary stoma

Transverse
colon

Ascending
colon

Descending
colon

Small
intestine

Opening of descending colon onto the surface
of the skin to form a permanent stoma

Figure 43.1   *Sites that may be chosen for colostomy*

A **jejunostomy** is an opening from the jejunum.

A **urostomy** is an opening from the bladder or ureter into a segment of the ileum, this being used as a channel for the urine to be diverted through an abdominal stoma. This is also known as an ileal conduit, and it may be required *for the treatment of malignant disease of the bladder* (Leaver 1994).

Equipment

Trolley or tray
Bowl of warm water
Tissues or paper towels
Material for protecting the skin area round the stoma, e.g. Stomahesive or
    karaya gum
Suitable appliance (stoma pouch)
Scissors
Measuring jug
Gloves (non-sterile)
Barrier cream for protecting the skin around the stoma
Deodorant as required
Receptacle for soiled disposable items.

Stoma appliances

There is a wide range of appliances available, and, with the guidance of a stoma care nurse, the patient will choose the one most suitable for his or her needs. Bags may have pre-cut apertures or may have to be cut to fit individually.

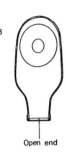

Figure 43.2
Examples of disposable stoma bags
A *Closed pouch*
B *Open lower end to permit emptying of the contents*

They may be closed pouches or open ended to allow emptying (Fig. 43.2). Some are two-piece appliances with a semi-rigid circular aperture onto which a bag can be clipped, allowing for changing or emptying (Black 1994a).

Immediately postoperatively, the surgeon will place a clear plastic appliance over the stoma, probably incorporating a suitable backing to protect the skin. This allows the observation of the stoma and its function. The protective backing also allows the removal of the appliance without too much discomfort for the patient during the postoperative period; it may be 2–5 days before the appliance needs to be changed for the first time.

Karaya gum-backed appliance   Such an appliance may have a circle of karaya gum pre-cut, when the appropriate size to fit the stoma should be chosen; otherwise, a hole should be prepared by cutting the karaya backing to a suitable size. The gum must be moistened before applying to the skin (see the manufacturer's instructions).

Skin protective wafer, for example Stomahesive   This is a square wafer in which a hole is cut to fit snugly round the stoma. A pouch with an adhesive backing is prepared to fit over the stoma and adhere to the wafer (see the manufacturer's instructions).

Protective cream   Protective barrier creams or gels are occasionally prescribed for patients who have particularly sensitive skin. These should be massaged into the skin until it is dry and non-greasy, any surplus cream being wiped off before the new appliance is fitted.

Deodorants   These can range from sprays to concentrated deodorants, only one drop being needed. The stoma care nurse should be consulted about the preparations most suitable for the patient's needs.

Guidelines and rationale for this nursing practice

- explain the nursing practice to the patient *to gain consent and co-operation, and encourage participation in care* (Kelly 1994)
- ensure the patient's privacy *to maintain self-esteem and prevent embarrassment*
- wash hands *to reduce the risk of cross-infection* (Horton 1995)
- collect and prepare the equipment *so that everything is ready*
- help the patient into a comfortable position *to reduce any distress and to help him or her see the area of the stoma*
- help to adjust the clothing to expose the patient's abdomen in the area of the stoma *for easy access and so that the patient can observe the practice* (Allison 1995)
- apply gloves *to prevent any contamination from body fluids*
- place a paper towel appropriately *to protect the surrounding area from spills or leakage*
- observe the patient throughout this activity *to monitor any adverse effects*
- empty the appliance and, if required, measure its contents *for an evaluation of the elimination fluid balance*
- gently remove the appliance and the protective backing *to expose the stoma area*

- wash the skin around the stoma with warm water only: *soap may cause skin irritation*
- encourage the patient to look at the stoma and explain what you are doing *so that he or she gradually accepts the change of body image and to encourage early independence* (MacGinley 1994)
- observe the colour and condition of the stoma and the surrounding skin *to evaluate the wound healing process*
- dry the skin around the stoma thoroughly *to maintain healthy intact skin and prevent excoriation*
- prepare the appliance as required by cutting the aperture of the bag and the skin protective wafer if necessary *so that it is tailored to fit the individual stoma*
- apply any prescribed protective creams if required and remove the surplus cream *to prevent any excoriation of the surrounding skin*
- place the new appliance in position *so that it fits comfortably and permits no leakage round the stoma* (Fig. 43.3)
- seal an open-ended bag with an appropriate closure *to prevent leakage*
- ensure that the patient is left feeling as comfortable as possible *to limit distress and promote the healing process*
- dispose of any waste products and soiled appliances according to health authority policy *to prevent the transmission of infection*
- wash the hands *to reduce the risk of cross-infection* (Horton 1995)
- document the nursing practice appropriately, monitor the after-effects and report any abnormal findings immediately. *This will ensure safe practice and enable prompt, appropriate medical and nursing intervention to be initiated*
- in undertaking this practice, nurses are accountable for their actions, the quality of care delivered and record-keeping according to the *Code of Professional Conduct* (UKCC 1992), *Guidelines for Professional Practice* (UKCC 1996) and *Guidelines for Records and Record Keeping* (UKCC 1998).

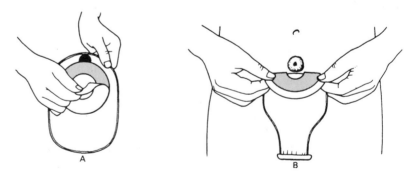

Figure 43.3 *Positioning an appliance over a stoma*
A *Removing the protective covering from the adhesive ring before placing the appliance over the stoma*
B *Applying a stoma pouch. The open-ended pouch is sealed with a clip ready for use; when the clip is removed, the stoma pouch can be emptied without removing the appliance from the skin*

Relevance to the activities of living	Observations on and further rationale for this nursing practice will be included within each activity of living as appropriate.

Maintaining a safe environment

In the postoperative period, the abdominal wound should be cared for separately and covered with plastic sealant spray or a sterile dressing before stoma care is performed (*see* 'Aseptic technique', p. 407).

Care of the stoma itself is not a sterile practice, but high standards of cleanliness should be maintained. Stoma care should be regarded as a form of toileting and appropriate handwashing performed to reduce the incidence of cross-infection (Horton 1995). Patient education should reflect this as patients are helped to look after their own stoma under the guidance of the stoma care nurse and others involved with their care.

The contents of the stoma bag should be emptied into the toilet or Clinamatic. The soiled bags should be treated as clinical waste. Once home, the patient will be instructed to wrap the bags in newspaper when they have been emptied and rinsed. They should be placed in the dustbin for disposal, although in some health authority areas, a special service is available for removal and disposal of soiled bags.

Communicating

An important part of patients' pre- and postoperative care should be to help them to care for the stoma themselves. It is helpful for all nursing staff to know the level of counselling given to each patient before the operation and the involvement of the stoma care nurse in this instruction. The nurse should encourage patients to talk about the stoma and create an environment for them to ask questions about any of their worries, initially while performing stoma care for them and then while helping them learn to care for the stoma themselves. Effective listening skills can be used to ensure that both the physical and psychological needs of the patient are met (Metcalf 1998).

Howie et al (2000) and Metcalf (1999) highlight the complex process involved in teaching patients the skills of stoma care and state that patients who are satisfied with the amount of preoperative information they receive are less likely to develop psychological problems. There should be good liaison between the ward staff and the stoma care nurse so that patients feel that they can discuss their concerns freely. Literature about the particular type of stoma should be readily available from the stoma care nurse, and discussions can be a useful aid for communication and patient education (Black 1994b). Details of local support groups and a visit from someone successfully coping with a stoma can also help the patient with his or her own adjustment to the stoma.

The patient may initially find the smell of flatus and excreta from the stoma difficult to accept. It should be explained that once a normal diet has been established, they will soon find out which foods appear to make the flatus worse, and exclude them. Once the stoma is established and functioning normally, unpleasant odour will be less of a problem. Local deodorant can be used, some appliances being fitted with deodorant filters to cope with the problem. Advice should be sought from the stoma care nurse. The most important way of helping the patient is for nurses to indicate by their non-verbal communication that they are not upset by a normal bodily function taking place in a different area of the body.

If patients normally use spectacles, they should be encouraged to wear them initially to watch while stoma care is performed, and later so that they can see properly to do it themselves.

Eating and drinking

Once the patient is allowed a normal diet, the stoma will discharge faecal material more frequently. By a process of observation, the patient should be encouraged to notice the effect that different foods have on faecal elimination. In this way, the diet can probably be adjusted so that a more solid stool is formed. This process may take several weeks, and the stoma care nurse will continue to give help and advice about an appropriate diet when the patient is at home.

Eliminating

The presence of a stoma completely changes the way in which faecal material is eliminated from the body, and the patient has to be helped to adjust to this.

Preoperatively, the patient should be involved in the discussion and decision surrounding the siting of his or her stoma. The stoma care nurse, the surgeon and the ward nursing staff should all, in their appropriate roles, take part in this important preoperative preparation.

In the immediate postoperative period, patients have no control over the faecal material eliminated through a stoma; this is an added problem about which they have to learn. The faecal material is initially fluid when expelled through the stoma, as the water absorption function of the colon may have been bypassed. After 2–3 weeks, when the patient is able to eat a normal diet, a semi-solid stool may be formed, especially when the stoma is a colostomy in the transverse or descending colon. The frequency of bowel function can eventually be reduced and controlled, almost resembling a normal bowel movement, to the extent that a stoma bag need not be worn continuously.

Drainage from an ileostomy is, on the other hand, liquid and rich in digestive enzymes, which can cause excoriation and erosion of the skin. The discharge flows almost continuously, requiring the constant wearing of an appliance unless an ileal pouch (a reservoir below the skin surface) has been constructed. Odour problems, a fear of soiling and skin complications are more common with an ileostomy, and an open-ended bag that can be regularly emptied is the most suitable appliance. Eventually, however, there is usually some control over the frequency of bowel function.

Appliances should be emptied or changed as often as necessary to prevent overfilling and leakage onto the surrounding skin area. This is usually when they are between one-third and one-half full, to prevent their becoming heavy and unwieldy. Any redness, swelling or abnormality of the stoma or the surrounding skin area should be reported.

The faecal fluid should initially be measured and observed for any abnormalities. Abnormal excreta should be kept for observation and reported.

An urostomy is formed to allow urine to be excreted through an abdominal stoma. This may be collected directly into a suitable stoma bag, or a catheter may be incorporated so that a closed drainage system may be used. Whichever system is used, the bag chosen should have facilities for frequent emptying (*see* 'Catheter care', p. 102). The principles of stoma care remain the same.

Personal cleansing and dressing

The patient may feel that the stoma is a threat to cleanliness. Shower or bathing facilities should be available as soon as the patient's condition allows, a bed bath being given as often as required prior to that. Stoma care should whenever possible be co-ordinated with showering or bathing; the appliance can be emptied and removed and the skin area washed first, the new appliance being fitted afterwards. This may not be possible with an ileostomy or urostomy so in these instances the appliance should be emptied, or changed and replaced, before showering or bathing.

While the patient is learning how to care for the stoma, comfortable clothes that give easy access to the stoma should be worn. Modern appliances are comfortable and unobtrusive so no permanent change in clothing style should be needed. Advice from the stoma care nurse and the appropriate support group can be helpful.

Working and playing

Once the patient has recovered from the operation and is able to cope with the stoma, it is hoped that he or she will return to a normal lifestyle. Even swimming is possible, using a small temporary appliance. Helpful advice can be obtained from the stoma care nurse and support groups.

Expressing sexuality

A stoma, especially if it is permanent, is a major insult to the patient's body image, and he or she may become withdrawn and depressed. Patients' acceptance by the hospital staff will be the first step in giving them confidence in themselves. They should choose which of their friends and relatives they tell about the stoma, their acceptance helping the patient's rehabilitation. Counselling before the operation and constant support from all concerned will boost self-esteem and help the patient to overcome the almost inevitable initial revulsion that he or she feels (Crooks 1994).

Patients who have a stoma following a resection of the lower bowel may have problems with sexual function. Men may become impotent, and women may have dyspareunia; sexual partners should therefore be included in counselling both before and after surgery. The presence of an abdominal stoma appliance inevitably calls for additional thoughtfulness and ingenuity during sexual intercourse. Counselling from the stoma care nurse, the surgeon and the appropriate support group will help in this situation, which may only be temporary (Black 1994c). The formation of a colostomy for a homosexual man will generate different emotional responses; this requires sensitive discussion and guidance in terms of the lifestyle changes required (Corless 1992).

The nurse should be aware of cultural beliefs that may affect how the patient adapts and adjusts to the formation of a stoma.

Sleeping

Stoma care should be performed prior to the patient settling for the night as this will prevent the need to empty or change an appliance, which will disturb sleep.

Once the patient is eating a normal diet, and has adjusted to his or her own requirements, it is unlikely that the stoma will need any attention during the night. A larger bag can be used overnight, which may be helpful for patients who have an ileostomy.

Patient/carer education: key points	In partnership with the patient and/or carer, ensure that they are competent to carry out any practices required. Information should be given on an appropriate point of contact for any concerns that may arise.

Before, during and after admission, patient education will be shared with the stoma care nurse, who should have very close links with the nursing staff in both the institution and the community. Patient education begins prior to stoma surgery, with counselling and decision-making on the site of the stoma related to the patient's individual problems and the activities of living.

The decision of which is the most appropriate stoma appliance should be shared between the stoma nurse and the patient. The method of application, retention and changing of the appliance should be explained and supervised until the patient is confidently self-caring.

The importance of adjusting the diet to suit the changed elimination process should be explained, advice being given to help the stoma to operate efficiently as soon as possible.

The patient should understand the importance of immediately reporting any redness, swelling or pain at the site, or any general feeling of illness or distress, which may need medical help. A telephone help-line can reduce anxiety in the first few weeks.

The address of a local support group should be given to the patient; a visit from a member who has a functioning stoma can help to increase the patient's confidence in his or her own self-care.

References

Allison M 1995 Comparing methods of stoma function. Nursing Standard 9(24): 25–28

Black P 1994a Choosing the correct stoma appliance. British Journal of Nursing 3(11): 545–550

Black P 1994b Management of patients undergoing stoma surgery. British Journal of Nursing 3(5): 211–216

Black P 1994c Problems in stoma care. British Journal of Nursing 3(14): 707–711

Corless R 1992 Caring for a homosexual man undergoing a colostomy formation. British Journal of Nursing 1(10): 501–506

Crooks S 1994 Foresight leads to improved outcome. Stoma care nurse's role in siting stomas. Professional Nurse 10(20): 89–92

Horton R 1995 Handwashing: the fundamental infection control principle. British Journal of Nursing 4(16): 926–933

Howie E, Miller M, Murchie M 2000 The gastrointestinal system, liver and biliary tract. In: Alexander M, Fawcett J, Runciman P (eds) Nursing practice – hospital and home: the adult. 2nd edn. Churchill Livingstone, Edinburgh

Kelly M 1994 Patients' decision making in major surgery. The case of total colectomy. Nursing Times 90(42): 48–51

Leaver R 1994 The Mitrofanoff pouch. A continent urinary diversion. Professional Nurse 9(11): 748–753

MacGinley K 1994 Nursing care of the patient with altered body image. British Journal of Nursing 3(22): 1098–1102

Metcalf C 1998 Stoma care: exploring the value of effective listening. British Journal of Nursing 7(6): 311–315

Metcalf C 1999 Stoma care: empowering patients through teaching practical skills. British Journal of Nursing 8(9): 593–600

United Kingdom Central Council for Nursing, Midwifery and Health Visiting 1992 Code of professional conduct. UKCC, London

United Kingdom Central Council for Nursing, Midwifery and Health Visiting 1996 Guidelines for professional practice. UKCC, London

United Kingdom Central Council for Nursing, Midwifery and Health Visiting 1998 Guidelines for records and record keeping. UKCC, London

44 Suppositories

Learning outcomes

By the end of this section, you should know how to:

- prepare the patient for this nursing practice
- collect and prepare the equipment
- administer rectal suppositories
- describe some of the types of suppository and their function.

Background knowledge required

Revision of the anatomy and physiology of the colon, rectum and anus
Revision of medicine administration, particularly checking the medication against the prescription (*see* p. 1).

Indications and rationale for administering suppositories

A suppository is a cone or cylinder of a medicinal substance that can be introduced into the rectum, will eventually dissolve and may be absorbed through the rectal mucosa. It is used:

- *to relieve constipation*
- *to evacuate the bowel prior to surgery or certain investigations*
- *to treat haemorrhoids or anal pruritis*
- *to administer medication*, e.g. antibiotics, bronchodilators or analgesics.

Equipment

Tray
Disposable gloves
Medical wipes/tissues
Water-soluble lubricant
Protective covering
Receptacle for soiled disposable items
Prescribed suppository.

Suppositories are of value in evacuating the rectum. Glycerine suppositories lubricate dry, hard stools and have a mild stimulant effect on the rectum. Other suppositories with a stimulant effect are Beogex and Bisacodyl.

Medication is well absorbed through the rectal mucosa. This route has for many years been a common way to administer medication in Europe, but it is only recently that it has become acceptable to patients in the UK.

Guidelines and rationale for this nursing practice

Moppett (2000) discusses the latest guidance on the insertion of suppositories, suggesting that, for physiological reasons, the suppository should be inserted blunt end first into the anus. It is proposed that this will aid the retention of the suppository, as the anal sphincter muscles will close tightly round the apex of the suppository, propelling it inwards. If it is inserted apex first, as is traditional, the sphincter closes incompletely over the blunt end, and the muscles are stimulated to expel the suppository. The introduction of the blunt end of the suppository also reduces the need to insert the full length of a finger.

- explain the nursing practice to the patient *to gain consent and co-operation*
- ensure the patient's privacy and assist him or her into the left lateral position with the buttocks near the edge of the bed *to allow ease of access to the rectal sphincter*
- observe the patient throughout this activity *for any signs of distress or discomfort*
- place the protective covering under the patient's buttocks *in case of soiling by faecal matter*
- check with the prescription sheet and with a qualified member of staff that the suppository is the correct one and is being administered to the correct patient, *in order to avoid mistakes*
- squeeze some lubricating gel onto a medical wipe or tissue and lubricate the blunt end of the suppository *for ease of insertion*
- put on disposable gloves *for your protection*
- part the patient's buttocks with the non-dominant hand *to allow easier access to the anal sphincter*
- with the dominant hand, insert the blunt end of the suppository into the rectum in an upwards and slightly backwards direction *to follow the natural line of the rectum* (Fig. 44.1)

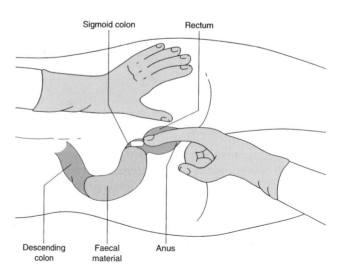

Figure 44.1 *Insertion of a rectal suppository*

- push the suppository in gently as far as possible with the middle finger *to optimise the effect*
- withdraw the gloved finger
- wipe the patient's anal area with a medical wipe or tissue *to clean any soiling*
- remove the protective covering
- remove the gloves
- provide a bedpan or commode, or assist the patient to the toilet, when this is required. *To reduce embarrassment* for the patient, try to provide as much privacy as possible, remembering that curtains do not act as sound or smell filters
- ensure that the patient is left feeling as comfortable as possible, *maintaining the quality of this practice*
- dispose of the equipment safely *to prevent the transmission of infection*
- document this nursing practice appropriately, monitor the after-effects and report any abnormal findings, *ensuring safe practice and enabling prompt, appropriate medical and nursing intervention to be initiated*
- in undertaking this practice, nurses are accountable for their actions, the quality of care delivered and record-keeping according to the *Code of Professional Conduct* (UKCC 1992), *Guidelines for Professional Practice* (UKCC 1996) and *Guidelines for Records and Record Keeping* (UKCC 1998).

Relevance to the activities of living

Communicating

It is important to explain clearly to the patient the reason for and method of action of the suppository.

Eliminating

If the suppository is being given to evacuate the rectum, the patient must have ready access to a bedpan, commode or toilet, and any necessary assistance should be given. Bedpans should be used as a last resort as patients may find it difficult to use a bedpan, which can aggravate an existing problem of constipation.

Expressing sexuality

Many patients find the administration of suppositories embarrassing so an adequate explanation should be given and maximum privacy must be provided (Roper et al 2000).

Patient/carer education: key points

In partnership with the patient and/or carer, ensure that they are competent to carry out any practices required. Information should be given on an appropriate point of contact for any concerns that may arise.

The patient should be told the reasons for administering his or her medication via the rectal route as this route of administration may be unknown to the patient. The patient may also require education in the self-administration of suppositories.

If suppositories are being prescribed to relieve constipation, it may be appropriate to discuss ways in which increased exercise, fluid and diet may relieve this problem. The development of a habit that encourages the bowel to empty at the same time each day and allows adequate time for this to happen is also worth discussing. A self-completion bowel chart may be useful for helping to resolve the problem of constipation.

References

Moppett S 2000 Which way is up for a suppository? Nursing Times Plus 96(19): 12–13
Roper N, Logan W, Tierney A 2000 The Roper–Logan–Tierney model of nursing. Churchill Livingstone, Edinburgh
United Kingdom Central Council for Nursing, Midwifery and Health Visiting 1992 Code of professional conduct. UKCC, London
United Kingdom Central Council for Nursing, Midwifery and Health Visiting 1996 Guidelines for professional practice. UKCC, London
United Kingdom Central Council for Nursing, Midwifery and Health Visiting 1998 Guidelines for records and record keeping. UKCC, London

45 Toileting

Learning outcomes

By the end of this section, you should know how to:

- prepare the patient for this nursing practice
- collect and prepare the equipment
- provide facilities for the patient to empty his or her bladder or bowel, at home or in an institutional setting.

Background knowledge required

Revision of the anatomy and physiology of the urinary system, with special reference to micturition

Revision of the anatomy and physiology of the rectum and anus, with special reference to defaecation

Review of health authority policy regarding the disposal of excreta and the control of infection in both community and institutional care

Revision of continence management.

Indications and rationale for toileting

Toileting aims *to provide the appropriate facilities for the patient to micturate or defaecate.* This may be a toilet, a commode, a bedpan or a urinal. A bedpan, urinal or commode should be provided for patients who are confined to bed or allowed up only for short periods. Assistance to the toilet should be provided for those who are too frail or immobile to be self-caring in relation to toileting.

Equipment

Bedpan, urinal, commode or toilet, as appropriate
Toilet paper
Disposable cover for the bedpan or urinal
Gloves
Measuring jug
Bedpan disposer, e.g. Clinamatic
Bedpan washer for non-disposable equipment
Facilities for handwashing
Facilities for communicating the patient's need for toileting to the nurse, e.g. a bell
Appropriate aids for moving and handling
Receptacle for soiled disposable items.

Bedpan

For female patients, a bedpan may be used for micturition and defaecation. For male patients, it may be used for defaecation, but a urinal should be offered at the same time for micturition. Toilet ware may be disposable or non-disposable, non-disposable equipment usually being made of plastic. Disposable equipment is, however, increasingly being used. A traditional or a slipper bedpan may be used, the latter having the advantage of being easier to insert and more comfortable to use.

Disposable bedpan   This should be placed in a rigid bedpan holder and taken to the bedside under a disposable cover. The used bedpan should be flushed in the bedpan disposer according to the manufacturer's instructions. The holder should be washed and dried before storage.

Plastic bedpan   This should be covered with a disposable cover and the used bedpan placed in the bedpan washer according to the manufacturer's instructions. The bedpan should be washed and dried before storing, and regular sterilisation should be performed according to health authority policy. In the community, waste should be disposed of in the toilet and the equipment cleaned according to local infection control policy.

Urinal

This is used for male patients for micturition and should be covered with a disposable cover when taken to and from the patient. Like a bedpan, it may be disposable or non-disposable; after use, it is processed in the same way. A female urinal is available and may be suitable for some patients (Fader et al 1999).

Commode

This is a mobile chair constructed to hold a bedpan, which can be taken to the bedside for the patient's use. It may also be built to transport the patient to the toilet so that the commode seat fits over the toilet seat. Many mechanical lifting aids incorporate a commode seat so that the patient may be taken safely to the ward toilet or use it as a conventional commode (see the manufacturer's instructions) (Professional Development Unit 1995). A commode can be made available for patients at home to maintain their independence, or as a temporary help for toileting if access to the bathroom is difficult.

Guidelines and rationale for this nursing practice

Guidelines are given for the provision of a bedpan to a female patient and a urinal to a male patient.

The provision of a bedpan for a female patient

- explain this nursing practice to the patient *to gain consent and co-operation, and encourage participation in care*
- ensure that the patient knows how to request a bedpan when needed *to reduce anxiety about this activity of living*
- respond immediately to the patient's request for a bedpan *to prevent incontinence and patient distress*
- don a plastic apron after washing the hands *to prevent contamination*
- don plastic gloves *to prevent contamination from body fluids*

- collect and prepare the bedpan, carrying it to the bedside under a disposable cover *to maintain self-esteem and reduce embarrassment*
- ensure the patient's privacy *to respect her individuality* (Glen & Jownally 1995)
- observe the patient's condition throughout this activity *to monitor any adverse effects*
- help the patient into a comfortable sitting position, supporting her back with pillows *so that she will be in the best position for micturition*
- help the patient to adjust her clothing *to expose the buttocks and perineum*
- if the patient's condition allows, ask her to lift her buttocks. A monkey pole or similar equipment may be used to facilitate this procedure, and two nurses may be required depending on the patient's condition. A hoist with a toileting sling may be used. The patient's moving and handling plan should be followed *to ensure safe technique* (RCN 1999)
- slide the bedpan into position with the shaped rim under the patient's buttocks *so that it is safely in place*
- adjust the patient's pillows *to ensure that she is sitting comfortably*
- leave the patient to use the bedpan, ensuring privacy *to maintain her self-esteem*
- remain in the vicinity *to be available when the patient is ready*
- assist with wiping the perineum and/or anus if necessary *to maintain healthy skin in the area*
- remove the bedpan *once toileting is complete*
- give the patient a bowl to wash her hands *for her own personal hygiene and to prevent cross-infection*, or help her to the washbasin if it is more appropriate
- ensure that the patient is left feeling as comfortable as possible *to minimise any distress*
- observe the contents of the bedpan *for any abnormalities*; these should be reported and the bedpan saved for inspection
- measure the urine and retain a labelled specimen *for ward testing if required* (*see* 'Urine testing', p. 377) (Daffurn et al 1994)
- dispose of the equipment safely *to prevent the transmission of infection*
- wash the hands using a good handwashing technique *to maintain a safe environment*
- document the nursing practice appropriately and report any abnormal findings immediately. *This will ensure safe practice and enable prompt, appropriate medical and nursing intervention to be initiated*
- in undertaking this practice, nurses are accountable for their actions, the quality of care delivered and record-keeping according to the *Code of Professional Conduct* (UKCC 1992), *Guidelines for Professional Practice* (UKCC 1996) and *Guidelines for Records and Record Keeping* (UKCC 1998).

Guidelines for providing a commode

These are in principle the same as those for using a bedpan. Once the prepared and covered commode has been taken to the bedside, the patient should be helped out of bed *to sit on the commode in privacy*, and the guidelines as for a bedpan followed. Help from one or two nurses may be needed *to assist the patient in and out of bed*, depending on the patient's condition and the mechanical aids being used for safe moving and handling (NPBA and RCN 1997).

The provision of a urinal for a male patient

- explain this nursing practice and *gain the patient's consent and co-operation*
- ensure that the patient knows how to request a urinal when needed *to reduce anxiety about this activity of living*
- collect and prepare the urinal and take it to the bedside under a disposable cover *to maintain self-esteem and reduce embarrassment*
- ensure the patient's privacy *to respect his individuality*
- help the patient to place the urinal in position if required *so that no urine is spilled*
- remain in the vicinity *to be available when the patient is ready*
- remove the urinal and proceed as for the guidelines for providing a bedpan.

Principles of continence assessment

The key principles of continence assessment are outlined in this section. Problems of continence can apply to both urine and faeces, and the majority of people with a continence problem can be cured, or have their condition improved, if they are assessed and managed appropriately (Bradley & Moran 1998). Evidence shows, however, that nursing intervention could be improved in this area of care (Bayliss et al 2000). It is also important to remember that continence is not just a problem for the older patient.

There are five main types of incontinence – stress, urge, overflow, neurogenic/reflex and functional – a detailed structured assessment being the key to the development of a management and treatment plan for the patient. The Department of Health (2000) recommends that all patients with a continence problem receive an initial assessment undertaken by a suitably qualified person that includes the following areas:

- a detailed description of the symptoms with regard to continence
- the effect on lifestyle and motivation for treatment
- a physical examination of the abdomen for a palpable mass or bladder distension; of the perineum to identify prolapse and excoriation, and to assess pelvic floor contraction; and of the rectum to check for faecal impaction
- urinalysis to exclude infection or identify potential underlying disease such as renal disease or diabetes
- an assessment of manual dexterity
- an assessment of the physical and social environment, for example the toilet and laundry facilities
- the use of an activities of living diary (including diet, exercise and bowel and urinary habits)
- an identification of the underlying conditions or medication that may exacerbate the problem.

A frequency–volume chart may be used to identify the patient's usual voiding pattern. This records the number and types of drink taken, the volume of urine passed at each voiding and the number of incontinent episodes. This is recorded over 24 hours for 3–5 days (Bardsley 2000). A variety of continence assessment forms are available, and health authorities will have developed one as part of their continence management protocol.

Following the initial assessment, it will be possible to determine the possible causes for the continence and from this establish a treatment plan – using locally developed protocols – that is acceptable to the patient. The role of the continence advisor is important in educating staff and auditing continence services.

Relevance to the activities of living

Observations on and further rationale for this nursing practice will be included within each activity of living as appropriate

Maintaining a safe environment

To prevent cross-infection and to maintain adequate standards of hygiene, a separate area should be designated for the storage and disposal of equipment used for toileting. Adequate handwashing facilities should be available for both patients and staff in this area and beside the patients' toilets. A good handwashing technique should be maintained to prevent cross-infection, and gloves should be worn to prevent contamination from body fluids. Nurses should be knowledgeable about related health authority practices.

All equipment should be washed and dried immediately after use in order to prevent cross-infection.

Plastic aprons should be worn by nursing staff when providing toilet facilities; these should be removed or changed after this nursing practice to prevent cross-infection.

Maintaining the patient's privacy during elimination sometimes conflicts with the need to maintain the safety of his or her environment. The nurse must make sure that there is no danger of the patient falling when using a bedpan or commode and ensure that he or she can be safely left on the ward toilet. The decision of which facilities are used for toileting depends not only on patients' conditions, but also on their orientation and mobility.

Safe moving and handling practices should be followed at all times according to the patient's individual plan. Hoists with toileting slings are available.

Communicating

Good communication skills on the part of the nursing staff can prevent patients worrying about toileting arrangements. They should be shown the patients' toilets or told how to ask for a bedpan, urinal or commode by the nurse who admits them, the reason for these arrangements being explained. A bell or other means of requesting assistance should be available as required, and requests for toilet facilities should be acted on immediately.

Eliminating is a private activity of living: the nurse's attitude and non-verbal communication when performing this nursing practice can affect the way in which the patient accepts the need for particular toilet arrangements.

Embarrassment and a fear of discovery are among the greatest concerns for patients with continence problems (Clayton et al 2000) so nurses should be sensitive to this as they are often the person with whom the patient will discuss the problem.

Eating and drinking

For the patient's own comfort and for the maintenance of personal hygiene, toilet facilities followed by handwashing should be offered before meals for all patients who are not self-caring.

A healthy diet that is high in fibre should be recommended in order to prevent constipation, which may exacerbate problems of continence. Some patients restrict their fluid intake to avoid incontinence, but this may aggravate an unstable bladder, causing increased frequency (Bardsley 2000). Certain drinks such as tea, coffee, carbonated drinks and alcohol can have an irritant effect on the bladder so should be restricted where appropriate without compromising the overall daily fluid intake (Dowse & McKender 2000).

A review of medicines is an important management strategy as some drugs, for example diuretics, sedatives, alcohol and analgesics, may affect continence either directly or indirectly (Getliffe & Dolman 1997).

Eliminating

The volume of urine should be measured and the results recorded for patients whose fluid balance is being monitored. Patients who are self-caring but whose urine is to be measured should be shown how to place a bedpan over the toilet seat and use that for micturition so that the nurse can measure the urinary volume. Urine should be observed for any abnormalities and tested as required (*see* 'Urine testing', p. 377).

Patients' bowel movements should be recorded so that problems of constipation or diarrhoea can be monitored. Any abnormalities should be immediately reported (*see* 'Specimen collection', p. 317).

The patient's condition will dictate whether a bedpan or commode is used when he or she is confined to bed. The stress of using a bedpan may, however, be considerable for some patients, and a commode should if possible be available. Male patients should be given a urinal for micturition whenever they require a bedpan or commode for defaecation.

Patients with problems of continence should be helped to use the appropriate toilet facilities at frequent intervals; any request for toileting should be answered immediately, so that the patient may regain adequate bladder control (Pomfret & Haslam 1994). If the patient is mobile, the bed and chair should be within easy reach of an available toilet to encourage continence. The assistance of one or two nurses may be needed. Patients with a continuing continence problem

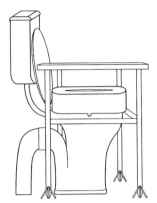

Figure 45.1 *Use of hand rails and a raised seat to promote independence at home*

should have a full continence assessment carried out (refer to the health authority policy).

At home, the toilet area can be adapted to promote independence, for example by rails, by raising the seat or by using a toilet frame (Fig. 45.1). The arrangements will be discussed and implemented by the primary health-care team (White 1994).

Personal cleansing and dressing

The nurse may have to help the patient to wipe or wash and dry the anus, vulval area and perineum following defaecation. This should always be done so that the wiping or washing is directed from front to back, away from the urethra, the paper towel being renewed after each wipe. For women in particular, it is important that no bacteria from the rectal area reach the urethra as this may cause a urinary tract infection; careful perineal toileting should prevent this (*see* 'Bed bath', p. 31).

To maintain independence, clothes can be adapted for ease of access for toileting, using folding skirts and extra Velcro fastenings (Fig. 45.2). The community team can help with appropriate advice.

Controlling body temperature

During toileting, the patient should be kept warm with adequate clothing and covers as well as footwear. This is particularly important in the ward toilet or on the bedside commode. Elderly people in particular become cold very quickly, and the nurse should ensure that patients are not left exposed for more than the minimum time required for toileting. The temperature of ward areas and toilet areas should remain at an environmentally comfortable level.

Mobilising

The choice of toilet arrangements for a particular patient, and the decision to use mechanical aids, may depend on the patient's individually assessed activity

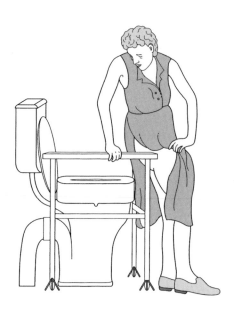

Figure 45.2 *Adaptation of clothing for ease of access when toileting*

of mobilising. The choice of arrangements should be discussed with and accepted by the patient. At home, special adjustments such as using rails or a raised seat may be made to the toilet area (Barker et al 1994).

Expressing sexuality

Help with toilet requirements is an invasion of a patient's privacy. The nurse may have to touch areas of the body that would normally be socially unacceptable to touch, which may embarrass the patient. The nurse's attitude and good communication skills will help to alleviate some of the embarrassment felt by the patient, although he or she may never be completely happy with this nursing practice. Urinary incontinence can also have an adverse effect on body image and be associated with sexual dysfunction (Winder 1994).

Sleeping

Toilet facilities should be offered just before the patient settles down for the night so that maximum comfort is achieved. The nurse should also assure the patient that if he or she needs help for toileting during the night, it will be readily available, ensuring that the bell or other means of communication is at hand.

Patient/carer education: key points

In partnership with the patient and/or carer, ensure that they are competent to carry out any practices required. Information should be given on an appropriate point of contact for any concerns that may arise.

The importance of regular toileting should be explained and if necessary reinforced with simple aids such as adapted clothing and the help of carers.

The reason for the use of mechanical aids for help with toileting should be explained.

Maintaining a healthy perineal area, and the efficient, safe cleaning of the area, should be emphasised. This may be achieved using something as simple as wet wipes or as specialised as a bidet.

The availability of special equipment to aid continence should be discussed with the patient according to his or her individual needs, as part of continuing care in an institutional setting or included in the goals for discharge to community care. This may include adaptations to the toilet area in the patient's home.

When a patient has had a full continence assessment, a plan of care should be discussed with the patient and mutually agreed with the community team.

References

Bardsley A 2000 Assessment of incontinence. Elderly Care 11(9): 36–39
Barker A, Cassar S, Gabbett J et al 1994 Handling people: equipment, advice and information. Disabled Living Foundation, London
Bayliss V, Cherry M, Lock R, Salter L 2000 Pathways for continence care: background and audit. British Journal of Nursing 9(9): 590–596
Bradley S, Moran R 1998 Better continence care through the use of research in clinical practice. Nursing Times 94(34): 52–53
Clayton J, Laycock J, Scott C 2000 What do users really think of continence care? Nursing Times Plus 96(19): 19–23
Daffurn K, Hillman K, Bauman A et al 1994 Fluid balance charts; do they measure up? British Journal of Nursing 3(16): 816–820
Department of Health 2000 Good practice in continence services. HMSO, London
Dowse J, McKender J 2000 Back to basics: continence. Nursing Times Plus 96(30): 7–9
Fader M, Petterson L, Dean G, Brooks R, Cottenden A 1999 The selection of female urinals: results of a multicentre evaluation. British Journal of Nursing 8(14): 918–925
Getliffe K, Dolman M (eds) 1997 Promoting continence: a clinical and research resource. Baillière Tindall/RCN, London
Glen S, Jownally S 1995 Privacy: a key nursing concept. British Journal of Nursing 4(2): 69–72
National Back Pain Association and Royal College of Nursing 1997 Guide to the handling of patients. 4th edn. NBPA, Middlesex
Pomfret I, Haslam J 1994 Continence management (a beneficial partnership). Community Outlook (Mar): 23–26
Professional Development Unit 1995 Lifting and handling, knowledge and practice. Nursing Times 91(1 suppl): 1–4
Royal College of Nursing 1999 Manual handling assessments in hospitals and the community. RCN, London
United Kingdom Central Council for Nursing, Midwifery and Health Visiting 1992 Code of professional conduct. UKCC, London
United Kingdom Central Council for Nursing, Midwifery and Health Visiting 1996 Guidelines for professional practice. UKCC, London
United Kingdom Central Council for Nursing, Midwifery and Health Visiting 1998 Guidelines for records and record keeping. UKCC, London
White H 1994 Choosing continence aids. British Journal of Nursing 3(22): 1158–1163
Winder A 1994 Incontinence and sexuality. Community Outlook (Aug): 21–22

46 Tracheostomy Care

There are two parts to this section:

1 Removal of respiratory tract secretions via a tracheostomy tube
2 Changing a tracheostomy tube.

The concluding subsection, 'Relevance to the activities of living', refers to both practices.

Learning outcomes

By the end of this section, you should know how to:

- prepare the patient for this nursing practice
- collect and prepare the equipment
- care for a patient who has a tracheostomy tube in situ.

Background knowledge required

Revision of the anatomy and physiology of the larynx, trachea and bronchus
Revision of 'Aseptic technique' (*see* p. 407)
Review of health authority policy on the care of a patient with a tracheostomy.

Indications and rationale for tracheostomy care

Tracheostomy is the surgical procedure of creating an artificial opening into the trachea *to relieve an obstruction of the airway* (caused by, for example, tumour or acute infection). This procedure is almost always performed in an operating theatre. The artificial airway is maintained with a suitable tube, which needs to be aspirated, cleaned and changed:

- *to ensure that the tube remains patent*
- *to reduce the risk of respiratory infection.*

1 Removal of respiratory tract secretions via a tracheostomy tube

Equipment

Tray
Sterile disposable gloves
Sterile suction catheters with a thumb control
Sterile container and water for flushing the catheter and tubing
Receptacle for soiled disposable items
Suction apparatus, e.g. a portable machine or centralised suction.

Guidelines and rationale for this nursing practice

- tracheal suction should be carried out only when secretions are audible in the tracheostomy tube or when the patient feels that the tube is blocked. *This reduces the risk of trauma to the mucosa*
- if possible, explain the nursing practice to the patient *to gain consent and co-operation.* Patients should be encouraged to participate actively in their care
- ensure the patient's privacy *to maintain dignity and a sense of self*
- collect the equipment *for efficiency of practice*
- assist the patient to a suitable position *for ease of access to the tracheostomy tube*
- observe the patient throughout this activity *for any signs of discomfort or distress*
- fill the sterile container with sterile water *to flush the suction catheter*
- open the end of the pack containing the connecting end of the suction catheter and connect it to the tubing of the suction machine. The diameter of the catheter should not exceed half the diameter of the tracheostomy tube *to ensure that hypoxia does not occur*
- put a disposable glove on the dominant hand
- slide the cover off the catheter and rinse it through with sterile water *to lubricate it*
- insert the catheter into the tracheostomy with the gloved hand but without any suction (Fig. 46.1) for the length of the tracheostomy tube

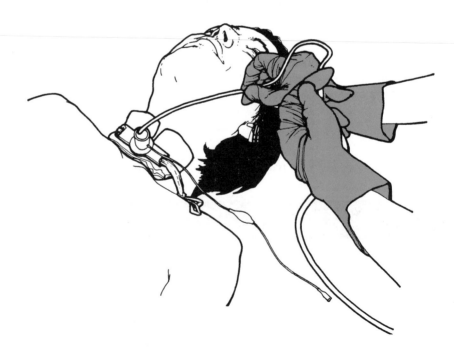

Figure 46.1 *Aspirating respiratory tract secretions via a tracheostomy tube. Reproduced from Chilman & Thomas (1987), with permission*

- withdraw the catheter, applying suction by covering the thumb control hole and rotating the catheter while this is being done. If the secretions are tenacious and difficult to remove, nebulised saline or mechanical humidification may be administered. *This loosens the secretions for easier removal.* Intermittent humidification helps the patient *to expectorate spontaneously*
- allow the patient to rest and re-oxygenate before repeating insertion of the catheter
- dispose of the catheter at the end of the practice after rinsing both the catheter and the tubing with sterile water
- ensure that the patient is left feeling as comfortable as possible
- dispose of the equipment safely *for the protection of others*
- document the nursing practice appropriately, monitor the after-effects and report any abnormal findings immediately *to provide a written record and enable prompt intervention should an adverse reaction to the procedure be noted*
- in undertaking this practice, nurses are accountable for their actions, the quality of care delivered and record-keeping according to the *Code of Professional Conduct* (UKCC 1992), *Guidelines for Professional Practice* (UKCC 1996) and *Guidelines for Records and Record Keeping* (UKCC 1998).

2 Changing a tracheostomy tube

Equipment

Tray or trolley
Sterile dressings pack
Sterile tracheostomy tube, taped and with an obturator, and a tube one size smaller in case of difficulty recannulating the stoma
Sterile KY jelly
Sterile tracheal dilators
Sterile scissors
Tracheostomy dressing, e.g. Lyofoam
Container of sodium bicarbonate solution in which to put the soiled silver tracheostomy tube
Disposable gloves
Instrument brush
Receptacle for soiled disposable items.

Plastic disposable or single-patient tracheostomy tubes are usually used in the management of both temporary and long-term tracheostomies. They normally incorporate an inner tube that can be changed and cleaned regularly, reducing the need to perform a complete change of the tracheostomy tube. A patient may occasionally have a silver tube in situ that also incorporates an inner tube, although this is now rare because of the extensive range of plastic tubes available (Fig. 46.2).

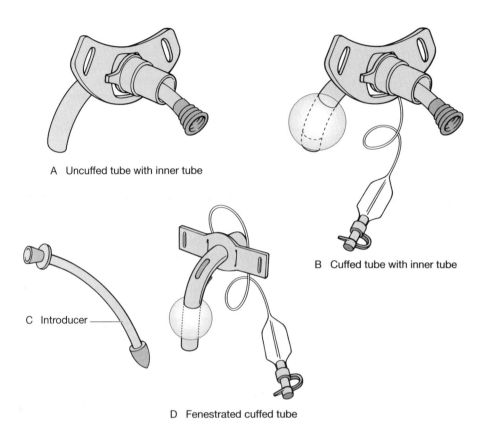

A   Uncuffed tube with inner tube

B   Cuffed tube with inner tube

C   Introducer

D   Fenestrated cuffed tube

Figure 46.2
*Tracheostomy tubes
in common use
A Uncuffed tube with
inner tube
B Cuffed tube with
inner tube
C Introducer
D Fenestrated
cuffed tube*

**Guidelines and
rationale for this
nursing practice**

- explain the nursing practice to the patient *to gain consent and co-operation. Patients should be encouraged to be active participants in care*
- ensure the patient's privacy *to maintain dignity and a sense of self*
- collect and prepare the equipment *for efficiency of practice*
- assist the patient to a suitable position *to allow this practice to be carried out*
- observe the patient throughout this activity *for any signs of discomfort or distress*
- open the dressings pack and the tracheostomy tube pack
- check that the obturator fits. Check in particular that it can be easily removed *as it blocks the airway once the tube is in situ*
- lubricate the end of the tube and obturator *for ease of insertion*
- make a slit in the end of the protective pad *so that it will easily wrap round the tube*
- put on the disposable gloves *for your own and the patient's protection*
- remove the soiled tube with a smooth outward and downward motion, discarding it into the receptacle for disposable items if it is plastic, or putting it into a container of sodium bicarbonate solution if it is silver. *The sodium bicarbonate loosens any dried areas of secretion.* Ensure that the tube is well rinsed after sodium bicarbonate has been used

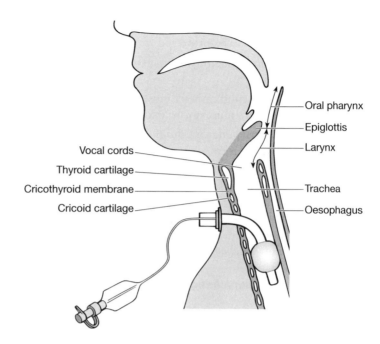

Figure 46.3 *The anatomical position of a tracheostomy tube*

Labels in figure: Oral pharynx, Epiglottis, Larynx, Vocal cords, Thyroid cartilage, Cricothyroid membrane, Cricoid cartilage, Trachea, Oesophagus

- remove the gloves *to allow more dextrous hand movements*
- hold the new tube by the tapes and insert it smoothly from below in an upwards, inwards and downwards movement into the trachea (Fig. 46.3). *This follows the line of the stoma*
- immediately remove the obturator while holding the tube in place *to free the airway*
- tie the tapes at the side of the patient's neck. *This is a more comfortable position than the back*
- slide the protective pad into position round the stoma
- ensure that the patient is left feeling as comfortable as possible
- dispose of the equipment safely *for the protection of others*
- if a silver tube has been used, clean the soiled tube using the brush and gloved hands
- record this nursing practice appropriately, monitor the after-effects and report any abnormal findings immediately, *providing a written record and enabling prompt intervention should an adverse reaction to the practice be noted*
- in undertaking this practice, nurses are accountable for their actions, the quality of care delivered and record-keeping according to the *Code of Professional Conduct* (UKCC 1992), *Guidelines for Professional Practice* (UKCC 1996) and *Guidelines for Records and Record Keeping* (UKCC 1998).

Relevance to the activities of living

Maintaining a safe environment

All precautions must be taken for the prevention of infection as the air inhaled via the tracheostomy tube bypasses the protective ciliated epithelium of the nose, the risk of pulmonary infection therefore being increased. The wound must also be protected from sources of infection.

Thorough handwashing should be carried out, preferably using an antiseptic detergent.

The suction catheter must be inserted gently (Buglass 1999). The prescribed suction pressure must not be exceeded or the tracheal mucosa may be traumatised.

Tracheal dilators should be available when changing the tube of a patient with a newly formed tracheostomy in case there is difficulty inserting the new tube. This is, however, a rare occurrence.

Care must be taken to maintain a clear airway at all times as the tube interferes with the normal cough reflex. The need for suctioning may be detected visually (the appearance of laboured breathing, an increase in the rate or a change in the pattern of breathing), aurally (moist, gurgling sounds) or by auscultation (low-pitched, loose rattling noises) (Griggs 1998).

Communicating

A tracheostomy reduces the function of the vocal cords so the patient may have a problem with verbal communication; the use of a pad of paper and pencil may partially overcome this. A bell must always be available for the patient to summon assistance.

Once the cuff on the tube has been deflated or the tube changed for an uncuffed one, the patient will be able to speak by breathing in, obstructing the tube with a finger and forcing the air up through the vocal cords to produce sound. If the tracheostomy is permanent or mechanical respiration is not required, a tube with a speaking valve may be used.

If it is envisaged that the tracheostomy will be permanent, a teaching programme to educate the patient to change his or her own tube may be planned and implemented by suitably qualified staff (Serra 2000).

Breathing

The purpose of a tracheostomy is to aid the patient's breathing so the nurse must be vigilant in ensuring the patency of the tube at all times.

Most tubes currently used incorporate an inner tube. This can be changed daily or more frequently if the patient produces a copious amount of secretions. The inner tube should be removed and a spare one inserted immediately to prevent a build-up of secretions in the outer tube, which will compromise the patient's airway and necessitate changing the whole tube. The dirty inner tube should be cleaned with sodium bicarbonate solution and stored dry ready for the next change.

Eating and drinking

As the trachea is anatomically in close proximity to the upper alimentary organs, the presence of a tracheostomy tube may cause apprehension about swallowing. This can be exacerbated if a cuffed tracheostomy tube is being used to prevent aspiration. The presence of the cuff in the trachea can press back against the oesophageal wall, giving the patient a sense of something in his or her throat; this may hinder swallowing. Education and encouragement should be given to the patient to maintain a good dietary intake.

Personal cleansing and dressing

Advice may be required on the most suitable type of clothing to wear around the stoma and on skin care of the stoma area, especially if the tracheostomy is permanent. The tapes should be tied at the side of the neck rather than over the cervical spine where the knot causes discomfort.

Expressing sexuality

A permanent tracheostomy may give the patient psychological problems as the result of an altered body image: any disfigurement or deviation from the normal appearance can alter a person's sexual self-image (Roper et al 2000). A talk with someone who has successfully adjusted to life with a tracheostomy can help.

Adapting to breathing through one's neck is likely to take time for the patient and his or her partner. The sensation of feeling moist air from the stoma on one's neck while kissing the patient may take some time to get used to.

A person with a tracheostomy has to learn that, when coughing, it is the stoma that needs to be covered rather than the nose or mouth.

Sleeping

The patient may initially be frightened to sleep, fearing that the tube may become blocked; reassurance that staff are available and observing him or her may have to be given to relieve such anxiety. A speaking valve attachment should not be left in situ at night in case secretions build up behind the flap and prevent it opening.

Patient/carer education: key points

In partnership with the patient and/or carer, ensure that they are competent to carry out any practices required. Information should be given on an appropriate point of contact for any concerns that may arise.

Patients require planned education to help them cope with the anxiety that most people experience when they first have a tracheostomy. If the tracheostomy tube does not have a speaking flap, they will need help and advice about alternative ways of communicating.

Patients who have permanent tracheostomies will require a structured teaching programme of self-care.

References

Buglass E 1999 Tracheostomy care: tracheal suction and humidification. British Journal of Nursing 8(8): 500–504

Chilman A, Thomas M 1987 Understanding nursing care. 3rd edn. Churchill Livingstone, Edinburgh

Griggs A 1998 Tracheostomy: suctioning and humidification. Nursing Standard 13(2): 49–53, 55–56

Roper N, Logan W, Tierney A 2000 The Roper–Logan–Tierney model of nursing. Churchill Livingstone, Edinburgh

Serra A 2000 Tracheostomy care. Nursing Standard 14(42): 45–52

United Kingdom Central Council for Nursing, Midwifery and Health Visiting 1992 Code of professional conduct. UKCC, London

United Kingdom Central Council for Nursing, Midwifery and Health Visiting 1996 Guidelines for professional practice. UKCC, London

United Kingdom Central Council for Nursing, Midwifery and Health Visiting 1998 Guidelines for records and record keeping. UKCC, London

47 Transfer of Patients Between Care Settings

Learning outcomes

By the end of this section, you should know how to:

- prepare the patient and carer for transfer to another care setting
- complete patient transfer documentation.

Background knowledge required

Carers (Recognition and Services) Act 1996
Revision of health authority policy on the transfer of patients
Discharge of Patients from Hospital (UKCC 1995)
The Hospital Discharge Workbook (DoH 1994).

Indications and rationale for patient transfer

Health-care reform has resulted in a much greater focus on the appropriate use of the services available for patient care. Thus, the patient may be transferred between institutional and community settings within the statutory health and social care agencies or in the voluntary or private/independent sectors, *as is judged appropriate for his or her individual needs and benefit.*

Outline of the procedure

'Patient transfer' (rather than discharge) is the term used in this section as it demonstrates a continuum rather than a cessation of care. The procedure may be simple or complex, depending on the needs of the patient and carer. The systematic approach to care – namely assessment, planning, implementation and evaluation – may, however, be used as a framework for the patient transfer process:

- The assessment phase involves the collection of data pertinent to the patient and/or carer. A variety of sources may be used to build up an holistic picture of the patient and the caring environment. Some of this information will already have been collected during the patient admission assessment.
- The planning stage utilises the assessment data to provide a plan of transfer. Liaison with other agencies to request and discuss their input will also be carried out at this stage of the process.
- The implementation phase involves putting the plan into action and completing patient transfer documentation.
- The evaluation stage of the transfer procedure is essential in order to assess the effectiveness of the process and to identify any difficulties or problems.

Guidelines and rationale for this nursing practice

General principles will be given, followed by guidelines for planning and implementing the transfer process. Some of the guidelines may not be applicable to patients transferring from community to institutional settings.

Multidisciplinary working has been shown to be challenging because of different practice goals and levels of professional power (Penhale 1997), assessment often being fragmented (Audit Commission 1997), and care roles and responsibilities becoming blurred between what is classed as nursing and social care. A new form of assessment is planned to differentiate between nursing and social care needs (DoH 2000). Poorly co-ordinated transfer arrangements have an enormous emotional and financial costs for families and care services, with an increased risk of readmission (Nazarko 1998).

Principles

- the patient and carer should be involved in all stages of the transfer process, *enabling a consideration and discussion of their needs prior to the transfer plan being completed and implemented* (DoH 1995, Worth & Tierney 1994). Older people in particular often find it difficult to adjust to early discharge (Nazarko 1999)
- patient transfer is normally a multidisciplinary procedure that may involve social, voluntary and independent care agencies as well as different health-care professionals, *ensuring an holistic approach to patient transfer*
- good communication is an essential part of the patient transfer process *as poor communication patterns affect continuity of care* on transfer from community to institutional settings as well as from institutional to community care (Evers 1991, Sollitt 1992)
- it is essential that there be an early involvement of and liaison with staff from the receiving care setting (which may be a hospital ward, an intermediate care facility, a nursing home or the patient's own home). Some areas have a designated liaison nurse who provides a link between institutional and community care *to promote continuity of care* (Worth & Tierney 1994)
- at least 48 hours' notice of transfer from institutional to community care should be provided. In addition, patients should not be transferred immediately prior to a weekend or public holiday *in order that adequate community care support services can be organised* (Saville & Bartholomew 1994, Worth & Tierney 1994)
- an evaluation system should be in place *to judge the effectiveness of the patient transfer process* (McHale 1995).

Planning patient transfer

- discuss care needs with the patient and carer *to ascertain their views and requirements, and involve them in the decision-making process*
- plan and initiate any teaching programmes for the patient and/or carer. Examples include a self-medication programme for patients being transferred from institutional to community care (Fuller 1995) and a moving and

handling teaching session for carers *to prepare the patient and carer for tasks that they will be required to undertake in the community*

- consult, liaise with and refer to the appropriate care agencies (health, social, voluntary or independent). If the patient has complex care needs, it may be necessary to invite all the relevant personnel, including the patient and/or carer, to a case conference *to ensure that support services are in position prior to transfer*
- order any equipment or patient aids *to ensure that the receiving care setting meets the patient's needs*
- if the patient has complex needs and is being transferred from institutional care, it is valuable to organise a home assessment visit prior to transfer. This will involve the patient, carer and district nurse as well as other relevant personnel such the occupational therapist, physiotherapist and social care staff *to enable the patient's needs to be assessed within his or her own environment and to enable an assessment of the carer's ability to provide care*
- arrange for transport between care settings *to ensure that the transport is appropriate for the patient's needs*
- order any medicines and assess the patient's ability to administer medication. If deficits are identified, a teaching programme may have to be initiated for the patient and carer, and/or patient compliance devices can be introduced. This should be carried out in conjunction with the pharmacist *to ensure that a small supply of medicines is available for the immediate transfer period and that the patient and carer are able to administer the medicines correctly*
- consult with the carers about access arrangements to the patient's home on the day of transfer *to enable access arrangements to be made in advance of the transfer*
- give an approximate expected time of arrival to the patient, carer and any other personnel who require this information (for example, the district nurse and home-help, or the continuing care facility) *to enable the caring network to be organised.*

Implementing the transfer process

- complete the patient transfer documentation (Box 47.1) and retain a copy *to provide a permanent record of the transfer process*
- ensure that the medical staff have completed a transfer form to give to the patient's general practitioner. This usually comprises a summary of diagnoses, treatments and medication and *provides a permanent summary of admission details*
- send the documentation to the personnel in the receiving care setting. This should be carried out according to local health authority policy but may involve an internal mailing system, the postal service, delivery by the patient/carer, faxing or a computer network. In the future, patient-held records (which stay with the patient as he or she moves between care areas) may be the way in which information is communicated, *thus enabling the sharing of information between care settings*

Box 47.1   Checklist of contents for transfer documentation

Social data
- Patient details – name, date of birth, address, telephone number, occupation, housing and any dependants
- Carer details – name, address, telephone number, occupation, any relevant health problems or disabilities, other dependants and ability/willingness to care

Health data
- Diagnosis (including patient/carer's knowledge and understanding of the diagnosis)
- Disability/impairment
- Prognosis (if applicable)
- Medication (including any specialised instructions or medicine aids)
- Treatment (this might include details of procedures such as wound care or catheter management)
- Investigations carried out and results if known

Patient/carer's needs
- These will be specific to the service user and should be decided in conjunction with the patient/carer (for more information, *see* 'Relevance to the activities of living' in the text)

Support services
- Details of care/therapy provided by professionals from other services (such as dietitians, physiotherapists or occupational therapists) in the current care setting
- Information – name, contact number and type of input – on any support services arranged for the post-transfer period (including the date of commencement)
- Most care settings will have a directory of services in the local area. For information on national services, contact the NHS Helpline (*see* text)

Financial data
- Details of welfare benefits (either in place or applied for)

Equipment data
- Details of equipment, either in place or requested (indicating the source of the equipment)
- Equipment should be in place prior to transfer

Health promotion/patient education
- Provide a summary of:
  — health promotion activities
  — information on any education programmes
- Enclose a copy of the patient education or health promotion literature given to the patient

All documentation should be signed and dated by the named nurse responsible for the patient's care.

- discuss any medication with the patient. This includes reinforcing information provided by the medical staff such as the reason for the drug, its dosage, timing or frequency and route of administration, and any special instructions. The use of a personal medical record card may be of value to some patients (Whyte 1994) *to reinforce the information given on the container label and to facilitate understanding*

- check that the patient has all his or her personal belongings *to ensure that no property is lost during transfer*
- arrange any follow-up outpatient appointment *so that the patient and carer are aware of follow-up care*
- provide details of the receiving care setting (the named nurse and contact number)
- in undertaking this practice, nurses are accountable for their actions, the quality of care delivered and record-keeping according to the *Code of Professional Conduct* (UKCC 1992), *Guidelines for Professional Practice* (UKCC 1996) and *Guidelines for Records and Record Keeping* (UKCC 1998).

Relevance to the activities of living	The material provided under each of the activities gives an indication of the type of information that could be shared between care settings.

Maintaining a safe environment

Information related to any risk factors should be recorded. This might include:

- difficulties related to the self-administration of medication
- the patient being at risk of falls
- any infection that may put the patient or carers at risk. If appropriate, the MRSA status of the patient should be given (*see* 'Isolation nursing', p. 201)
- any sensory deficit that may put the patient at risk.

Whereas patients may function effectively within their existing environment, they may be at risk (for example by becoming disorientated) in a new care setting.

Communicating

The patient's ability to communicate and understand information, as well as any deficits such as of hearing, sight or speech, should be noted. Information on equipment such as hearing aids or spectacles that the patient may require to communicate effectively should be provided.

It is essential that staff communicate with the patient/carer to ensure that they are fully informed and understand all aspects of the transfer. Any anxieties or concerns should be discussed and documented.

If transfer is taking place to a continuing care facility, the emotional feelings experienced by patients are often neglected (Cotter et al 1998), hospital nursing staff knowing little about care homes (Reed & Morgan 1999). The patient should whenever possible visit the facility prior to discharge.

Breathing

Record any difficulties that the patient has with breathing, as well as treatments such as inhalers or oxygen therapy. For the patient being transferred to the community, arrangements should be made for the delivery of oxygen cylinders or a concentrator, teaching being given to the patient and carer on its use and precautions.

Eating and drinking

The nutritional status of the patient can affect the healing process so any problems should be documented. Information should be provided on any special dietary requirements and whether there has been input from a dietitian. Information is also needed on patients' ability to feed themselves and on the equipment required to aid this activity.

Equipment and feeding regime details should be provided for patients with enteral feeding requirements. Carers or patients will usually be taught this procedure prior to leaving hospital.

Eliminating

Bladder and bowel function are essential activities. Like nutrition, they may be affected by a change in environment or illness. A record of the patient's current bladder and bowel pattern should therefore be given, together with a note of any difficulties related to function, including abnormal patterns such as diarrhoea, constipation or urinary incontinence. Any investigations should be documented, and a record of necessary continence aids or toilet equipment should be given.

The patient may have begun a teaching programme (such as bladder training) that requires to be continued in the receiving care setting.

Personal cleansing and dressing

The patient's ability to carry out this activity should be described, a record being given of the assistance the patient requires as well as of equipment such as bathing aids (Seymour 1995).

The patient may be at risk of pressure sores. The risk factors and score (*see* 'Skin care', p. 309) should be documented, along with the plan of care and any special equipment required. If pressure sores are present, a full description (including tracings) should be documented as baseline data for the staff in the receiving care setting.

The condition of the patient's mouth may affect his or her health. Thus, any problems such as ulceration, oral infection or problems with dentition, plus details of treatment, should be described.

Mobilising

The following should be documented:

- deficits in the patient's ability to mobilise
- information on any rehabilitation programmes
- the equipment required to aid mobility
- the level and type of assistance required from another person
- any active or passive exercises that need to be followed up in the receiving care setting.

Working and playing

Information on the patient's social activities may be of importance. The patient's employment status may also be relevant if, because of the illness, time off is required or unemployment is a possibility.

Day care attendance and/or activities should be recorded.

Expressing sexuality

Concerns regarding a change in body image caused by the illness should be discussed and documented.

Sexual issues require sensitivity and diplomacy. The patient may discuss issues of a highly confidential nature, and it may not always be appropriate to document this information. Advice on how to approach the issue of sexuality is given by Van Ooijen (1995).

Sleeping

A change in environment or anxiety about his or her health is likely to have an impact on the patient's normal sleep pattern. Any difficulties and treatments should be recorded.

Dying

Patients may contemplate death during an episode of illness. Such thoughts may be transitory or may be longer lasting when the patient has a life-threatening or terminal illness. It is important that the staff in the receiving care environment are aware of the information and understanding that the patient has about his or her condition and prognosis. Counselling initiated with the patient should be outlined.

Patient/carer education: key points

In partnership with the patient and/or carer, ensure that they are competent to carry out any practices required. Information should be given on an appropriate point of contact for any concerns that may arise.

Education for the patient and carer will depend on the needs identified in the planning phase of transfer. Patient education may take the form of:

- health promotion initiatives
- the teaching, demonstration and supervision of a practical procedure such as the administration of insulin
- literature on a specific illness or disease such as myocardial infarction. This will be used in conjunction with discussion
- verbal discussion to evaluate understanding (for example of an illness or medication) as verbal advice is not always assimilated by patients.

Information on support groups is available from local health, social and voluntary agencies or at a national level from the National Health Service

Telephone Helpline Scotland (0800 224488) or NHS Direct (not available in Scotland; 0845 4647), or via the Internet.

Details of patient education programmes should be recorded in the transfer documentation.

References

Audit Commission 1997 The coming of age: improving care services for older people. Audit Commission, London

Cotter A, Meyer J, Roberts S 1998 Transition from hospital to long term institutional care. Nursing Times 94(34): 54–56

Department of Health 1994 The hospital discharge workbook: a manual on hospital discharge practice. HMSO, London

Department of Health 1995 The patient's charter. HMSO, London

Department of Health 2000 The NHS National Plan. HMSO, London (Applies to England; different plans have been developed within the other countries of the UK)

Evers HK 1991 Issues in community care services. Nursing Standard 5(21): 29–31

Fuller D 1995 Simplifying the system: assessing drug administration methods. Professional Nurse 10(5): 315–317

McHale SA 1995 Implementation of a patient discharge policy. Professional Nurse 10(9): 590–592

Nazarko L 1998 Improving discharge: the role of the discharge coordinator. Nursing Standard 12(49): 35–37

Nazarko L 1999 Paying the price for early discharge. Nursing Times 95(12): 51–52

Penhale B 1997 Towards effective discharge planning. Health Care in Later Life 2(1): 46–56

Reed J, Morgan D 1999 Discharging older people from hospital to care homes. Journal of Advanced Nursing 29(4): 819–825

Saville R, Bartholomew J 1994 Planning better discharges. Journal of Community Nursing 8(3): 10–14

Seymour J 1995 Bathing aids: handling and lifting in the home. Nursing Times 91(8): 53–54

Sollitt L 1992 Working together. Journal of Community Nursing 6(3): 9–11

United Kingdom Central Council for Nursing, Midwifery and Health Visiting 1992 Code of professional conduct. UKCC, London

UKCC 1995 Discharge of patients from hospital. Registrar's letter 18/1995. UKCC, London

United Kingdom Central Council for Nursing, Midwifery and Health Visiting 1996 Guidelines for professional practice. UKCC, London

United Kingdom Central Council for Nursing, Midwifery and Health Visiting 1998 Guidelines for records and record keeping. UKCC, London

Van Ooijen E 1995 How illness may affect patients' sexuality. Nursing Times 91(23): 36–37

Whyte LA 1994 Medication cards for elderly people: a study. Nursing Standard 8(48): 25–28

Worth A, Tierney A 1994 Community nurses and discharge planning. Nursing Standard 8(21): 25–30

48 Unconscious Patient

Learning outcomes	By the end of this section, you should know how to:
	▪ maintain an adequate airway for the unconscious patient
	▪ care for the unconscious patient in such a way that his or her activities of living are appropriately maintained despite almost total dependency.

Background knowledge required	Revision of the anatomy and physiology of the nervous system, with special reference to the brain
	Review of health authority policy relating to the care of the unconscious patient.

Indications and rationale for care during a state of unconsciousness	Nursing intervention is required when a patient's level of consciousness is such that, unaided, he or she can no longer maintain a clear airway, the normal protective reflexes are so reduced that the patient can no longer maintain the safety of the environment, and the patient is unable to perform the everyday activities of living (Hickey 1997).

The unconscious state is most commonly associated with:

▪ patients who have a cerebral vascular accident, *when areas of brain tissue will be damaged and have a diminished blood supply*, e.g.:
  — cerebral haemorrhage
  — cerebral embolus or ischaemia
  — subarachnoid haemorrhage
▪ patients who have taken an overdose of analgesic drugs, *which will affect the function of the brain cells*
▪ patients who have a traumatic head injury *as brain cells may be damaged by the injury*
▪ patients who have a brain tumour *causing pressure on and damage to the brain*
▪ patients who are in a comatose state caused by:
  — severe infection *as hyperpyrexia may affect brain cell function*
  — hypothermia *because a severe temperature change reduces brain cell activity* (Toulson 1994)
  — metabolic disturbances, i.e. uncontrolled diabetes mellitus (hyperglycaemia or hypoglycaemia), *which may result in reduced brain cell function*
▪ patients who have received prescribed anaesthetic medication during and following surgery, *which affects the patient's neurological state*
▪ patients in the terminal stage of illness *when cerebral function is diminished.*

Equipment

Bed with a detachable head
Padded cot sides
Disposable airway – either Guedel oropharyngeal or nasopharyngeal
Ambubag with valve and mask
Equipment for assessing the level of consciousness
Equipment for oral, pharyngeal or tracheal suction
Equipment for oxygen therapy
Equipment for a nasogastric, PEG or total parenteral nutrition feeding system
Mouth care tray
Eye care tray
Catheter care tray
Equipment for endotracheal intubation if required.

Details of the equipment for specific nursing practices can be found in the relevant sections of this book.

Equipment for assessing the level of consciousness

Pencil torch to assess eye pupil size and reaction
Level chart of consciousness, e.g. the Glasgow coma scale.

The Glasgow coma scale   This enables an assessment of level of consciousness to be made, using a numbered scale. The assessment is of motor activity, for example limb movements, verbal responses, reaction to pain and pupillary reactions to light (Fig. 48.1). This scale is now used in many health authorities, although each area may have documentation of the scale of recordings presented in a different way and may incorporate other recordings on the same chart (Ellis & Cavanagh 1992); this has been permitted without infringement of copyright (Allan 1984). A total score of 15 indicates full consciousness.

Guidelines and rationale for this nursing practice

The most important aspect of nursing is the maintenance of a clear airway while the reason for the patient's unconsciousness is being diagnosed and treated *so that the patient's respiratory function is as efficient as possible in the circumstances.*

- remove any dentures that may be present *to avoid obstruction of the airway*
- turn the patient into a semi-prone position or onto his or her side, the neck extended, *to prevent the tongue slipping back and occluding the airway, and also to prevent any secretions flowing into the trachea as the swallowing reflex is absent*
- observe the patient throughout this activity *to monitor any adverse effects*
- perform oral and pharyngeal suction – endotracheal suction being carried out only by an appropriately skilled practitioner – *to prevent the aspiration of bronchial or oral secretions* (*see* 'Tracheostomy care', p. 351)
- insert an airway if required, *to help to maintain an adequate airway*
- administer oxygen therapy as prescribed *to prevent hypoxia* (*see* 'Oxygen therapy', p. 271)

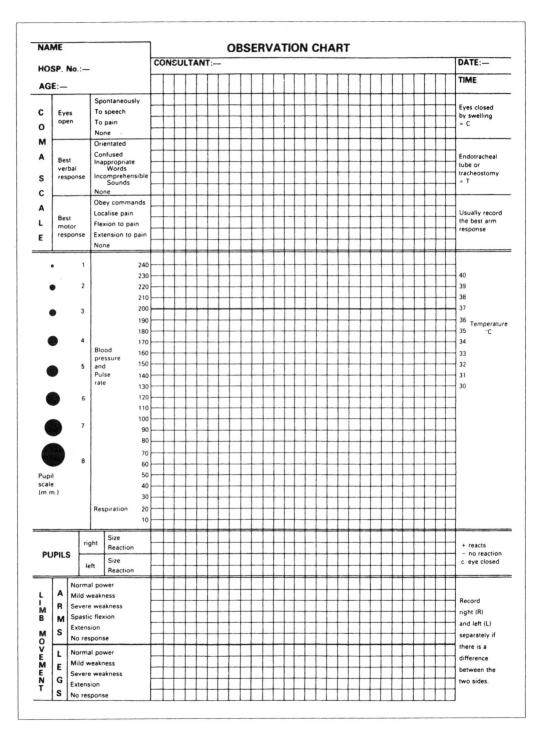

Figure 48.1 *Glasgow coma scale: chart for documenting the assessment of patient's level of consciousness*

- position the patient's limbs *to maintain his or her position comfortably and to allow an adequate flow of blood to the extremities*
- assess and record the level of consciousness at appropriate intervals between quarter and 4 hourly as advised by the medical practitioner *to monitor and evaluate the patient's progress*
- perform oral and pharyngeal suction every 2 hours or as frequently as required, either directly or through the airway as appropriate, *to reduce the volume of secretion to a minimum, thus preventing any danger of aspiration*
- nurse the patient on a high-dependency pressure-relieving mattress system, and alternate the patient's side of lying every 2 hours *to maintain healthy tissue at the pressure areas and to aid the expansion of each lung* (*see* 'Skin care', p. 309)
- provide all nursing care as frequently as required, explaining the care to the patient despite the unconscious state and ensuring privacy before commencing care. The patient will be completely dependent for all his or her needs, and the nurse must *respect the patient's individuality and maintain his or her dignity at all times* (Hancock 1992)
- record the temperature, pulse, respiration rate and blood pressure as frequently as required *to maintain the observations and record any change in the patient's condition*
- document all nursing practices appropriately and report abnormal findings immediately *to ensure safe practice and enable prompt, appropriate medical and nursing intervention to be initiated*
- in undertaking this practice, nurses are accountable for their actions, the quality of care delivered and record-keeping according to the *Code of Professional Conduct* (UKCC 1992), *Guidelines for Professional Practice* (UKCC 1996) and *Guidelines for Records and Record Keeping* (UKCC 1998).

Relevance to the activities of living

Observations on and further rationale for this nursing practice will be included within each activity of living as appropriate.

A patient who is unconscious is at or near the totally dependent end of the dependence–independence continuum. Nursing staff have to assist, or perform for the patient, the various activities of living until he or she fully regains consciousness (Pemberton 2000).

Maintaining a safe environment

The patient should be nursed on a firm bed in an area where he or she can be constantly observed. This may be in a single cubicle with a nurse to provide special care, or in a bed near the nurses' station so that frequent observations can be maintained.

The area should be well lit so that any change in the patient's colour can be noted and any abnormal findings reported. Diurnal variations in the light level should, however, be maintained.

Cot sides should be in position expect when nursing practices are being performed. This will prevent the patient falling if he or she is restless or in a semi-conscious state. The cot sides should be padded to prevent patients damaging themselves on any hard equipment; appropriately placed pillows can be effective.

Communicating

Before beginning the assessment, the nurse should ensure that the patient is as comfortable as possible in the circumstances. The response to verbal commands and the movement of limbs may be impaired if the patient is uncomfortable or in pain, which may also affect pupillary reactions (Chudley 1994).

It is essential to make sure that the patient has no major hearing deficit: a profoundly deaf patient will not respond to any verbal instructions and may be less comatose than the nurse realises. Such a patient may become restless and frightened when regaining consciousness as explanations of his or her surroundings and the nursing interventions have not been heard.

The nursing assessment of the patient should be obtained from his or her family, especially if the patient is unconscious on admission; this should also include the social and family background. It is a great help to communication if the nurse knows the patient's forename or nickname as he or she may not readily respond to a formal approach such as 'Mr or Mrs Smith'. It is also a help to know something about the patient's family and interests. Individualised care is enhanced when the nurse is able to chat about the grandchildren, or the dog or the music charts even when there is no immediate response from the patient. This also helps the family to feel that the nursing remains individualised and personal.

The nurse should talk to the patient at every opportunity, using touch to reassure the patient even if he or she appears to be deeply unconscious (Smith 1997). The nurse must try to orientate patients to their surroundings even when there appears to be no response: they should be told where they are and why, as well as the day, date and time as appropriate.

Before commencing any nursing intervention, nurses should introduce themselves and explain what is to happen, reinforcing this throughout the time they spend with the patient.

The use of touch as a means of communication is helpful to both the patient and the nurse when caring for an unconscious patient. Physical contact with friends or relatives can help to reorientate a patient as he or she regains consciousness. Relatives should be encouraged to sit beside an unconscious patient, holding a hand as well as talking to him or her, whenever they visit (Carruthers 1992).

The patient's response to pain should be noted as part of the assessment of the level of consciousness. This can be achieved by squeezing the trapezius muscle or supraorbital region only. This will not cause any damage, but the patient will react if the pressure is felt as pain. The way the limbs move in response to pain should be noted and recorded on the assessment chart.

Eye care should be carried out 2 hourly. The inability to blink prevents the eyes being bathed in lacrimal fluid, and the unconscious patient is at risk of developing corneal ulcers if the eyes are not treated regularly (*see* 'Eye care', p. 151). The lids can be taped shut to prevent drying.

The nursing plan should indicate how and when nursing care is carried out and needs to include the position of the patient during each period of turning.

Breathing

A clear airway should be maintained until the patient has fully recovered consciousness and has an adequate swallowing and cough reflex.

The respiration rate should be recorded as frequently as necessary but at least every 4 hours. The depth and the pattern of respiration should also be noted, as should any evidence of a cough or cough reflex.

The blood pressure and pulse rate should be recorded at least every 4 hours or as frequently as necessary as any abnormality may indicate a change in intracranial pressure.

Oral and pharyngeal suctioning should be performed every 2 hours or as required to clear the airway of secretions. It should be carried out before turning the patient as this will prevent secretions draining into the trachea when the patient is moved. The amount and consistency of the secretions should be noted and any purulent or bloodstained secretions reported. If the airway is not adequately maintained with such routine measures, and the patient has excess secretions that are difficult to clear, the medical practitioner may intubate the trachea with an endotracheal tube, the patient then breathing through this.

The patient's position should be changed 2 hourly so that he or she lies on alternate sides. This helps to ensure an equal expansion of each lung over 24 hours and aids with the drainage of any bronchial secretions.

Eating and drinking

Nutrients and fluids may have to be given by nasogastric tube or intravenously. The nasogastric route is used when possible, and a nasogastric tube should initially be passed to prevent any inhalation of the stomach contents. When the presence of bowel sounds has been established, the medical practitioner may prescribe nasogastric feeds (*see* 'Nutrition', p. 253).

The patient should have 2 hourly mouth care to maintain a healthy oropharyngeal mucosa (*see* 'Mouth care', p. 225).

Fluid intake should be recorded and fluid balance charts maintained to monitor the level of hydration and prevent dehydration.

Eliminating

The unconscious patient is incontinent of both faeces and urine.

Male patients may be fitted with an external sheath catheter, observation for any sign of bladder distension being maintained. Catheterisation should be performed for female patients to prevent incontinence, which increases the risk of tissue damage to the pressure areas. Catheterisation may also be prescribed for male patients who have a prolonged period of unconsciousness. Catheter care should be performed regularly, and bladder washouts may also be prescribed (*see* 'Catheterisation: urinary', p. 95).

The urinary output should be recorded and fluid balance charts maintained as this helps to monitor the patient's renal function.

Bowel movements should be noted and recorded. Constipation may be more of a problem than diarrhoea for the unconscious patient so suppositories or enemas may be prescribed regularly (*see* 'Suppositories', p. 337).

Personal cleansing and dressing

The nursing plan should include a daily bed bath and any additional washing as required to keep the patient clean and comfortable, and the skin in good condition. The nails should be cut short to prevent abrasions caused by scratching, and the hair should be kept clean and tidy (*see* 'Bed bath', p. 31).

Clothing may have to be adapted to suit the patient's requirements, depending on the reason for the condition. It may not be suitable for patients to wear their own clothes, but they should be worn if possible to retain individuality, this often being a source of comfort to relatives.

The patient's position should be changed every 2 hours to maintain the skin in good condition. An appropriate pressure-relieving mattress system will be needed in addition to positional changes (*see* 'Skin care', p. 309).

Controlling body temperature

The temperature should be recorded 4 hourly or more frequently if required. Any abnormality should be reported immediately. Damage to the hypothalamus and its temperature-regulating centre can lead to an abnormal temperature.

The bed covers should be adapted to keep the patient comfortably warm. Unconscious patients may show signs of hypothermia so the nurse should feel the temperature of the feet and hands, and note the colour of the skin, when observing or working with the patient (*see* 'Body temperature', p. 59).

Mobilising

The unconscious patient should be turned every 2 hours so that the tissues under the pressure areas are kept healthy (Johnson 1994) and the blood circulation to all areas of the body is maintained (*see* 'Skin care', p. 309).

Passive exercises may be performed three times a day, if possible under the guidance of the physiotherapist (*see* 'Exercises: active and passive', p. 145). This helps to prevent muscle contractions. In addition, light splints may be applied to the lower limbs for patients who are unconscious for a period of time; these are made individually for each patient by the physiotherapist. The nurse should if possible consult the physiotherapist for guidance on the most suitable method of helping to maintain the patient's musculoskeletal system in good condition so that when he or she regains consciousness mobility is not impaired by any muscular or skeletal abnormalities.

Figure 48.2
Unconscious patient: the semi-prone position. Reproduced from Roper et al (1985), with permission

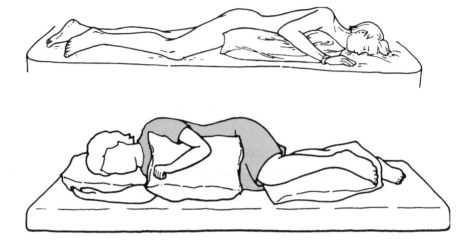

Figure 48.3
Unconscious patient: the lateral position

The feet should be supported to prevent foot drop. This can be done with well-placed sandbags, but specialised splints are more efficient; the guidance of the physiotherapist is essential here.

The semi-prone position (Fig. 48.2) is the most suitable position for maintaining a clear airway, but it is not as suitable for carrying out various nursing activities. The lateral position is preferable, it still being possible to maintain an adequate airway with this.

In the lateral position (Fig. 48.3), the patient is turned onto his or her side; the head may be placed on a low pillow with the neck extended. The spine should be extended and pillows placed at the back to maintain the position. The uppermost leg should be flexed and brought forwards to be supported on a pillow clear of the extended lower leg; this prevents internal rotation of the hip and any constriction of blood flow to the lower leg. Pillows should not be placed between the legs. The lower arm should be flexed with the palm facing up, the uppermost arm being brought forwards and supported on a pillow.

Working and playing

It is important for those looking after unconscious patients to learn as much as possible about their interests; it may even be possible to arrange for tapes of their favourite music, or messages from their family and friends, to be played in an attempt to evoke a response. When suitable, visits from friends and relatives should be encouraged so that they can talk to patients about their hobbies or particular interests.

Expressing sexuality

Although expressing sexuality may not at first seem relevant to an unconscious patient, ensuring that, for example, the hair is combed and that a male patient is shaved shows respect for the patient's personal identity and can be of inestimable comfort to the family; they may in fact wish to assist with these activities.

Sleeping

The nursing of a dependent patient can appear to be constant, but nursing interventions should if possible be arranged to coincide with the time of changing the patient's position. This is particularly important for individuals who show signs of cerebral irritability when handled. It may be beneficial to all unconscious patients to adapt the care so that a period of activity is followed by a long rest period.

Dying

Although an unconscious patient is not necessarily expected to die, the family often associates the apparent unresponsiveness with the imminence of death. It is important to listen to the family's concerns and to explain the cause of the unconsciousness and the prognosis in terms appropriate to the circumstances. When a patient's death is imminent, the family should be encouraged to share their feelings with the nursing staff.

Patient/carer education: key points

In partnership with the patient and/or carer, ensure that they are competent to carry out any practices required. Information should be given on an appropriate point of contact for any concerns that may arise.

Education primarily involves the family. Explanations of the rationale for the nursing interventions and the expected outcome should therefore be shared with them.

The family should be encouraged to talk to the patient about his or her interests and hobbies, this being reinforced with tapes and music if appropriate. They should understand that hearing is the first avenue of communication that returns as the patient recovers consciousness.

The family should also be encouraged to touch the patient and hold his or her hand; they may even wish to help with some of the nursing care. The family should be made to feel welcome at the bedside.

References

Allan D 1984 Glasgow coma scale. Nursing Mirror 158(23): 32–34

Carruthers A 1992 A force to promote bonding. Therapeutic touch and massage. Professional Nurse 7(5): 297–300

Chudley S 1994 The effects of nursing care on intracranial pressure. British Journal of Nursing 3(9): 454–459

Ellis A, Cavanagh S 1992 Aspects of neurological assessment using the Glasgow coma scale (research into the pattern of errors made by nurses when assessing neurological patients). Intensive and Critical Care 8(2): 94–100

Hancock K 1992 Caring is a gift of the heart (personal account of sub-arachnoid haemorrhage). Journal of Neuroscience Nursing 24(2): 110–112

Hickey JV 1997 The clinical practice of neurological and neurosurgical nursing. 4th edn. JB Lippincott, New York

Johnson J 1994 Pressure area risk management in a neurological setting. British Journal of Nursing 3(18): 926–935

Pemberton L 2000 The unconscious patient. In: Alexander M, Fawcett J, Runciman P (eds) Nursing practice – hospital and home: the adult. 2nd edn. Churchill Livingstone, Edinburgh

Roper N, Logan W, Tierney A 1985 The elements of nursing. 2nd edn. Churchill Livingstone, Edinburgh

Smith S 1997 The outer edge of consciousness. Nursing Times 93(39): 28–32

Toulson S 1994 Treatment and prevention of hypothermia. British Journal of Nursing 3(13): 662–666

United Kingdom Central Council for Nursing, Midwifery and Health Visiting 1992 Code of professional conduct. UKCC, London

United Kingdom Central Council for Nursing, Midwifery and Health Visiting 1996 Guidelines for professional practice. UKCC, London

United Kingdom Central Council for Nursing, Midwifery and Health Visiting 1998 Guidelines for records and record keeping. UKCC, London

49 Urine Testing

Learning outcomes	By the end of this section, you should know how to: ■ prepare the patient for this nursing practice ■ collect the equipment required ■ carry out testing of the urine.
Background knowledge required	Revision of the anatomy and physiology of the urinary system, with special reference to the formation of urine Revision of the manufacturer's instructions for the chemical reagents to be used.
Indications and rationale for testing urine	Testing urine involves assessing the constituents of the urine by observational, biochemical and mechanical means: ■ *to aid in the diagnosis of disease* ■ *to assist in the monitoring of disease and treatment* ■ *to assist in the assessment of the health of an individual* ■ *to exclude pathology.*
Equipment 	Clean, dry container for the urine sample Bottle of reagent strips Jug for volume measurement Bedpan or urinal Watch with a second hand Trolley, tray or adequate surface for equipment Receptacle for soiled disposable items Disposable gloves.
Guidelines and rationale for this nursing practice 	■ explain the nursing practice to the patient and obtain consent and co-operation *to inform the patient about the practice and ensure that he or she is aware of a person's rights as a patient* ■ wash the hands *to reduce cross-infection and contamination by the nurse's and patient's hands* (Horton 1995) ■ instruct or assist the patient to collect urine in the clean, dry container the next time he or she empties the bladder *as this will ensure that the urine specimen is fresh and uncontaminated before testing* ■ collect and prepare the equipment *to ensure that the equipment is available and ready for use*

- wash the hands *to reduce cross-infection and contamination by the nurse's and patient's hands* (Horton 1995)
- apply gloves *to protect the nurse's hands from contamination by body fluids*
- measure the volume of urine if the patient has a fluid balance chart *as this will ensure accurate fluid balance monitoring*
- observe and note any sediment present in the urine *as this may indicate an abnormality of the patient's renal tract*
- observe and note the colour of the urine *as an unusual colour of the urine may indicate an abnormality*
- note any smell *as this may suggest an infection*: infected urine has a foul, fishy odour
- check the expiry date on the container of reagent strips *to prevent inaccurate results from using out-of-date reagents*
- remove a reagent strip, being careful not to touch the test squares on the strip *as contamination of the reagent strip may give a false reading*
- immerse the reagent strip fully in the urine. Note the time *to permit an assessment of the results after the correct interval*
- withdraw the strip, removing any excess urine by gently tapping the strip on the rim of the container (Torrance & Elley 1998a); *this will reduce the risk of contamination to the tester*
- hold the strip at an angle *to prevent cross-contamination from one reagent pad to another* (Mallett & Dougherty 2000)
- hold the strip vertically or horizontally against the results guidance chart *to ensure an accurate interpretation of the colour change* (Cook 1996)
- read the reagent strip after the recommended time has elapsed *to ensure an accurate result*
- note the result, *providing an accurate written record*
- dispose of the equipment safely, *reducing any risk to staff and other equipment*
- document the nursing practice appropriately and report any abnormal findings immediately *to provide a written record and assist in the implementation of any action should an abnormal result be noted*
- in undertaking this practice, nurses are accountable for their actions, the quality of care delivered and record-keeping according to the *Code of Professional Conduct* (UKCC 1992), *Guidelines for Professional Practice* (UKCC 1996) and *Guidelines for Records and Record Keeping* (UKCC 1998).

| Relevance to the activities of living | *Maintaining a safe environment* |

Although testing urine does not require an aseptic technique, all equipment should be clean or disposable, and all precautions should be taken to prevent cross-infection (Horton 1995). Nurses should wash their hands before commencing and on completing this nursing practice.

When a patient is asked to collect a specimen of urine for routine testing, the container to be used must be clean and dry. It is essential that the container is free from contaminating substances as this may lead to an inaccurate result. Once the urine sample has been obtained, it should be tested immediately. Urinary constituents can alter when left exposed to the environment, which may predispose to an inaccurate reading.

All the chemical reagents should be stored in a cool dry place (Cook 1996), within a locked cupboard or drawer to comply with Health and Safety at Work regulations and the Control of Substances Hazardous to Health Regulations.

The manufacturer's instructions for care and storage should be followed precisely. The chemical reagents are liable to degradation over a period of time or when storage conditions are not adequate. Reagent strips must be stored in their original container and kept dry using the dessicant provided (*Nursing Standard* 1999). It is essential that the lid of the container is replaced quickly and securely following the removal of a reagent strip. The strips are particularly sensitive to changes in temperature and humidity, which will affect the accuracy of the result recorded (Nicol et al 2000). The chemical reagents should be handled carefully as touching the test square may introduce contaminants that can affect the results obtained.

When using a reagent strip, hold the strip horizontally or place it over the urine container. This will prevent any excess urine dripping onto the nurse's hand and proving a health hazard to the member of staff. Holding the strip horizontally will also prevent mixing of the urine between the test squares, which could lead to inaccuracy.

It is important that the reagent strip is read at the time specified by the manufacturer. Reading the test too late or too soon will give an inaccurate reading.

Communicating

The patient will require a full and easily understood explanation of why the specimen of urine is required and of how to collect it.

The nurse should be aware of different cultural attitudes towards handling and collecting body fluids and be sensitive to patients' individual needs (Cook 1996).

Nurses should familiarise themselves with any medications the patient may be taking, as certain drugs can affect the test.

Eliminating

Fresh urine from a healthy individual should not have an offensive odour, but decomposing urine will smell like ammonia. A patient whose urine is found to have a 'sweet' smell may be investigated further for diabetes mellitus. Urine smelling of fish can be an indication of infection of the urinary system.

The normal colour of urine ranges from pale straw to dark amber and will vary according to the amount of fluid that has been taken into the body (Marieb 1990). The type and amount of urinary constituents also affect the colour of urine; a dark-coloured urine can, for example, be an indication of dehydration or the presence of bile pigments, a manifestation of liver or biliary tract disease.

Certain foods and drugs alter the colour of a patient's urine: beetroot can cause the urine to take on an orangy-red hue.

'Haematuria' is the term used to describe blood in the urine. This can vary from microscopic haematuria, i.e. that detected only by testing, to frank haematuria, with an obvious red colouration. Blood in the urine is suggestive of disease or damage to the renal system (Selfe 2000).

Glycosuria refers to the presence of glucose in the urine. This is suggestive of diabetes mellitus.

'Proteinuria' is the term used when there is protein in the urine, which can be a manifestation of acute or chronic renal disease.

When the body metabolises fat, ketones are one of the products of this metabolism. Ketones are acidotic so if the excessive metabolism of fat persists, a state of metabolic acidosis develops, which can, if untreated, lead to coma and death. At a certain stage of acidosis, the ketones are excreted by the urinary system; when they are identified in the urine, they may be indicative of excessive fasting or uncontrolled or poorly controlled diabetes mellitus.

The specific gravity is a measure of the concentration of the substances dissolved in the urine, the normal range being 1.005–1.025. A single measurement of the specific gravity of the urine provides little information as the specific gravity varies with the state of hydration of the body. Urine that continually has a low specific gravity indicates renal damage or diabetes insipidus. The pH of a urine sample reflects the function of the kidney in maintaining the acid–base balance within the body.

Expressing sexuality

Micturition is an activity associated with privacy so collecting a specimen of urine is an unfamiliar and embarrassing experience for the patient (Torrance & Elley 1998b). Providing privacy and giving an adequate explanation of the practice will thus be conducive to an uncomplicated collection of the specimen.

When asking a female patient for a urine specimen, it is necessary to ask whether she is menstruating as the menstrual flow may give a false-positive result for blood in the urine (Bowker 1986).

Patient/carer education: key points

In partnership with the patient and/or carer, ensure that they are competent to carry out any practices required. Information should be given on an appropriate point of contact for any concerns that may arise.

Should the patient be collecting the urine specimen unassisted, ensure that he or she is aware of the importance of placing the urine in a clean, dry, leakproof container for transport to the doctor's practice or hospital.

Inform the patient of the results and any action required should an abnormality be detected.

A patient or carer may need to be taught this nursing practice so the nurse should therefore devise a suitable educational programme.

References

Bowker C (ed.) 1986 Focus on urinalysis.
1. Anatomy and physiology of renal tract. Nursing Times 81(17 suppl): 1–6
2. Collection of urine samples. Nursing Times 81(20 suppl): 1–6
3. Urine testing. Nursing Times 81(23 suppl): 1–6
4. Case history – diabetes: urine tests for glucose and ketones. Nursing Times 81(26 suppl): 1–6
5. Proteinuria. Case history – liver function tests: differential diagnosis of jaundice: urine tests for bilirubin and urobilinogen. Nursing Times 81(29 suppl): 1–6
6. Regulation of water balance-specific gravity: urinary pH: urinary tract infection: haematuria. Nursing Times 81(32 suppl): 1–6
Cook R 1996 Urinalysis: ensuring accurate urine testing. Nursing Standard 10(46): 49–54
Horton R 1995 Handwashing: the fundamental infection control principle. British Journal of Nursing 4(16): 926–933
Mallett J, Dougherty L 2000 The Royal Marsden manual of clinical nursing procedures. 5th edn. Blackwell Science, Oxford
Marieb E 1990 Human anatomy and physiology. Benjamin Cummings, New York
Nicol M, Bavin C, Bedford-Turner S, Cronin P, Rawlings-Anderson K 2000 Essential nursing skills. CV Mosby, London
Nursing Standard 1999 Urine testing. Nursing Standard 13(50): 2
Selfe L 2000 The urinary system. In: Alexander M, Fawcett J, Runciman P (eds) Nursing practice – hospital and home: the adult. 2nd edn. Churchill Livingstone, Edinburgh
Torrance C, Elley K 1998a Urine testing. 2. Urinalysis. Nursing Times 94(5 suppl): 1–2
Torrance C, Elley K 1998b Urine testing. 1. Observation. Nursing Times 94(4 suppl): 11–12
United Kingdom Central Council for Nursing, Midwifery and Health Visiting 1992 Code of professional conduct. UKCC, London
United Kingdom Central Council for Nursing, Midwifery and Health Visiting 1996 Guidelines for professional practice. UKCC, London
United Kingdom Central Council for Nursing, Midwifery and Health Visiting 1998 Guidelines for records and record keeping. UKCC, London

50 Vaginal Examination

Learning outcomes	By the end of this section, you should know how to:
	▪ prepare the patient for this procedure
	▪ collect and prepare the equipment
	▪ describe the various positions that enable this examination to be carried out most easily
	▪ assist the examiner as necessary.

Background knowledge required	Revision of the anatomy and physiology of the female reproductive system
	Revision of infection control procedures.

Indications and rationale for a vaginal examination	The vagina can be examined visually or digitally for the following reasons:

▪ *to assess the position, size, texture or appearance of the cervix and vagina*
▪ *to obtain a swab from the cervix or vagina*
▪ *to obtain a cervical smear for cytological examination* (*see* 'Specimen collection', p. 317)
▪ *to administer treatment to the cervix or vagina*
▪ *to determine the site of a haemorrhage*
▪ *to insert an intrauterine contraceptive device.*

Outline of the procedure

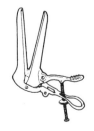

Figure 50.1
Cusco's vaginal speculum. Reproduced from Chilman & Thomas (1987), with permission

The examiner puts on a pair of disposable gloves and applies some water-soluble lubricant to the dominant hand. Two or three fingers of the dominant hand are then inserted into the vagina, and the uterus is palpated through the abdominal wall with the non-dominant hand. This is known as a digital or bimanual examination.

For a visual examination of the vagina and cervix, the examiner will insert a lubricated speculum – usually a Sims' or Cusco's speculum (Fig. 50.1) – into the vagina. The speculum is gently opened to separate the vaginal walls and enable an inspection of the vagina and cervix; a good light is required for this. A pair of vulsellum forceps may be used to hold the cervix while it is examined. A pair of swab-holding forceps and some swabs may be necessary to wipe away any blood or vaginal discharge that might be obstructing the inspection of the mucosa. After the examination, the speculum is closed and removed gently from the vagina.

Equipment

Tray or trolley

For digital examination:
— disposable gloves
— water-soluble lubricant
— medical wipes or tissues
— receptacle for soiled disposable items.

For visual examination, in addition to the above:
— sterile vaginal speculum
— sterile vulsellum forceps
— sterile swab-holding forceps
— swabs
— light source.

Additional equipment may be required depending on the purpose of the examination.

The position of the patient

There are several suitable positions for this procedure, the position of choice usually being the one most convenient for the medical practitioner and patient.

The recumbent position   The patient lies on her back with her knees drawn up and separated and the sides of her feet resting on the bed (Fig. 50.2).

The left lateral position   The patient lies on her left side with her knees flexed and her buttocks near the edge of the bed.

The knee–chest position   The patient kneels on the bed with her thighs vertical. Her head is turned to one side and her chest rests on a pillow.

The lithotomy position   The patient's buttocks are positioned at the end of the table or couch (Fig. 50.2). The thighs are flexed on the trunk and the legs flexed on the thighs, supports attached to the table or couch keeping the patient's legs in the correct position. To avoid injury to the patient, both legs must be lifted gently into position at the same time.

Guidelines and rationale for this nursing practice

- help to explain the procedure to the patient *to gain her consent and co-operation*. Ensure that the woman is aware of her pelvic anatomy and physiology
- ensure as much privacy as possible for the patient *as the majority of patients are very embarrassed about having this examination*
- collect and prepare the equipment *for efficiency of practice*
- assist the patient into the agreed position *for ease of examination*
- observe the patient throughout this activity *to detect any signs of discomfort or distress*
- assist the examiner and the patient as necessary
- ensure that the patient is left feeling as comfortable as possible afterwards with protection for her underwear if there is any risk of discharge from her vagina

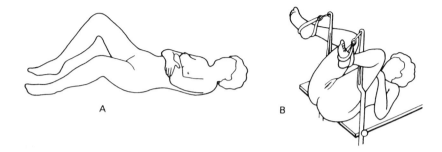

Figure 50.2 *Two common positions used for vaginal examination* A *Recumbent position* B *Lithotomy position*

- ensure that the patient is aware of the location of toilet or washroom facilities *so that she can freshen up and remove traces of water-soluble gel*
- dispose of the equipment safely *for the protection of others*
- dispatch any specimens to the laboratory with the completed form and in a plastic specimen bag
- document this procedure, monitor the after-effects and report any abnormal findings immediately *to provide a written record and assist in the implementation of any action should an abnormal result be noted*
- in undertaking this practice, nurses are accountable for their actions, the quality of care delivered and record-keeping according to the *Code of Professional Conduct* (UKCC 1992), *Guidelines for Professional Practice* (UKCC 1996) and *Guidelines for Records and Record Keeping* (UKCC 1998).

Relevance to the activities of living

Maintaining a safe environment

Examiners are advised to use a disposable vaginal speculum to prevent any possibility of infecting staff or subsequent patients with human immunodeficiency virus (HIV), which leads to acquired immunodeficiency syndrome (Wright 1999). Because of the currently limited knowledge on HIV, the nurse should wear disposable gloves if there is a risk of contact with vaginal discharge or soiled equipment.

Elderly patients may have problems adopting a position appropriate to the examination; help may be required and support necessary to promote comfort, ease of examination and safety. Care must be taken when handling joint areas such as hips and knees so that injury is not inflicted.

Communicating

If the patient can co-operate by relaxing as much as possible, it is easier for the examiner to carry out the examination and also reduces the patient's discomfort. A clear explanation of why the examination is necessary and how the patient can relax, for example by deep breathing, will help to ensure relaxation.

Breathing

Slow, regular, concentrated deep breathing will help the patient to relax the abdominal and perineal muscles.

Eliminating

The patient should be given the opportunity to empty her bladder before the examination. This makes it easier for the examiner to palpate the uterus and also more comfortable for the patient, who is usually feeling apprehensive.

Personal cleansing and dressing

If treatment that may result in vaginal discharge is to be given during the examination, the patient should have prior information so that appropriate underwear can be worn. The provision of washroom facilities after the procedure or examination has been completed is important to help patients maintain their self-esteem (Roper et al 2000). Assistance with dressing and undressing should be offered.

Expressing sexuality

Many patients find this examination stressful and embarrassing so the best privacy possible should be provided and the patient covered up as much as is feasible. The surroundings need to be as calm and relaxed as possible (Tomlinson 1998). Some patients may appreciate the opportunity to observe the examination by means of a mirror, or by a small camera fixed to the examiner's head that transmits pictures onto a screen.

Women who have had no heterosexual experiences and women who have suffered from abuse should be offered extra time, support, information and counselling before and after this examination. Nurses should also demonstrate an awareness of the significance and implications of vaginal examination for women from a variety of cultural and lifestyle backgrounds (Bell 1999) and following pelvic surgery (Marquiegui & Huish 1999) and plan for this when caring for these patients.

Patient/carer education: key points	In partnership with the patient and/or carer, ensure that they are competent to carry out any practices required. Information should be given on an appropriate point of contact for any concerns that may arise. Encourage an open discussion with the patient about her vaginal anatomy and the details of the practice. Appropriate written information given to patients prior to attendance at the examination may help to reduce their anxiety and embarrassment.

References

Bell R 1999 Homosexual men and women. British Medical Journal 318: 452–455
Chilman A, Thomas M (eds) 1987 Understanding nursing care. 3rd edn. Churchill Livingstone, Edinburgh
Fogel C, Woods N 1995 Women's health care. Sage, London
Marquiegui A, Huish M 1999 A woman's sexual life after an operation. British Medical Journal 318: 178–181

Roper N, Logan W, Tierney A 2000 The Roper–Logan–Tierney model of nursing. Churchill Livingstone, Edinburgh

Tomlinson J 1998 Taking a sexual history. British Medical Journal 317: 1573–1576

United Kingdom Central Council for Nursing, Midwifery and Health Visiting 1992 Code of professional conduct. UKCC, London

United Kingdom Central Council for Nursing, Midwifery and Health Visiting 1996 Guidelines for professional practice. UKCC, London

United Kingdom Central Council for Nursing, Midwifery and Health Visiting 1998 Guidelines for records and record keeping. UKCC, London

Wright S 1999 Sexually transmitted diseases. Nursing Standard 13(46): 37–42

51   Vaginal Pessary Insertion

Learning outcomes	By the end of this section, you should know how to: ■ prepare the patient for this nursing practice ■ collect and prepare the equipment ■ administer the prescribed pessaries to the patient.
Background knowledge required	Revision of the anatomy and physiology of the cervix and vagina Revision of infection control procedures Revision of guidelines on administering medicines (*see* p. 1).
Indications and rationale for administering medicinal vaginal pessaries	Vaginal pessaries are cones or cylinders of medication that are inserted into the vagina, where they dissolve and have their effect topically or after absorption. They are used *to administer medication* such as antibiotics (Wright 1999).
Equipment 	Tray Prescribed pessaries Medicine prescription chart Disposable gloves Water-soluble lubricant Medical wipes or tissues Protective pad Receptacle for soiled disposable items.
Guidelines and rationale for this nursing practice 	■ explain the nursing practice to the patient *to gain her consent and co-operation.* The woman should ideally be taught to insert the pessary herself *and thereby increase her participation in her care* (Fig. 51.1) ■ collect, check and prepare the equipment *for efficiency of practice* ■ ensure maximum privacy and assist the patient into the position that she and the nurse have agreed (*see* 'Vaginal examination' for a description of suitable positions, p. 384) ■ observe the patient throughout this activity *to detect signs of discomfort or distress* ■ lubricate the end of the pessary *to ease insertion into the vagina*

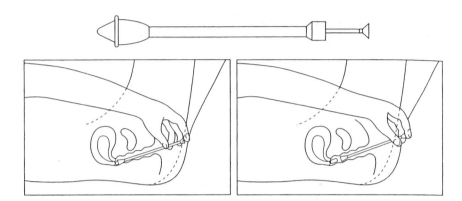

Figure 51.1 *Patient inserting a vaginal pessary using an applicator*

- put on the disposable gloves
- part the labia majora with the non-dominant hand and, on locating the vagina, insert the pessary in an upward and backward direction with the dominant hand for the length of the index finger if possible. *This should ensure that the pessary is deposited in the posterior fornix to dissolve and obtain maximum absorption*
- put a protective pad over the patient's vulval area *to protect the patient's underwear from being stained by the dissolving pessary*
- ensure that the patient is left feeling as comfortable as possible, *with the underwear adequately protected*
- dispose of the equipment safely *for the safety of others*
- document this nursing practice appropriately, monitor the after-effects and report any abnormal findings immediately *to provide a written record and assist in the implementation of any action should an abnormal result be noted*
- in undertaking this practice, nurses are accountable for their actions, the quality of care delivered and record-keeping according to the *Code of Professional Conduct* (UKCC 1992), *Guidelines for Professional Practice* (UKCC 1996) and *Guidelines for Records and Record Keeping* (UKCC 1998).

Relevance to the activities of living

Maintaining a safe environment

Although this practice does not require an aseptic technique, the equipment should be disposable and nurses should wash their hands before commencing and on completing the nursing practice.

Communicating

A clear explanation should be given to gain the patient's consent and co-operation (Tomlinson 1998), which should make administering the pessary easier. Encourage the patient to familiarise herself with the size and texture of the pessary prior to insertion to help to reduce her anxiety and increase her sense of control. The majority of women should be able to insert the pessary themselves if adequate information and support are given.

Eliminating

The patient should be given the opportunity to empty her bowel and bladder before the pessary is administered. This gives the pessary time to dissolve and be absorbed before the patient's next visit to the toilet.

Mobilising

It should be suggested to the patient that she move around as little as possible for half an hour after the insertion of the pessary so that it can dissolve and be absorbed.

Expressing sexuality

This can be an embarrassing practice for some patients, and maximum privacy is important (Roper et al 2000). Self-administration of the pessary can help to reduce embarrassment and increase the woman's sense of control.

Patient/carer education: key points

In partnership with the patient and/or carer, ensure that they are competent to carry out any practices required. Information should be given on an appropriate point of contact for any concerns that may arise.

Encourage an open discussion with the patient of her vaginal anatomy. This should promote confidence in administration and reduce anxiety. Diagrams or models may be helpful.

References

Roper N, Logan W, Tierney A 2000 The Roper–Logan–Tierney model of nursing. Churchill Livingstone, Edinburgh

Tomlinson J 1998 Taking a sexual history. British Medical Journal 317: 1573–1576

United Kingdom Central Council for Nursing, Midwifery and Health Visiting 1992 Code of professional conduct. UKCC, London

United Kingdom Central Council for Nursing, Midwifery and Health Visiting 1996 Guidelines for professional practice. UKCC, London

United Kingdom Central Council for Nursing, Midwifery and Health Visiting 1998 Guidelines for records and record keeping. UKCC, London

Wright S 1999 Sexually transmitted diseases. Nursing Standard 13(46): 37–42

52 Vaginal Ring Pessary Insertion

Learning outcomes

By the end of this section, you should know how to:

- prepare the patient for this practice
- collect and prepare the equipment
- assist the qualified practitioner in the insertion of a ring.

Background knowledge required

Revision of the anatomy and physiology of vagina, cervix and uterus
Revision of infection control procedures.

Indications and rationale for the insertion of vaginal ring pessaries

Ring pessaries are made of a PVC type of material that is flexible and compressible by hand but springs back into shape when in situ (Fig. 52.1). The pessaries are supplied individually wrapped and sterile. There is a range of sizes; the experienced practitioner will select the most appropriate size for the patient.

Ring pessaries are used *to relieve the symptoms caused by a degree of uterine prolapse* (Alexander et al 2000) when the patient:

- is unfit for a surgical repair of her prolapse
- does not wish to undergo surgery
- requires a temporary treatment to alleviate problems while awaiting surgery.

Equipment

Selected pessary
Disposable gloves
Water-soluble lubricant
Protective pad
Receptacle for soiled disposable items.

Guidelines and rationale for this nursing practice

- explain the nursing practice to the patient *to gain her consent and co-operation*
- collect, check and prepare the equipment
- ensure maximum privacy for the patient and assist her into the position she has agreed with the person inserting the pessary (*see* 'Vaginal examination' for a list of appropriate positions, p. 384)
- observe the patient throughout this activity *to detect any signs of discomfort or distress*

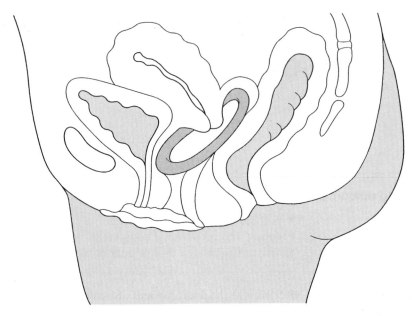

Figure 52.1 *Vaginal ring pessary in position*

Ring pessary in situ

- put on the disposable gloves *for protection*
- lubricate the pessary and, using the thumb and forefinger of the dominant hand, squeeze the pessary into an oval shape *for ease of insertion*
- with the non-dominant hand, part the labia *to expose the entrance to the vagina*
- slide the pessary into the posterior part of the vagina and gently push it downwards and backwards until it settles in the posterior fornix
- once it is in this position, it will spring into its normal shape. The person inserting the pessary then needs to hook the front portion of the pessary into the anterior fornix behind the symphysis pubis
- ensure that the patient is left feeling comfortable
- dispose of the equipment safely
- document this nursing practice appropriately, monitor the after-effects and report any abnormal findings immediately *to provide a written record and assist in the implementation of any action should an abnormal result be noted*
- in undertaking this practice, nurses are accountable for their actions, the quality of care delivered and record-keeping according to the *Code of Professional Conduct* (UKCC 1992), *Guidelines for Professional Practice* (UKCC 1996) and *Guidelines for Records and Record Keeping* (UKCC 1998).

Relevance to the activities of living

Maintaining a safe environment

Although this practice does not require an aseptic technique, the equipment used should be sterile and nurses should wash their hands before commencing and on completing the nursing practice. Gloves should be worn for protection.

The importance of good personal hygiene practices to avoid the risk of infection should be explained to the patient: the pessary is a foreign body in the vagina and therefore a possible focus for infection.

Communicating

If a clear explanation is given, and the woman understands the reasons for the insertion of the pessary and has sufficient knowledge of her anatomy to know exactly where it will be positioned, the insertion should be made easier.

Eliminating

The patient should be given the opportunity to empty her bladder prior to the insertion of the vaginal ring pessary. Micturition and bowel movements should not be hindered by the presence of the pessary; it may in fact improve any micturition and bowel problems that the patient has been experiencing.

Mobilising

It should be suggested to the patient that she move around as much as possible after the pessary has been inserted to ensure that it is correctly fitted. The patient should be unaware of its presence.

Expressing sexuality

The pessary will not interfere with sexual intercourse. Personal hygiene is important to prevent infection. In older women, the lining of the vagina may be dry so an oestrogen cream may be prescribed to help avoid any irritation of the mucosal lining.

A slight watery discharge from the vagina is common, but patients should be advised to seek help if the discharge becomes purulent or bloodstained, or develops an offensive smell.

Patient/carer education: key points

In partnership with the patient and/or carer, ensure that they are competent to carry out any practices required. Information should be given on an appropriate point of contact for any concerns that may arise.

An explanation of the reasons for the insertion of the pessary will help to gain the patient's co-operation. Assurance about the normal functions of micturition, bowel movement and sexual activity should be given.

It is essential to teach the patient the importance of good personal hygiene habits to reduce the risk of infection. Advice, and a contact name and telephone number, should be given in case the patient experiences problems related to the pessary.

Ensure that full details of any follow-up care are given to the patient, and encourage attendance at check-up appointments for an assessment of vaginal health.

References

Alexander M, Fawcett J, Runciman P 2000 Nursing care – hospital and home: the adult. 2nd edn. Churchill Livingstone, Edinburgh

United Kingdom Central Council for Nursing, Midwifery and Health Visiting 1992 Code of professional conduct. UKCC, London

United Kingdom Central Council for Nursing, Midwifery and Health Visiting 1996 Guidelines for professional practice. UKCC, London

United Kingdom Central Council for Nursing, Midwifery and Health Visiting 1998 Guidelines for records and record keeping. UKCC, London

53 Venepuncture

Learning outcomes	By the end of this section, you should know how to: ■ prepare the patient for this procedure ■ collect and prepare the equipment ■ obtain a sample of blood from the patient ■ educate the patient on selfcare following this procedure.
Background knowledge required	Anatomy and physiology of the venous blood system and upper limb Principles of infection control with respect to blood-borne infection Different devices used in venepuncture *The Scope of Professional Practice* (UKCC 1992a) Health authority policy for this procedure Understanding of routine blood investigations and their results.
Indications and rationale for venepuncture	Venepuncture is carried out in order: ■ *to obtain a specimen of blood for clinical analysis.* This may include measuring electrolyte, haemoglobin or antibody levels within the blood ■ *to cross-match blood for transfusion.*
Outline of the procedure	Venepuncture is performed by the medical practitioner or phlebotomist, or by a qualified nurse who has undertaken specialised education and is competent in this practice. The non-specialist nurse may be asked to assist with this procedure. Blood may be withdrawn from the vein using a closed vacuum system or the traditional method of a needle and syringe, or alternatively a butterfly infusion set, which may be more appropriate for some elderly patients (Black & Hughes 1997). Hoeltke (1995) advises that the syringe method be used when the veins are fragile or when the superficial veins in the back of the hand are used. The value of the vacuum system is that several different samples may be taken as only the tube (rather than the syringe, as may be necessary in the traditional method) needs to be changed, thus protecting the nurse from blood spillage. There is also a reduced risk of needle-stick injury because blood flows directly from the vein to the specimen bottle and does not have to be transferred to individual

containers. If the veins are too small or fragile to tolerate these techniques, Hoeltke (1995) advises that a butterfly infusion device be used to gain venous access.

The traditional or manual method is outlined in this section as the same general principles apply regardless of the system. Additional information is given where the procedure differs if a vacuum system is used. It is important to note that the technique may vary slightly depending on the type of vacuum device used in the clinical area so the nurse should adhere to local policy and follow the manufacturer's instructions. For further reading on two different types of vacuum system, see Griffiths (1999) and Black & Hughes (1997).

Equipment

Clean tray for equipment
Disposable gloves
Alcohol-impregnated cleansing swab
Sterile needle(s) or infusion device (20–21 G)*
Sterile syringe(s)*
Disposable drape
Sterile adhesive plaster
Sterile gauze swab or cotton wool balls
Tourniquet
Sharps box
Receptacle for soiled material
Appropriate specimen containers*
Venepuncture vacuum system
Completed laboratory form(s)
Plastic envelope for transferring the specimen.

If a vacuum container system is used, the items marked with an asterisk are not required. Special equipment is available for use with this system. Alternatively, normal needles can be used with an adaptor produced by the manufacturer.

Guidelines and rationale for this nursing practice

- discuss the procedure with the patient and ascertain whether he or she has an allergy to adhesive plaster, *informing the patient about the procedure, discussing any concerns or queries and identifying any previous difficulties experienced with venepuncture*
- obtain consent from the patient to undertake the procedure *to ensure that the patient is aware of a person's rights as a patient*
- select a suitable clean surface and lay out the equipment. If the procedure is being undertaken in the patient's own home, cover the surface with a waterproof cover *to provide a suitable, protected work surface*
- check that the laboratory forms have been completed and select the appropriate specimen containers *to ensure that the documentation is correct and that the samples are put into the correct specimen containers*
- cleanse the hands using a bactericidal solution *to reduce the risk of cross-infection* (Gould 1995)

- open the sterile packs and attach a needle to the syringe (or assemble the vacuum system) *to ensure that equipment is ready for use*
- position the patient in a supine position on a bed, trolley or couch. If these are not available, the patient should be seated *to ensure patient comfort and prevent injury should the patient feel faint during the procedure*
- observe and palpate the veins on both arms. The vessels most commonly used are the cephalic, basilic and median cubital veins (in the forearm; Fig. 53.1), followed by the superficial veins on the dorsal aspect of the hand (Fig. 53.2). The nurse should be aware of the location of the brachial artery and median nerve (*see* Fig. 53.1) *as injury to either will cause pain and may lead to temporary or permanent damage*

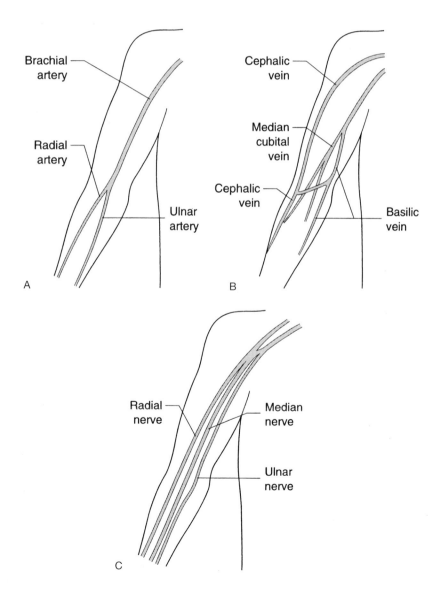

Figure 53.1
Anatomical features of the forearm
A *Arteries*
B *Veins*
C *Nerves*

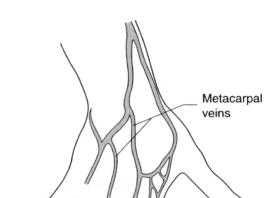

Metacarpal
veins

Digital
veins

Figure 53.2 *Superficial
veins on the dorsal
aspect of the hand*

- select a vein that is visible and firm to the touch. If there is lymphatic impairment or the patient has had an illness, disease or surgery affecting the limb, an alternative site should be selected. Take into account the patient's own past experience of venepuncture *to identify the vein most likely to provide the best venous access*
- place the tourniquet or sphygmomanometer cuff approximately 5–12 cm above the proposed puncture site *to promote vasodilatation*. This should not remain in situ for any longer than 2 minutes
- ask the patient to clench the fist *to promote vasodilatation*
- put on gloves *to protect both patient and nurse from potential blood-borne infection* (Black & Hughes 1997, Clulow 1994)
- select a firm visible vein and cleanse the skin with an alcohol-impregnated cleansing swab for a minimum of 5 seconds before allowing the site to air dry, thus *reducing the skin flora by* 97% (Lawrence et al 1994) (*see* 'Personal cleansing and dressing', below)
- place the thumb or index finger below the proposed puncture site and pull the skin in a downward direction *to stabilise the vein*
- with its bevel facing upwards, gently and slowly insert the needle at an angle of 15° (Hoeltke 1995) *to ensure the correct angle of entry into the vein*
- when the vessel wall has been punctured and blood appears in the barrel of the syringe, level off the needle and advance it slightly further into the vein (some vacuum systems do not allow a flash back to be seen, the needle being felt to enter the vein by a slight change in resistance) *to ensure that the opposite side of the vessel is not punctured*
- gently pull back the plunger of the syringe and collect the required amount of blood *to prevent collapse of the vein and to obtain a specimen of blood.*

The vacuum system allows blood to flow directly from the vein into the specimen container

- release the tourniquet *to prevent further compression of the blood supply and excessive bleeding at the puncture site on removal of the needle*
- if blood does not appear, the needle should be removed and, adhering to health authority policy, the nurse should either undertake the procedure using another vessel or seek assistance from another practitioner *to prevent undue distress to the patient and excessive trauma to the vein*
- remove the needle (keeping it straight) and cover the puncture site with cotton wool or a gauze swab *to prevent leakage of blood from the puncture site*
- apply pressure directly over the puncture site for 2–3 minutes (3–5 minutes if the patient has a clotting defect) after the needle has been removed. The patient may be able to undertake this activity. The patient should not bend the arm as this may enlarge the puncture wound, causing more bleeding (Campbell 1995). This pressure will *reduce trauma to the vein and discomfort for the patient, and stop the bleeding from the vein, thus reducing the risk of formation of a haematoma*
- as soon as possible after collection, transfer the blood to the appropriate specimen container(s). This is not required for vacuum systems. If additives are present in the container, rotate it gently several times *to prevent clotting of the blood*
- complete the label on the specimen container(s) *to ensure that correct investigations are carried out and that the results are returned to the correct patient*
- place the specimen container and laboratory form in the plastic bag (or follow health authority policy) *to ensure that the laboratory receives the correct specimen*
- inspect the puncture site for bleeding and/or haematoma formation and apply adhesive plaster over the site *to ensure that clotting has occurred and that the puncture site is protected from infection and trauma.* If the patient has an allergy to sticking plaster, apply a gauze swab and secure it firmly with hypoallergenic tape
- dispose of contaminated equipment according to health authority policy *to prevent the transmission of infection*
- remove the gloves and dispose of as above. Wash the hands or cleanse them with bactericidal solution *to prevent cross-infection*
- ensure that the patient is feeling well *to ensure that the patient does not feel unwell as a result of the procedure.* This is especially important if the procedure is being carried out in the patient's own home
- discuss the points raised under 'Patient/carer education: key points' below. If the patient is unable to participate in this stage of the procedure, monitoring should be undertaken by the nurse or by an appropriate adult carer *to ensure that the patient, carer or nurse is aware of, and understands, the follow-up self care*
- in undertaking this practice, nurses are accountable for their actions, the quality of care delivered and record-keeping according to the *Code of Professional Conduct* (UKCC 1992b), *Guidelines for Professional*

Practice (UKCC 1996) and *Guidelines for Records and Record Keeping* (UKCC 1998).

Relevance to the activities of living	***Maintaining a safe environment***

Maintaining a safe environment

All precautions should be maintained to prevent potential complications, such as damage to nerves or other blood vessels, during venepuncture (Campbell et al 1999). The puncture site and surrounding area should be observed for signs of infection, for example inflammation and pain. Any symptoms, including swelling, pain, tingling in the arm and excessive bruising or bleeding at or around the puncture site should be reported to a medical practitioner.

The nurse should adhere to health authority policy on the safe preparation, use and disposal of all equipment. Although the use of vacuum systems reduces the risk of spillage and needle-stick injury, it does not completely eliminate it so protocols on the handling of blood products and the use of sharps should always be followed (Griffiths 1999).

Communicating

The nurse should be aware of the information the patient needs about the practice of venepuncture, encouraging the patient to discuss his or her understanding of why the blood specimen is being obtained. The nurse must therefore be familiar with routine blood investigations and the interpretation of their results (Bratt-Wyton 1998).

The nurse should also respond to the patient's need for information regarding the reason for venepuncture; this should be carried out in consultation with the medical practitioner who authorised the investigation. Selective health education may be carried out in relation to any underlying disease, for example with a diabetic patient attending for blood glucose monitoring.

Counselling may be required following diagnosis of any disease as a result of the blood test.

Personal cleansing and dressing

There has been some debate over the cleansing of puncture sites. A study carried out by Lawrence et al (1994) found that cleansing the skin for 5 seconds with a swab impregnated with 70% isopropanol reduced the number of skin flora by 97%. The value of skin cleansing for invasive procedures such as venepuncture is, however, inconclusive so local policy should always be followed. Franklin (1999) advises to err on the side of caution and cleanse the skin until more evidence is available.

Patient/carer education: key points	In partnership with the patient and/or carer, ensure that they are competent to carry out any practices required. Information should be given on an appropriate point of contact for any concerns that may arise.

When preparing the patient for the procedure:

- advise the patient of any dietary restrictions that may be required for blood glucose or cholesterol investigations
- check with the medical practitioner whether there is any information that you require from the patient for more specialist investigations, for example drug doses and times or menstrual cycle dates (Black & Hughes 1997).

With aftercare of the puncture site:

- report any bleeding oozing from under the adhesive plaster
- if itching or a rash occurs at the plaster site, remove the plaster and apply a gauze swab secured with hypoallergenic tape
- remove the adhesive plaster 24–48 hours after venepuncture.

There are potential complications following venepuncture:

- the patient should report excessive bruising radiating from the puncture site as this could relate to haematoma formation
- the patient should report any tingling, pain or swelling in the arm as this may indicate pressure on a nerve.

Inform the patient when the test results will be available and how to obtain them.

References

Black F, Hughes J 1997 Venepuncture. Nursing Standard 11(41): 49–55

Bratt-Wyton R 1998 Interpretation of routine blood tests. Nursing Standard 13(12): 42–48

Campbell J 1995 Making sense of venepuncture. Nursing Times 91(31): 29–31

Campbell H, Carrington M, Limber C 1999 A practical guide to venepuncture and management of complications. British Journal of Nursing 8(7): 426–431

Clulow M 1994 A closer look at disposable gloves. An assessment of the value of vinyl, latex and plastic gloves. Professional Nurse 9(5): 324, 326–329

Franklin L 1999 Skin cleansing and infection control in peripheral venepuncture and cannulation. Nursing Standard 14(4): 49–50

Gould D 1995 Now please wash your hands. Practice Nurse 10(3): 188–190

Griffiths E 1999 Venepuncture. Practice Nursing 10(1): 23–25

Hoeltke LB 1995 Phlebotomy. The clinical manual series. Delmar, New York

Lawrence JC, Lilly HA, Kidson A, Davies J 1994 The use of alcoholic wipes for disinfectant of injection sites. Journal of Wound Care 3(1): 11–14

United Kingdom Central Council for Nursing, Midwifery and Health Visiting 1992a The scope of professional practice. UKCC, London

United Kingdom Central Council for Nursing, Midwifery and Health Visiting 1992b Code of professional conduct. UKCC, London

United Kingdom Central Council for Nursing, Midwifery and Health Visiting 1996 Guidelines for professional practice. UKCC, London

United Kingdom Central Council for Nursing, Midwifery and Health Visiting 1998 Guidelines for records and record keeping. UKCC, London

54 Wound Care

There are four parts to this section:

1 Wound assessment
2 Aseptic technique
3 Wound drain care
4 Removal of stitches, clips and staples.

The concluding subsections, 'Patient/carer education: key points' and 'Relevance to the activities of living' refer to the four practices collectively.

Learning outcomes

By the end of this section, you should know how to:

- prepare the patient for these four nursing practices
- collect and prepare the equipment
- carry out these nursing practices.

Background knowledge required

Revision of wound assessment
Revision of the physiology of wound healing and the factors that affect wound healing
Review of health authority policies regarding all four parts of wound care technique
Review of the common classification of wound dressing materials and their individual properties.

1 Wound assessment

Indications and rationale for wound assessment

Wound assessment is the process used by the nurse to determine the appropriate management of individual patients who have a wound (Bale 2000). The main aims of wound assessment are:

- *to provide baseline information about the state of the wound, allowing progress to be monitored* (Dealey 1994)
- *to ensure that the appropriate wound management product has been chosen* (Dealey 1994)
- *to allow the nurse to set realistic and measurable goals*

The assessment process should assess:

- the patient
- the wound
- the patient's environment
- the appropriateness of the wound dressing materials.

Equipment

Material to record assessment details, e.g. a wound assessment chart (Morison 1992)
Clean ruler to measure the wound size
Grid to record the shape of the wound
Vascular flow detector, e.g. Doppler ultrasound, commonly used with leg ulcers by skilled personnel
Camera or grid camera.

Guidelines and rationale for this nursing practice

This full assessment of the patient and the wound will not be required every time the wound is dressed, weekly wound measurement usually being sufficient (CREST 1998).

- explain the nursing practice to the patient *to gain consent and co-operation*
- collect and prepare the equipment required *to ensure that it is available and ready for use*
- ensure the patient's privacy *to reduce anxiety*
- wash the hands *to reduce cross-infection* (Horton 1995)
- help the patient into a comfortable position *to create a sense of well-being*
- using an appropriate nursing model, assess the patient *to identify any factors that may interfere with wound healing*, such as poor nutritional status or dehydration, underlying disease, prescribed medication or the amount of pain experienced by the patient, smoking, sleep disturbances, stress, anxiety or advancing age
- classify the wound as chronic, acute or postoperative *as the classification will determine the subsequent management* (Dealey 1994)
- assess the wound dimensions using the ruler, which should come into direct contact with the wound. *This provides baseline data that can be used to monitor the progress of wound healing* (Peters 2000)
- assess and record the shape of the wound using a measured grid tracing *to permit changes to the wound shape to be noted* (Benbow & Dealey 1995). A camera or camera grid may, with the patient's permission, be used
- note the amount of wound exudate *as this may determine the choice of dressing*
- assess the wound condition and appearance, which may be epithelialising, granulating, sloughy, infected or necrotic (Thomas et al 1994) *to provide information regarding the stage of healing*
- assess the condition of the surrounding skin *to provide information on the underlying disease and the effectiveness of the current treatment* (CREST 1998)

- assess wound odour *to establish whether infection may be present.* This symptom is particularly unpleasant for both patients and carers (CREST 1998)
- carry out a pain assessment *to determine the analgesic requirement and the timing of any medication required*
- note the position of the wound on the patient's body *as this may guide the choice of dressing*
- record where the patient is being cared for – in hospital, at home or in a long-term care institution – *as this may alter the initial wound management regime* (Bale 2000)
- for leg ulcers, assist a skilled practitioner in the assessment of the venous flow of the limb (including the use of Doppler measurement) *as this will help in identifying the underlying cause of the ulcer, which will then determine the management of the wound* (Morison & Moffat 1994)
- discuss with the patient previous treatments and their effect, allergies and dressing preferences *to increase concordance with the treatment regime*
- following the initial assessment, evaluate the wound at regular intervals *to monitor the overall progress of the wound*
- reassess the appropriateness of the choice of wound dressing at regular intervals *as one wound may require different dressing materials at the various stages of healing*
- ensure that the patient is left feeling as comfortable as possible, *maintaining the quality of this nursing practice*
- dispose of the equipment safely *to reduce any health hazard*
- document the nursing practice appropriately, monitor the after-effects and report any abnormal findings. *This provides a written record and assists in the implementation of any action should an abnormality or adverse reaction to the practice be noted*
- in undertaking this practice, nurses are accountable for their actions, the quality of care delivered and record-keeping according to the *Code of Professional Conduct* (UKCC 1992), *Guidelines for Professional Practice* (UKCC 1996) and *Guidelines for Records and Record Keeping* (UKCC 1998).

2 Aseptic technique

Indications and rationale for aseptic technique

This is the technique used to lessen the potential problem of introducing pathogenic micro-organisms into the body when the integrity and/or effectiveness of the natural body defences has been reduced. The details of the technique may be modified according to the particular dressing pack used, but the principles are the same. The equipment, lotions and dressing used are sterile, the risk of contamination by air-borne pathogenic micro-organisms being kept to a minimum. Aseptic wound dressing is indicated:

- *to remove wound discharge*
- *to apply special treatments to a wound,* e.g. a venous leg ulcer
- *if signs of wound infection are present*

- *following trauma to the skin tissue*, e.g. a pressure sore
- *during an invasive procedure* such as catheterisation or the introduction of an intravenous cannula.

Equipment

Dressings trolley, or an appropriate clean surface if in the patient's home

Sterile dressing pack containing a gallipot or similar container, low-linting swabs, disposable forceps, a drape and a disposal bag

Sterile wound-irrigating lotion, e.g. normal saline, or sterile irrigating solution. It is important for cell function that the cleansing fluid is at body temperature *as it takes about 40 minutes for the cells to recover from irrigation with cold fluid and 3 hours for cell division to recommence* (Myers 1982)

10 ml syringe for irrigating the wound. This may not be required as some solutions are packaged to allow irrigation

Additional sterile dressing material, usually packed separately

Sterile disposable gloves

Hypoallergenic tape

Clean pair of scissors for cutting the tape

Clean disposable plastic apron

Alcohol-based hand preparation lotion

Primary and secondary dressings plus a securing bandage if required

Receptacle for soiled disposable items.

Characteristics of an ideal dressing

Nurses are accountable for administering topical preparations, as they are for the administration of all other medicines, so they must be familiar with the properties and side-effects of any wound care products they are using. Up-to-date information on these preparations is available from the *British National Formulary*.

Morison (1992) identified the characteristics of an ideal dressing, which the nurse should be aware of when choosing the most appropriate dressing for the patient's wound. The ideal dressing should be:

- non-adherent
- impermeable to bacteria
- capable of maintaining a high humidity while removing excess exudate
- thermally insulating
- non-toxic and non-allergenic
- comfortable and conformable
- protective of the wound from further trauma
- requiring infrequent dressing changes
- cost-effective
- long in shelf life
- available in both hospital and community settings.

In addition to the above, it is also important for the dressing to have the necessary physiological and biochemical properties to facilitate wound healing at a cellular level.

Tissue viability nurses may provide input if complex wounds are present or healing is impaired.

Continuity of wound care from hospital to home can present a problem for the community nurse because of the constraints of the drug tariff. As a result, the community nurse may need to review the wound management strategy with reference to the dressing materials available (Dealey 1994). Many district nurses have undertaken a nationally accredited course to enable them to prescribe a range of wound care products.

Guidelines and rationale for this nursing practice

Institutional

- explain the nursing practice to the patient *to gain consent and co-operation*
- use a treatment room for wound dressing *as this reduces the incidence of cross-infection*. If one is not available, prepare the environment around the patient's bed appropriately
- wash the hands *to reduce the risk of cross-infection* (Horton 1995)
- wash the dressings trolley thoroughly with detergent and water, and then dry it *to provide a socially clean surface*
- disinfect the dressings trolley with 70% ethyl alcohol immediately prior to every dressing undertaken *to reduce the number of micro-organisms on the trolley surface*
- collect and prepare the equipment, check the packaging for damage such as tears or leakage, and check the expiry dates of all the materials to be used, *ensuring that the equipment has not been contaminated*
- place all the equipment on the bottom shelf of the trolley, preferably in order of use, *to leave the top shelf free and clean during the practice and to permit easy access to the equipment*
- ensure the patient's privacy *to reduce anxiety*
- observe the patient throughout this activity, *noting any signs of distress*
- adjust the position of the bed *to ensure safe working practice and the most comfortable position to carry out this procedure* (Nicol et al 2000)
- help the patient into a comfortable position *to allow the position to be maintained during the practice*
- adjust the patient's clothing to expose the wound area *in order to give the nurse easy access to the wound*
- wash the hands *to reduce the risk of cross-infection*
- apply the plastic disposable apron *to prevent micro-organisms adhering to the nurse's uniform,* which could be a source of cross-infection
- open the outer packaging of the dressing pack and slip the contents on to the top shelf of the dressings trolley, *allowing the inner cover of the dressing pack to come into contact with a clean surface*
- loosen the outer dressing covering the patient's wound *to ease removal after the nurse has commenced the dressing*
- wash the hands using bactericidal soap or an alcohol-based hand lotion *to reduce the risk of cross-infection* (Horton 1995)

- open the dressing pack, touching the sterile covering as little as possible *in order to reduce contamination from the dresser's hands*
- open any additional equipment and drop it on to the sterile field. If using a sachet of skin cleansing lotion, pour the contents into the gallipot, *thereby preparing the equipment for use*
- wash the hands with alcohol-based lotion
- place one hand inside the disposal bag and arrange the contents of the dressing pack, *thus reducing the risk of contamination*
- with the hand still in the bag, remove the soiled dressing from the wound, *removing contaminated material from the wound site*
- turn the bag inside out with soiled dressing inside and attach it to the side of the trolley, below the level of the top shelf *to reduce the risk of contamination*
- apply gloves *to prevent contact with body fluids*
- drape the wound with the sterile drape
- note the condition of the wound and the surrounding skin *to assess and evaluate the healing rate and identify potential problems*
- if required, irrigate the wound, ensuring that the tip of the syringe or container does not come into contact with skin surface, *to remove debris without localised trauma*
- use the gauze swab to dry the surrounding skin, *aiding dressing adherence and preventing maceration of the skin*
- apply the primary dressing, which is part of the wound management strategy *to create the optimum wound healing environment*
- discard the gloves or forceps, *thus removing contaminated material*
- *to maintain the position of the dressing*, secure it by the chosen method
- apply any secondary material, such as compression bandaging for a patient with a venous leg ulcer, *to assist in the overall healing of the wound* (Morison & Moffat 1994)
- ensure that the patient is left feeling as comfortable as possible, *thus maintaining the quality of this nursing practice*
- dispose of all equipment safely *to reduce any health hazard*
- document this nursing practice appropriately, monitor the after-effects and report any abnormal findings immediately, *providing a written record and assisting in the implementation of any action should an abnormality or adverse reaction to the practice be noted*
- in undertaking this practice, nurses are accountable for their actions, the quality of care delivered and record-keeping according to the *Code of Professional Conduct* (UKCC 1992), *Guidelines for Professional Practice* (UKCC 1996) and *Guidelines for Records and Record Keeping* (UKCC 1998).

Community

- explain the nursing practice to the patient *to gain consent and co-operation*
- identify an adequate surface within the patient's home *to provide a working environment that is as clean and dry as possible*

- wash the hands *to reduce the risk of cross-infection* (Horton 1995)
- collect and prepare the equipment, check all packaging for damage such as tears or leakage and check the expiry dates of all the materials *to ensure that the equipment has not been contaminated*
- ensure the patient's privacy *to reduce anxiety*
- observe the patient throughout this activity, *noting any signs of distress*
- help the patient into a comfortable position *to allow the position to be maintained during the practice*
- adjust the patient's clothing to expose the wound area *to give the nurse easy access to the wound*
- wash the hands using the alcohol-based lotion *to reduce the risk of cross-infection* (Horton 1995)
- apply the plastic disposable apron *to prevent micro-organisms adhering to the nurse's uniform*, which could be a source of cross-infection
- open the outer packaging of the dressing pack and slip the contents on to the surface, *allowing the inner cover of the dressing pack to come into contact with a clean surface*
- loosen the outer dressing covering the patient's wound *to ease removal after the nurse has commenced the dressing*
- wash the hands using bactericidal soap or an alcohol-based hand lotion *to reduce the risk of cross-infection* (Horton 1995)
- open the dressing pack, touching the sterile covering as little as possible *in order to reduce contamination by the dresser's hands*
- open any additional equipment and drop it on to the sterile field. If using a sachet of skin cleansing lotion, pour the contents into the gallipot, *thereby preparing the equipment for use*
- wash the hands with the alcohol-based lotion
- place one hand inside the disposal bag and arrange the contents of the dressing pack, *to reduce the risk of contamination*
- with the hand still in the bag, remove the soiled dressing from the wound, *thus removing contaminated material from the wound site*
- turn the bag inside out with soiled dressing inside and attach it to a nearby surface *to reduce the risk of contamination*
- apply gloves *to prevent contact with body fluids*
- drape the wound with the sterile drape
- note the condition of the wound and the surrounding skin *to assess and evaluate the healing rate and identify potential problems*
- if required, irrigate the wound, ensuring that the tip of the syringe or container does not come into contact with skin surface, *in order to remove debris without localised trauma*
- use the gauze swab to dry the surrounding skin, *aiding dressing adherence and preventing maceration of the skin*
- apply the primary dressing, which is part of the wound management strategy *to create the optimum wound healing environment*
- discard the gloves or forceps *to remove contaminated material*
- *to maintain the position of the dressing*, secure it by the chosen method

- apply any secondary material, such as compression bandaging for a patient with a venous leg ulcer, *to assist in the overall healing of the wound* (Morison & Moffat 1994)
- ensure that the patient is left feeling as comfortable as possible, *thus maintaining the quality of this nursing practice*
- dispose of all equipment safely *to reduce any health hazard*
- document this nursing practice appropriately, monitor the after-effects and report any abnormal findings immediately, *providing a written record and assisting in the implementation of any action should an abnormality or adverse reaction to the practice be noted*
- in undertaking this practice, nurses are accountable for their actions, the quality of care delivered and record-keeping according to the *Code of Professional Conduct* (UKCC 1992), *Guidelines for Professional Practice* (UKCC 1996) and *Guidelines for Records and Record Keeping* (UKCC 1998).

3   Wound drain care

Indications and rationale for wound drain care

Wound drains are inserted at the time of surgical intervention by the medical practitioner *to prevent fluid collecting at the operation or wound site*, which may retard tissue healing. The extent and site of the surgery will influence the types and number of drains used. Drains may be inserted away from the original incision, to be dressed and to heal independently. *This will help to prevent the transmission of infection between the incision/operation site and the exit site for the wound drain.*

Drains are frequently stitched in position and attached to a closed-circuit drainage bag, or to portable suction if required (Nightingale 1989).

Types of wound drain

Hollow plastic tube   This is a deep drain with drainage holes at the proximal (drainage site) end, which is usually stitched in position and attached to a closed-circuit drainage bag. Such a drain may be used following major abdominal surgery to drain fluid collections.

Corrugated rubber drain   This is a superficial drain that usually drains directly into the dressing. It may be used to drain an incision site.

T-tube   A T-tube is a specialised tube inserted into the common bile duct following a cholecystectomy. It allows bile to drain into a closed circuit bag for 6–10 days postoperatively until normal drainage is re-established.

Portable vacuum suction drain   This is a perforated plastic catheter attached to a specialised sterile vacuum suction bag (Fig. 54.1). Two or more may be attached to the same vacuum bag with a Y-connection. This system is used *to prevent the formation of a haematoma, by maintaining gentle suction*. It may be used following joint replacement surgery or surgery to the face or neck area, where fluid may collect rapidly because of the efficient local blood supply.

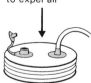

Use hand pressure to expel air

Replace stopper while maintaining pressure to create vacuum

Figure 54.1 *Wound care: a portable vacuum drain*

Equipment

As for 'Aseptic technique' above.

Additional equipment as required

- Sterile gloves
- Sterile scissors
- Sterile stitch-cutters
- Sterile drainage bag
- Portable wound suction equipment
- Sterile specialised keyhole dressing
- Extra sterile dressings material (Thomas et al 1993)
- Sterile safety pin
- Sterile wound pads
- Measuring jug
- Sterile specimen container.

Sterile gloves should be used when dressing wound drains to help to maintain asepsis and to protect nursing staff from infected body fluids.

Guidelines and rationale for this nursing practice

- explain the nursing practice to the patient *to gain consent and co-operation, and encourage participation in care*
- ensure the patient's privacy *to respect his or her individuality*
- help the patient into a comfortable position depending on the area of the wound drain *so that the area for dressing is easily accessible and the patient is able to maintain the position with minimum distress*. In some instances, carefully timed prescribed analgesia may be given *to ensure its maximum effect during the wound care*
- observe the patient throughout this activity *to monitor any adverse effect*s. This continual evaluation ensures that nursing or medical intervention can be altered as necessary
- collect and prepare the equipment *to ensure an efficient use of time and resources*
- remove clothes and covers from the area of the wound, ensuring that, with the exception of that area, the patient remains covered, *to expose only the site for wound care and respect the patient's dignity*
- perform the dressing for the surgical incision line first if necessary, maintaining asepsis. Dressings will usually be removed from the incision line after 24 hours and the wound may be covered by a plastic spray dressing *to encourage healing by first intention*. After this, only the drainage tube sites need to be dressed *to promote healing and prevent infection* (Guilding 1993)
- prepare the sterile field for dressing the drainage tube site *as an essential component of the aseptic technique*
- don sterile gloves after efficient handwashing *to prevent any contamination with body fluids*
- proceed as for 'Aseptic technique' above until the drainage tube has been exposed

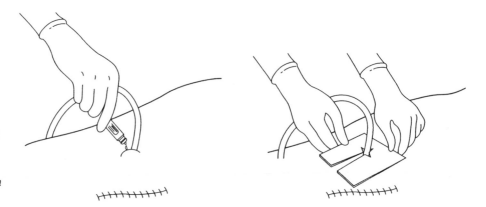

Figure 54.2 *Cleansing the skin round the wound drain*

Figure 54.3 *Applying a keyhole dressing*

- cleanse the skin round the wound drain with wound cleansing lotion if there is any exudate *to prevent any spread of infection* (Fig. 54.2)
- dry the skin round the wound drain *to reduce any infection*
- prepare a 'keyhole' dressing. *This allows the dressing to fit snugly round the drain* (Fig. 54.3)
- shorten the drain as ordered by the medical practitioner. This will depend on the healing process of the individual wound
- apply the keyhole or other dressing as required *to maintain asepsis and promote healing*
- secure the dressing *to prevent its slipping*
- change the drainage bag and secure it in such a position that *gravity will help the fluid to drain away from the wound efficiently*
- measure the drainage fluid and note its colour, consistency and smell *so that the process of healing can be monitored and any adverse condition reported*
- ensure that the patient is left as comfortable as possible *to create an environment that will promote healing*
- dispose of the equipment safely *to maintain a safe environment*
- document this nursing practice appropriately, monitor the after-effects and report any abnormal findings immediately *so that any nursing or medical intervention can be evaluated and altered as required*
- in undertaking this practice, nurses are accountable for their actions, the quality of care delivered and record-keeping according to the *Code of Professional Conduct* (UKCC 1992), *Guidelines for Professional Practice* (UKCC 1996) and *Guidelines for Records and Record Keeping* (UKCC 1998).

Shortening wound drains

Deep wound drains may be shortened, as ordered by the medical practitioner, once or twice during the postoperative period as healing proceeds.

- expose the drain site, maintaining asepsis and cleansing the skin as above. Sterile gloves should be worn after effective handwashing *to prevent contamination with body fluids*

- remove any stitches holding the drain in position (*see* 'Removal of stitches, clips and staples' on p. 416) *to release the drain*
- support the skin round the drain site with one hand using a sterile swab and gently withdraw the drain as far as ordered by the medical practitioner, e.g. 3–5 cm. Supporting the surrounding area *reduces discomfort and prevents damage to healthy tissue*
- insert a sterile safety pin through the drain near the entry site. *This prevents the drain falling back into the wound*
- cut off the extra length of drain if necessary *so that it lies neatly at the drain site and causes no discomfort.* Drains attached to drainage bags will not need to be cut
- apply one sterile keyhole dressing under the safety pin and another over it. *This helps to maintain the drain in position and prevents the safety pin damaging the skin*
- secure the dressing in position *to prevent any drag on the drain or contamination of the wound* (Pagget 1992)
- proceed as for the guidelines above.

Removing wound drains

This will be ordered by the medical practitioner when there is no longer any significant drainage from the wound.

- expose the drain site
- the skin should be cleansed only if this is needed *to ensure that the suture is visible*
- gloves should be worn *to prevent contamination with body fluids*
- release the vacuum or clamp the tubing *to prevent suction during removal*, which may cause tissue damage or pain (Nicol et al 2000)
- remove any stitches holding the drain in position
- support the skin round the drain site with one hand, using a sterile swab, and gently withdraw the drain using either a sterile gloved hand or sterile forceps held in the other hand. *This prevents damage to the surrounding tissues and helps to reduce discomfort as well as maintaining asepsis*
- maintain pressure over the wound after the drain has been removed (Smith et al 1999)
- the tip of the drain should be cut off with sterile scissors and placed in a sterile specimen container, maintaining asepsis, *if it is required for microbiological investigation*
- cleanse and dry the wound site again if necessary (Young 1995)
- apply and secure an appropriate sterile dressing *to maintain asepsis and promote healing*
- proceed as for the guidelines above
- immediately dispatch the labelled specimen to the laboratory along with the completed form *so that investigative procedures may be completed as soon as possible.*

Emptying the portable wound suction container

The containers should be emptied as soon as they are no longer maintaining a vacuum suction, or every 12 hours as required *to measure drainage and prevent ascending infection.*

- clamp the drainage tubing above the level of the wound drainage container *to prevent backflow*
- remove the stopper or bung from the container, maintaining asepsis, *to release the vacuum*
- obtain a specimen of drainage fluid *for microbiological investigation if required*
- pour the remaining contents into a measuring jug, *avoiding contamination*
- wipe the outside of the entry channel with an alcohol solution, e.g. Mediswab, *to remove any drainage fluid that might cause infection*
- press the two rigid surfaces of the container together and maintain the pressure until the stopper is firmly in position. Once the pressure is removed, a gentle vacuum suction is created
- secure the drainage bag in position as before
- document the amount and details of the drainage fluid in the patient's records *so that accurate monitoring of the healing process and an evaluation of treatment can continue*
- in undertaking this practice, nurses are accountable for their actions, the quality of care delivered and record-keeping according to the *Code of Professional Conduct* (UKCC 1992), *Guidelines for Professional Practice* (UKCC 1996) and *Guidelines for Records and Record Keeping* (UKCC 1998).

4   Removal of stitches, clips and staples

Indications and rationale for the removal of stitches, clips and staples

Following surgery, stitches, clips or staples are used *to place the skin edges in apposition and promote rapid healing.* These are removed when there is:

- evidence of the wound having healed
- infection in part of the wound.

If the wound is greater than 15 cm in length, or if healing is slow, alternate sutures or clips may be removed (Nicol et al 2000). The remaining sutures should be removed as directed by the medical practitioner.

Adhesive sutures are sometimes applied to the wound edges when healing is not complete. Some wounds are sutured using a subcuticular method that uses biodegradable material; these do not require manual removal.

Equipment

Sterile dressing pack
Sterile normal saline
Sterile stitch-cutter or scissors, clip or staple remover
Receptacle for soiled disposable items.

Guidelines and rationale for this nursing practice

- explain the procedure to the patient *to gain consent and co-operation*
- ensure the patient's privacy *to maintain dignity and a sense of self*
- collect the equipment *to help the efficiency of the practice*
- observe the patient throughout this activity *to detect any signs of discomfort or distress*
- clean the wound with solution only if it is necessary to gain access to the stitches, clips or staples as studies have shown that *unnecessary washing increases the risk of infection being introduced* (Harding 1992)
- examine the wound to ensure that it is appropriate to remove the sutures or clips (Smith et al 1999a).

Removing sutures

There are two main types of suture, continuous and individual (Fig. 54.4) – their method of removal being similar. For individual stitches:

- hold the stitch-cutter or scissors in the dominant hand and the dissecting forceps in the other hand *to lift the knot of the stitch gently* (Fig. 54.4A)
- cut between the knot and the skin so that no part of the stitch above the skin surface is pulled under the tissues; then gently pull out the cut stitch. This helps *to reduce the risk of introducing infection* (Smith et al 1999a)
- ensure that no piece of the stitch is left in the wound *as this could eventually form a wound sinus.*

For continuous stitches:

- hold the stitch-cutter or scissors in the dominant hand and the dissecting forceps in the other hand to lift gently the knot at one end of the suture line
- cut between the knot and the skin, so that no part of the stitch above the skin surface is pulled under the tissues. This helps *to reduce the risk of introducing infection* (Smith et al 1999a)
- grasp the knot at the other end of the suture line and pull gently away from the wound *to remove the total suture intact.*

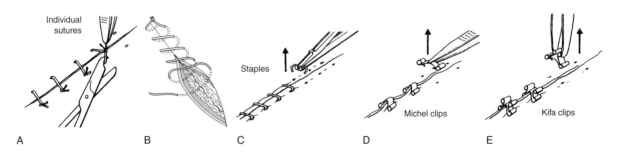

Figure 54.4   *Removal of sutures, clips and staples.* A *Individual suture;* B *Continuous suture;* C *Staples;* D *Michel clips;* E *Kifa clips*

Removing clips or staples

- hold the remover in the dominant hand and the dissecting forceps in the other hand when removing clips or staples (Fig. 54.4C–E)
- steady the clips or staples with the dissecting forceps. Depending on the type of clip or staple, either insert one blade of the remover under the centre of the clip or staple and the other blade over it, then gently squeezing the blades together, or place one blade of the remover on the outside of each wing on top of the clip and squeeze the blades together. Depending on the clip or staple type, one or other of these actions should lift the clip from the skin on either side of the wound
- follow health authority policy for the aftercare of a wound. The wound may be cleaned if necessary and then left exposed or covered with a dressing if discharge is present
- ensure that the patient is left as comfortable as possible
- dispose of all equipment safely *for the protection of others*
- document the nursing practice appropriately, monitor the after-effects and report any abnormal findings immediately
- in undertaking this practice, nurses are accountable for their actions, the quality of care delivered and record-keeping according to the *Code of Professional Conduct* (UKCC 1992), *Guidelines for Professional Practice* (UKCC 1996) and *Guidelines for Records and Record Keeping* (UKCC 1998).

Relevance to the activities of living	### Maintaining a safe environment

In a healthy individual, the skin and mucous membranes act as a natural defence against the entry of pathogenic micro-organisms. When the continuity of these tissues is lost, even temporarily, there is the potential for infection (Horton 2000), and infection of any kind is an extremely debilitating process. It can cause a great deal of discomfort and inconvenience to the patient, as well as increasing the length of stay in hospital, with its attendant alteration in lifestyle and huge health cost (Morison & Moffatt 1994).

In an institutional environment, the number of air-borne pathogenic micro-organisms can be reduced by working in a well-ventilated room used solely for procedures involving aseptic technique, or by performing procedures at least 30 minutes after the completion of ward cleaning and bed-making. This may not always be possible in the home setting, where the community nurse has little control over the environment (Bale 2000).

There is no need for the nurse to wear a disposable cap or face mask, but verbal communication should be kept to a minimum during the aseptic technique in order to reduce droplet contamination. When a number of aseptic wound dressings are to be performed, a known contaminated and/or infected wound should be treated last to reduce environmental contamination.

In an institutional setting, careful preparation of the equipment to be used can further reduce environmental contamination. The dressings trolley should be washed daily, using detergent and water, and then dried; immediately prior to its preparation for an aseptic technique, it should be disinfected with 70% ethyl alcohol. It is preferable that the dressings trolley be solely used for that purpose. All equipment packaging should be checked for damage and the date of expiry, which affect the equipment's sterility.

At home the nurse should assess each situation on an individual basis and, where possible, create a clean environment; he or she may therefore have to adopt an educative role (Bale 2000).

The member of staff who performs the aseptic technique also needs specific preparation. Because of the nature of nurses' work, their uniforms and hands can be a catchment area for pathogenic micro-organisms. A disposable plastic apron should be worn to provide a barrier to the transmission of micro-organisms.

Thorough handwashing *prior* to the dressing must be performed, further hand preparation being performed *during* the aseptic technique as stated in the guidelines above and when the nurse accidentally contaminates his or her hands. An alcohol-based hand rub is used for the subsequent hand preparation; it has the benefit that the nurse does not have to leave the patient during the practice.

It is preferable for the skin cleansing lotion to be supplied as an individual single-use sterile sachet or bottle. Once a bottle has been opened, environmental contamination can occur so any residual lotion should be discarded. If an aerosol can of irrigating fluid is used, the nurse should ensure that the dispensing nozzle does not become contaminated and therefore act as a source of infection.

The continual use of an aseptic skin cleansing lotion may have a detrimental effect on granulation tissue (Cameron & Leiper 1988). Adequate cleansing of an open granulating wound can be achieved with the use of sterile normal saline.

Thomlinson (1987) noted that, during the cleansing of a chronic wound, the micro-organisms were redistributed throughout the tissue rather than being removed from the wound bed.

A non-touch technique reduces the potential problem of contamination from the nurse's hands to the wound. Sterile forceps or gloves can be used, the latter having the benefit of easing manipulative skills and promoting comfort for the patient. As the soiled dressing and equipment used during removal may be contaminated, all items must be discarded before continuing with the aseptic technique. The wound should be irrigated only if required. These measures may reduce cross-infection from one part of the wound to another. The use of cotton wool balls has been found to be detrimental to the wound healing process as cotton fibres can be left within the wound surface.

On completion of the aseptic technique, discard all the equipment in the appropriate receptacles and seal them, before leaving the patient, to reduce environmental contamination from the soiled materials. In an institutional setting, the trolley should be washed, dried and returned to its place of storage; at home, the surface should be cleared of any visible contaminating materials. The nurse should thoroughly wash his or her hands using soap and water only.

Wound care is a dynamic and evolving process, especially as far as wound dressing materials are concerned; nurses have a legal, moral and professional responsibility to ensure that their knowledge and practice of wound care is based on recent research findings (Bennett & Moody 1995).

As a wound drain is in direct contact with the underlying tissues, pathogenic micro-organisms could gain entry to a wound through the drain site (Dealey 1994). The maintenance of a closed drainage system and aseptic technique may help to reduce the chance of wound infection.

The wound drain site should be dressed after the incision site to minimise the risk of cross-infection. Gauze swabs should not be cut for keyhole dressings as small pieces of cut gauze may remain within the wound. Commercial keyhole dressings with sealed edges can be purchased. If these are not available, any suitable sterile dressing may be placed around the drain and secured in position to cover the drain site.

During suture, clip or staple removal, care must be taken to prevent the sharp equipment causing accidental injury to the patient.

When infection is suspected, it is important to distinguish between colonisation and infection. Colonised wounds will heal, but infected ones will require antibiotic therapy (Donovan 1998).

Communicating

The nursing practice should be explained simply to the patient. Any discomfort or pain should be anticipated by the nurse and the appropriate analgesic offered, as prescribed by a medical practitioner. At home, the nurse should confirm with the patient the date and time of the next dressing change; this will allow the patient to administer a painkiller to reduce potential discomfort. Pain leads to a reduced blood supply and delayed healing at the wound site as a result of physiological and psychological responses (Hampton 2000). The nurse should also be aware of culturally determined responses to pain (Casey 1998c).

The nurse should inform the patient of his or her intended actions during the nursing practice as this may help to reduce anxiety.

An explanation for reduced verbal communication during aseptic technique should be given. Nurses must be alert to the fact that their non-verbal communication can often be interpreted by a patient; when faced with a malodorous or unsightly wound, for example, a reaction of disgust must not be evident. The patient's non-verbal communication may be an indicator of his or her acceptance of a change in body image if the wound is defacing.

The nurse should observe and note any sign of inflammation such as increased heat, redness or swelling around the wound as this may indicate the presence of infection.

Breathing

The patient's respiration and pulse rates may increase as a result of anxiety.

Eating and drinking

Nutritional requirements are increased following surgery or trauma, or in the presence of a chronic wound (Casey 1998a). Nutritional assessment is therefore essential to determine any deficiencies in the nutrients involved in the wound healing process (CREST 1998). Essential nutrients include additional carbohydrate, protein, vitamin C, zinc, iron, vitamins A, B, E and K, and trace elements such as manganese and copper (Casey 1998a). The nurse has an important role to play in the nutrition assessment of all patients, but the input of a dietitian may be required in the management of complex wounds.

Some medication, for example steroids, anticoagulants and cytotoxic agents, can have a significant effect on wound healing (Collier 2000).

Eliminating

The patient should empty his or her bladder prior to these nursing interventions to facilitate comfort. Constipation may delay wound healing as a result of abnormal internal pressure and the inability to absorb nutrients as usual. Diarrhoea will also affect absorption of nutrients.

Personal cleansing and dressing

Care must be taken during the performance of this activity of living that the wound dressing or drain comes to no harm.

In some hospital departments, surgical wounds are left exposed to the environment within the first few days of surgery. If this is practised, the dried blood along the suture line should not be removed because it acts as a protective barrier.

When securing a dressing with tape, allow for body movement when applying the tape, stretching out any natural skin creases during application. Wet wound dressings should be changed immediately except during the first 24 hours after surgery, when the dressing is used as an estimation of approximate fluid loss.

Even before the removal of sutures, clips or staples, an immersion bath or shower can usually be performed by the patient with assistance from the nurse or carer, but this will vary in different health-care settings. A bath in an institutional setting may increase the risk of cross-infection.

Following the removal of sutures, clips and staples, advice may have to be given to the patient about the aftercare of a healing wound and the most appropriate clothing to wear. The area should be washed and dried carefully each day. The clothing worn on top of the wound should not be tight but may be gently supportive if desired.

Wound dressing deodorants may be found to be useful in concealing the smell from a malodorous wound.

A patient with a chronic wound should be given advice regarding the appropriate care for this activity of living. For example, the patient with a venous leg ulcer who also has compression bandages in situ will require advice on the most suitable method of personal cleansing and the most appropriate form of hosiery to wear.

Controlling body temperature

A patient with an infected wound may develop pyrexia. The nurse should implement the appropriate nursing intervention to assist the patient if this complication occurs.

Mobilising

A wound dressing should not impede mobilisation, but discomfort caused by the presence of a wound drain or awkwardness of the site of the wound may interfere with the patient's normal form of mobilising.

A patient may fear that the sutures, clips or staples holding the wound may give way when moving. The nurse should allay these fears and explain the importance and benefit of adequate mobilisation.

The patient may also be afraid that the wound will open up following the removal of the wound closures. Some education and guidance may be necessary here: many surgical units have printed leaflets with advice and information that can be given to the patient to read at leisure.

Expressing sexuality

The adequate provision of privacy is essential in reducing patient anxiety during these interventions. The nurse should assist the patient in adjusting to the altered body image whether the disfigurement is temporary or permanent.

Sleeping

The patient's normal sleep pattern may be altered as a result of the discomfort caused by the wound and/or drain. The most appropriate nursing intervention may be to help the patient to find a more comfortable position, to listen to his or her concerns and help to allay anxiety, or to administer a prescribed analgesic to reduce discomfort and pain.

Patient/carer education: key points

In partnership with the patient and/or carer, ensure that they are competent to carry out any practices required. Information should be given on an appropriate point of contact for any concerns that may arise.

The nurse should discuss the identified factors that may interfere with wound healing for each patient and, where possible, agree realistic goals for these factors with the patient. The nurse should provide information and education for the patient and/or carer relating to the care of the wound between each dressing change. The community nurse should agree and confirm the place, date and time of the next dressing change with the patient.

At home, the patient or carer may assume some or all of the responsibility for wound care; the nurse therefore has an important role in the education of all concerned.

Some education and guidance may have to be given to allay patients' fears that the wound will open up once the clips or sutures have been removed. Advice and guidance should be given on any lifestyle restrictions. Smoking in particular should be discouraged as it delays wound healing by causing vasoconstriction and reduced prostaglandin and fibrinogen production (Hampton 2000).

References

Bale S 2000 Wound healing. In: Alexander M, Fawcett J, Runciman P (eds) Nursing practice – hospital and home: the adult. 2nd edn. Churchill Livingstone, Edinburgh

Benbow M, Dealey C 1995 Parameters of wound assessment. British Journal of Nursing 4(11): 647–651

Bennett G, Moody M 1995 Wound care for health professionals. Chapman & Hall, London

British National Formulary (current edition) British Medical Association/Royal Pharmaceutical Society of Great Britain, London

Cameron S, Leiper D 1988 Antiseptic toxicity in open wounds. Nursing Times 84(25): 77–79

Casey G 1998a The importance of nutrition in wound healing. Nursing Standard 13(3): 51–54, 56.

Casey G 1998b Three steps to effective wound care. Nursing Standard 12(49): 43–44

Casey G 1998c Management of pain in wound care. Nursing Standard 13(12): 53–54

Collier M 2000 Principles of wound drainage, healing and management. In Manley K, Bellman L (eds) Surgical nursing advancing practice. Churchill Livingstone, London

CREST 1998 Guidelines for wound management in Northern Ireland

Dealey C 1994 The care of wounds. Blackwell Scientific, London

Donovan S 1998 Wound infection and wound swabbing. Professional Nurse. 13(11): 757–759.

Guilding 1993 Dimensions of nursing knowledge in wound care. British Journal of Nursing 2(14): 712–716

Hampton S 2000 Choosing the right dressings for managing arterial ulcers. Community Nurse 6(8): 51–54

Harding K 1992 The wound programme. Centre for Medical Education, University of Dundee

Horton R 1995 Handwashing: the fundamental infection control principle. British Journal of Nursing 4(16): 926–933

Horton R 2000 Infection control: maintaining a safe environment. In Manley K, Bellman L (eds) Surgical nursing advancing practice. Churchill Livingstone, London

Morison M 1992 A colour guide to the nursing management of wounds. Wolfe, London

Morison M, Moffat C 1994 A colour guide to the assessment and management of leg ulcers. 2nd edn. Mosby-Times Mirror, London

Myers J 1982 Plastic surgical dressings. Social Services Journal 11(18): 336–337

Newton H 1999 Improving wound care through clinical governance. Nursing Standard 13(29): 51–52, 55–56

Nicol M, Bavin C, Bedford-Turner S, Cronin P, Rawlings-Anderson K 2000 Essential nursing skills. CV Mosby, London

Nightingale K 1989 Making sense of wound drainage. Nursing Times 85(27): 40–42

Pagget L 1992 Wound dressing packs, a simpler alternative. Journal of Tissue Viability 2(1): 18–21

Peters M 2000 Measuring and assessing wounds effectively. Community Nurse 6(7): 339–340

Plassmann P 1995 Measuring wounds. Journal of Wound Care 4(6): 269–272

Smith L, Baker F, McDougall C, Stead L 1999 Removal of a vacuum drain. Nursing Times 95(11 suppl): 1–2

Smith L, Baker F, Stead L 1999a Removal of sutures. Nursing Times 95(10 suppl): 1–2

Smith L, Baker F, Stead L 1999b Removal of staples. Nursing Times 95(9 suppl): 1–2

Thomas S, Loveless P, May N, Toyick N 1993 Comparing non-woven, filmated and woven gauze swabs. Journal of Wound Care 2(1): 35–41

Thomas S, Fear M, Humphreys J 1994 Assessment of patients with chronic wounds. Journal of Wound Care 3(3): 151–154

Thomlinson D 1987 To clean or not to clean. Nursing Times (Mar 4): 71–75

United Kingdom Central Council for Nursing, Midwifery and Health Visiting 1992 Code of professional conduct. UKCC, London

United Kingdom Central Council for Nursing, Midwifery and Health Visiting 1996 Guidelines for professional practice. UKCC, London

United Kingdom Central Council for Nursing, Midwifery and Health Visiting 1998 Guidelines for records and record keeping. UKCC, London

Young T 1995 Common problems in wound care: wound cleansing. British Journal of Nursing 4(5): 286–289

Index

Page numbers in **bold** indicate figures and tables